Clinical Aviation Medicine

Third Edition

Russell B. Rayman, MD, MPH, DAvMed (London)
Executive Director, Aerospace Medical Association
Alexandria, Virginia

John D. Hastings, MD
Federal Aviation Administration Consultant in Neurology
Tulsa, Oklahoma

William B. Kruyer, MD, FACC, FAsMA
Chief of Cardiology, Aeromedical Consultation Service
USAF School of Aerospace Medicine
San Antonio, Texas

Richard A. Levy, MD, MPH
Consultant in Aerospace Medicine
(Formerly Chief of the Neuropsychiatry Branch,
Aeromedical Consultation Service
USAF School of Aerospace Medicine)
Scarborough, Maine

Sponsored by a grant from
Aventis Pharmaceuticals

Aventis

The views expressed herein are those of the authors and not necessarily those of the U.S. Federal Aviation Administration or Department of Defense.

Published by
Castle Connolly Graduate Medical Publishing, LLC
133 East 58th Street
New York, NY 10022
(212) 644-9696

Library of Congress Cataloging-in-Publication Data

Rayman, Russell B.
      Clinical aviation medicine / Russell B. Rayman.– 3rd ed.
      Includes bibliographies and index

ISBN 1-883769-86-8

Cover illustration: The Cessna Citation X, the world's fastest business jet, which cruises at .92 Mach. Photo courtesy of the Cessna Aircraft Company.

PRINTED IN THE UNITED STATES OF AMERICA

Table of Contents

Preface to Third Edition

A viation was born almost a century ago. Today we have at our disposal an array of flying machines ranging from a single-prop driven to 8-engine jet aircraft. Some are used for commercial purposes, some for military operations, and some for pleasure and recreation. No matter the type of aviation, physiological stresses will always be imposed to varying degrees on the operators. Consequently, there must be established medical standards to ensure that only fit operators receive flight certification. Because commercial, military, and private (general) aviation are so different, medical standards for each must necessarily also be different.

It is the responsibility of the civil aviation medical examiner (AME) and military flight surgeon (FS) to determine fitness to fly or aeromedical disposition. In order to do so, it is necessary to have an understanding of the stresses of flight, aircraft operations, general medicine, and the appropriate medical standards. This book provides guidance to AMEs and flight surgeons, particularly inexperienced ones, who must determine aeromedical disposition, by discussing the more common disease entities and treatment modalities with particular emphasis on their significance in an aviation environment.

The first and second editions of *Clinical Aviation Medicine* were published in 1982 and 1990 respectively. Since that time, many physicians in the practice of aviation medicine or in teaching and administering aviation medicine programs have conveyed to me how useful the book was to them. Although this was very gratifying, perhaps the greatest reward was the many favorable comments from my intended audience: students as well as young, relatively inexperienced practitioners. It is for the continuing support of these readers, as well as all other AMEs and flight surgeons, that prompted this new revision of *Clinical Aviation Medicine*.

Because there have been so many advances in medicine as well as in aeromedical policy changes during the past decade, much of the material has been rewritten and updated. In particular, three new highly qualified authors were invited to write the chapters on cardiovascular disease (William B. Kruyer, MD), neurologic disease (John D. Hastings, MD), and psychiatric disease (Richard A. Levy, MD). Furthermore the book was further demilitarized so the principles could be applied not only to aviation in the armed forces, but also to civil aviation at home and abroad. As in the first two editions, painstaking efforts were taken not to dictate aeromedical disposition, but only to provide the AME and flight surgeon with the information that is clinically relevant when making decisions regarding flight certification.

Russell B. Rayman, MD, MPH, DAvMed (London)
Alexandria, Virginia

Acknowledgments

The authors express their deep appreciation to Dr. Michael D. Wolf, Executive Vice President, Castle Connolly Graduate Medical Publishing, whose professional assistance, guiding hand, and perseverance made this book possible.

The authors gratefully acknowledge Mike Shelton, whose editorial skills, attention to detail, and patience greatly facilitated the publication of this book.

Dedication

This book is dedicated to the thousands of civil aviation medical examiners and military flight surgeons throughout the world who serve those who fly.

Dear Doctor:

Aventis Pharmaceuticals is proud to sponsor the third edition of *Clinical Aviation Medicine*. This book is the only worldwide text dedicated to the clinical aspects of aviation medicine, and can be used as a reference in the aeromedical disposition of pilots and other crew.

We at Aventis Pharmaceuticals hope you find this edition of *Clinical Aviation Medicine* useful in your practice.

Sincerely,

Kim Carroll
Senior Product Director
Aventis Pharmaceuticals

Chapter 1
Introduction

The practice of aviation medicine has advanced remarkably since the days of Flanders fields and Verdun. It was then, approximately 80 years ago, that more aviators were lost due to poor medical selection techniques and practically nonexistent physical standards than to enemy fire. It was this stark realization that prompted the founding of the aeromedical laboratory in Mineola, Long Island, New York in 1917, to begin aeromedical research, to establish physical standards for military aircrewmen, and to investigate human factors as a cause of aircraft losses during World War I. In a few wooden buildings at Mineola, a small, dedicated staff, America's earliest flight surgeons, developed the first concepts of aircrew physical standards, concepts which, though primitive by today's standards, had an almost immediate effect in significantly reducing aircraft losses over the battlefields of France, Germany, and the Low Countries.

These early medical standards were only the beginning. As those flight surgeons who have preceded us accumulated experience and as aviation technology sired the *Spirit of St. Louis,* the *China Clipper,* the flying fortress, and the jet and space age, physical standards for aviators gradually evolved. Without recapitulating the fascinating stories of earlier flight surgeons, let it suffice to recognize here their initiative, innovation, and in many cases bravery, which paved the way for the opening of a new frontier in aviation medicine.

The development over the years of medical standards for civil and military aviation has been an evolutionary process based not only on scientific inquiry, but also on trial and error, accumulated experience, and, in some cases, intuition, all of which create a continuing evolution in the science. Do not let today's era of sophisticated jet and space travel create the illusion that aviation medicine has reached the end of this evolution. It will undoubtedly continue to change in the light of new knowledge. We must continue to implement medical standards which will assure the health of the aviator and do not compromise flying safety, but at the same time will not unnecessarily prevent trained individuals from flying. That is the essence of today's aeromedical challenge.

1

Aviation organizations must establish standards somewhere on the continuum between the extremes of overconservatism and overliberalism. Although in previous decades medical standards tended more toward conservatism—"It is better to err on the side of safety than sorrow"—that trend has slowly and cautiously reversed, tending toward a more liberal view today. Although this policy shift is still in a state of flux, it is certain that individual policies will differ from regulator to regulator.

The stresses of flight such as acceleration, vibration and noise, lowered barometric pressure, extremes of temperature and humidity, and fatigue among others, vary considerably depending on the type of aviation operation. Clearly, there is great diversity in commercial, military, and general aviation operations. Therefore, medical standards for such widely disparate operations rightfully should be, and are indeed, very different. Medical departments must adopt policies appropriate to their different types of aviation operations. The authors acknowledge these differences and do not intend in these pages to be dogmatic or to suggest rigid, universally applicable aeromedical disposition policy. Rather, it is the authors' sole purpose to describe those aspects of a disease and its treatment the AME or flight surgeon must consider when determining aeromedical disposition.

To begin, a few words about terminology are in order to avoid confusion. The terms **aviation medical examiner** (AME) and **flight surgeon** (FS) are used interchangeably keeping in mind that the former minister to civilian aviators while the latter cater to military aviators. The term **aviator** is meant to be all inclusive. Besides pilots and navigators, the reader should consider all other crew duty positions (eg, flight engineers, load masters, flight attendants, etc) to be aviators. Although this may be stretching the term **aviator** a bit, this was done for practical reasons, and the authors are confident that our readers will fully appreciate the differences in these crew duty positions and will apply the aeromedical principles herein accordingly. The terms **waiver** and **special issuance** are used interchangeably. The terms **flying status**, **flying or flight duty**, or simply **flying** also have identical meanings as used here, although the former two terms have a more military ring. In any event, these terms can be applied to all aviators (as defined above), civil (commercial and private) and military. And finally, a **flight**, **flying or flight operations**, or **mission** are likewise interchangeable whether applied to a military crew, commercial crew, or private pilot.

The following chapters are concerned with clinical aviation medicine. The reader is reminded that this is not a textbook of medicine, therefore the descriptions of diseases were kept abbreviated and elementary. The emphasis instead is on signs, symptoms, modes of therapy, prognosis, and aeromedical significance. Like any segment of the population, aviators, particularly those of advanced age, are not exempt from disease and therefore cannot be expected to enjoy perfect health throughout their entire aviation careers. When a doctor, plumber, or other laborer develops an infirmity, a decision is made as to whether the worker should remain on the job. However, with aviators, the nature of their profession necessitates exercising extreme caution when making such decisions. Although a pilot may become afflicted with an infirmity, this need not necessarily terminate his or her career. The essential question then becomes: Can the aviator afflicted with a disease continue to fly without jeopardizing health and compromising flying safety? It is from this occupational perspective that disease is surveyed in the following pages. The authors hope that all AMEs and flight surgeons will find the information in these pages useful in their practice of aviation medicine.

Chapter 2
Internal Medicine

Because internal medicine encompasses the broadest spectrum of disease, most medical waiver requests will fall within this specialty. Peptic ulcer disease, diabetes, the arthritides, and gastrointestinal disorders will have the highest incidence followed by a host of other entities. The discussion that follows will include only those conditions most likely to confront the AME/flight surgeon and also some conditions of special aeromedical interest.

Varicose Veins and Deep Venous Thrombosis

Varicose veins are dilated, superficial, and tortuous, and are most commonly found in the lower extremities. Although the exact etiology is unclear, it is thought that congenital factors and/or thrombophlebitis may damage and render incompetent the venous valves, particularly of the saphenous vein. In either case, the condition is exacerbated whenever the venous pressure of the legs is significantly elevated for sustained periods. Well-known examples include sitting or standing for hours at a time as well as excessive venous pooling secondary to $+G_z$ acceleration, all of which are stresses familiar to aviators. And with the admission of more women into aviation, varicose veins may take on added significance because of its association with pregnancy. Although varicosities may be asymptomatic, they can cause annoying symptoms such as aching, cramps, and edema, as well as the more serious long-term effects of stasis dermatitis, ulceration, and thrombus formation.

Once varicosities form, treatment can be conservative, with use of elastic stockings and leg elevation, while other patients may require sclerotherapy or surgical excision and stripping. No matter what treatment modality is selected, many patients will continue to have recurrences. In one study, 278 patients with varicose veins were followed for 10 years following surgery.[1] Eighty-five percent were reported to have had good to excellent results with 15% developing recurrences and other complications.

Varicose veins may correctly be called an occupational hazard for aviators in that cockpit conditions may cause or aggravate the condition. Crew members, particularly those flying transoceanic flights of 6-12 hours' duration, frequently remain seated for long periods. To help prevent varicose veins, a short walk periodically to the rear of the aircraft is advisable (for passengers as well as crew). Walking will prevent venous pooling through the squeezing action of the calf and thigh muscles on the venous system, and AMEs and flight surgeons should advise their patients to walk around the craft to prevent varicose veins from forming. However, should varicosities develop, flying status would have to be determined on an individual basis because of the broad spectrum of patient disability. For example, a patient with recurring symptoms should not be exposed to the accelerative forces of high-performance aircraft, while an airline captain should be able to continue flying with encouragement to avoid remaining seated in the cockpit without periodic walking breaks.

Deep venous thrombosis (DVT) and thrombophlebitis are more serious than varicosities because they may involve the deep venous system of the legs causing significant complications. For these conditions to exist, there must be thrombus formation followed by inflammation. As with varicose veins the etiology is not always known, although there is an association with immobilization possibly related to sitting for prolonged periods, postoperative recovery, or convalescence. Patients frequently complain of pain and swelling of the involved leg with some developing serious complications. Foremost is pulmonary embolism which can be incapacitating and life threatening; other cases may progress to chronic venous insufficiency with persistent pain, edema, and skin changes including ulceration. The cornerstone of medical treatment is anticoagulants which may be prescribed for several weeks to several months depending on the clinical circumstances. Surgery, such as insertion of an inferior vena cava filtering device or ligation/plication, has been reserved for more serious cases and has met with variable success. Prevention, especially for aviators on long flights, is best achieved by walking about the aircraft periodically when movement is possible.

Regarding aeromedical disposition, patients with uncomplicated DVT/thrombophlebitis should be able to return to the cockpit once there is complete recovery. In some cases it may be advisable to also wait until anticoagulant medication has been discontinued. However, these patients should be followed because recurrences are common. As for the unfortunate patient with chronic venous insufficiency or pulmonary embolism, a return to flying is more guarded. The patient with chronic insufficiency, besides being frequently symptomatic, may exacerbate the condition depending upon the nature of flying. Certainly, frequent long-duration missions and accelerative forces would not be advisable for these aviators. The seriousness of pulmonary embolism cannot be overstated not only because of its immediate effects, but also because of its propensity to recur. Perhaps such individuals could be safely returned to flying in a multicrew aircraft. In military aviation, particularly in single seat high-performance aircraft, disqualification would be most prudent.

Arthritides

The number of these joint disorders is large, and it is a subspecialty in its own right. Although granting medical waivers for degenerative arthritis and gout is usually not problematic, it often is for the more serious entities such as rheumatoid arthritis and the collagen vascular diseases because of the frequency and intensity of symptoms, their natural course of remissions and exacerbations with varying degrees of functional impairment, and the frequent need for medication.

Degenerative Joint Disease

Degenerative joint disease (DJD) or osteoarthritis can affect almost any joint of the body, but it most frequently involves those of the fingers, hips, knees, and cervical or lumbar spine. Although it may result from repeated trauma, there is evidence that it also results from a slowly progressive aging process beginning in the second decade of life. In either case, there is gradual degeneration of cartilage with osteophyte formation causing insidious pain of the involved joint, particularly noticeable after exercise. Permanent deformity and severe limitation of range of motion come only in the late stages of the process. The diagnosis must be made by history and x-ray changes as there are no diagnostic laboratory tests available.

Most aviators diagnosed with DJD are relatively young and have only occasional minimal discomfort which responds to conservative measures such as salicylates, other nonsteroidal antiinflammatory drugs (NSAIDs), and physical therapy. As long as the disease process is in its early stages and requires only infrequent use of mild analgesics and causes no limitation of motion which would interfere with the performance of the patient's duties, medical waivers can usually be granted. DJD of the spine can cause further difficulties for military aviators who fly high-performance aircraft because of the requirement to wear heavy parachutes, climb into small cockpits, and sustain high G loads in the course of normal operations or ejection. Therefore, return to the cockpit for these individuals should be given special consideration.

Rheumatoid Arthritis

It is of particular importance to differentiate DJD from rheumatoid arthritis since each has its own prognosis, therapeutic regimen, and aeromedical disposition. Without going into a description of rheumatoid arthritis, let it suffice to say that it is a more serious disease with graver implications than DJD. The patient is afflicted by inflammatory joint disease, usually involving the wrists, fingers, knees, or feet, which is painful, each episode is often of weeks' duration, and it is usually associated with systemic symptoms. As the disease progresses, the involved joints become deformed with resulting functional impairment. Besides the history, the diagnosis can be made by radiographic changes as well as a positive serologic test for the rheumatoid factor. Treatment consists of physical therapy as well as a host of drugs including nonsteroidal antiinflammatory agents (NSAIDs), gold, penicillamine, antimalarials, steroids, and immunosuppressive or cytotoxic drugs. NSAID COX-2 inhibitors have recently been added to the therapeutic armamentarium.

Although many medications are available for the treatment of rheumatoid arthritis, they only ameliorate rather than cure, and they can cause adverse reactions. The NSAIDs, which include salicylates, are frequently helpful even in low dosages, but their potential side effects including gastric irritation and bleeding and tinnitus would be of aeromedical significance. Gold and penicillamine are 2 medications that are often poorly tolerated (15%-30% of patients have to stop taking gold) and cause pruritic rashes, cytopenia, and nephrotic syndrome.[2] Caution must also be taken when prescribing antimalarials such as hydroxychloroquine because of occasional pigmentary retinitis and possible loss of vision. Eye examinations are therefore advisable every 6 months. Other medications on the more potent end of the spectrum include immunosuppressive and cytotoxic drugs and steroids, all of which have known significant side effects that could be incompatible with aviation. If patients require these stronger medications, the disease process may be reaching its more advanced stages.

For all these reasons, it is understandable why waivers cannot always be granted for aviators with rheumatoid arthritis. The frequency of the arthritic attacks, their severity and duration, and the necessity for therapeutic regimens requiring high doses of strong medication must be given serious consideration in determining aeromedical disposition.

Ankylosing Spondylitis

Ankylosing spondylitis or Marie-Strumpell arthritis, an inflammatory condition, is the third most common form of chronic arthritis.[3] It is an inherited disease that most commonly strikes males between 20 and 40 years of age. Hence, it is occasionally diagnosed in flight personnel who are in the midst of their aviation careers. In general, the disease causes an arthritic process most commonly of the spine, sacroiliac, and large peripheral joints. Furthermore, in its most serious forms, patients may develop systemic symptoms as well as uveitis, pulmonary fibrosis, and aortic insufficiency.

Early in the disease, the patient complains of mild lower back pain which progressively worsens, eventually causing limitation of motion. X-ray changes with disease progression may show calcification of the spinal ligaments and a "bambooing" of the vertebrae. However, the best clue in diagnosis, in addition to the history, is the presence of HLA-B27 antigen. The symptoms are caused by a process of slow fusion of the vertebrae which cannot be cured but can be retarded by daily exercise, physical therapy, and NSAIDs including aspirin and indomethacin. Care must be taken with these medications in that some may cause gastric irritation and hemorrhage.

The discomfort caused by ankylosing spondylitis, its natural course of remissions and exacerbations, the limitation of motion, and the frequent use of medication are important factors to consider in disposition. Long hours in a cramped cockpit as well as the possibility of ejection from a high-performance aircraft could be intolerable to military aviators with this disease. Certainly a medical waiver can be considered as long as the disease is in its early stages and causes only mild symptoms. The natural progressive course of the disease will probably not allow an aviator to enjoy a long and full career in aviation.

Gout

Gout is a disease most often afflicting males over 30 years of age. Although most cases present with severe and incapacitating acute arthritis involving the first metatarsophalangeal joint, others present with renal lithiasis. Besides arthritis and renal stone formation, a rarer but much more serious form of gout is renal nephropathy with failure due to urate depositions in the renal interstitial tissue. Although the precise pathophysiology of gout is not entirely understood, there appears to be an association with uric acid levels, tophus formation, and the inflammatory process.

Diagnosis of gouty arthritis is made by clinical impression, serum uric acid, 24-hour urine uric acid, synovial fluid aspirate, and x-ray; relief of symptoms with a therapeutic trial of colchicine provides further evidence for the diagnosis. Although nearly all patients with gout have hyperuricemia, it is not pathognomonic; elevated levels may be seen in other disease entities including sarcoid and myeloproliferative disorders. Once the diagnosis of gout is verified, the presence of hypertension, diabetes mellitus, and atherosclerosis should be sought because of gout's known association with them. The clinical course of gouty arthritis is extremely variable; some patients have only one episode while others suffer for many years.

Regarding treatment, colchicine and indomethacin are usually prescribed for several days during the acute attack. However, once the patient is back to normal, a decision must be made as to prophylactic management. Factors to consider are severity and frequency of gouty arthritis and the serum uric acid level. If medication is deemed necessary during the symptom-free period, colchicine, a uricosuric agent such as probenecid, and allopurinol, a xanthine oxidase inhibitor, should be considered. Although these medications are relatively benign, it should be kept in mind that colchicine commonly causes abdominal cramping and diarrhea and that allopurinol can cause a pruritic rash (in 2% of patients with 0.1% developing exfoliative dermatitis), as well as precipitate an acute gouty attack.[4] There is also a slight risk of probenecid causing renal colic due to urate crystal deposition in the kidney.

Several specific points must be considered before requesting a waiver for the diagnosis of gout:

- Are the gouty attacks frequent and severe?
- Is the patient free of renal involvement?
- Does the patient have hypertension, diabetes, atherosclerosis, or other disease associated with gout?
- Is the serum uric acid kept at normal levels with medication and is the patient free of untoward side effects of the medication prescribed?

All these factors must be considered when determining the flight status of an aviator with gout.

Systemic Lupus Erythematosus (SLE)

SLE most frequently afflicts individuals between 20 and 40 years old of either sex and has been reported in aviators.[5] Because the disease can cause multisystem dysfunction, the spectrum of signs and symptoms varies greatly. Approximately 50% of patients will have some degree of renal involvement as manifested by proteinuria and hematuria sometime during the course of the disease. Younger patients usually have more severe forms of renal disease which result in hypertension, nephrotic syndrome, and renal failure. Anemia, leukopenia, and thrombocytopenia are common laboratory findings and may cause related symptoms. If the nervous system is affected, a wide array of neurologic as well as psychiatric manifestations with varying degrees of disability will become apparent including headaches, seizures, depression, and cognitive dysfunction. A common complaint of patients is poly-arthralgias due to arthritis or synovitis, which can cause considerable discomfort as well as eventual deformity. Other major complications involve the heart and lungs with pericarditis, myocarditis, pleuritis, and interstitial pulmonary disease and fibrosis often reported. And finally, cutaneous lesions may appear anywhere on the body with the classical malar butterfly rash being best known to most physicians.

The diagnosis of SLE is primarily a clinical one with several laboratory tests available such as the antinuclear antibody tests and LE cell phenomenon for confirmation of the clinical impression. Other nonspecific findings may include leukopenia, thrombocytopenia, anemia, and an elevated sedimentation rate.

Treatment available today is not curative but does afford the patient some relief. Regimens prescribed include systemic steroids, nonsteroidal antiinflammatory agents, antimalarials, and immunosuppressive agents.

Although some cases of SLE have a benign course, the majority experience a course of remissions and exacerbations. Certification of flight status depends on what organ systems are involved, the severity, and the frequency of exacerbations. The need for medication, particularly steroids with their host of side effects (hyper-glycemia, edema, hypertension, osteoporosis, electrolyte imbalance, peptic ulcer, and changes in mentation) must be taken into account. The unpredictable course of the disease and its multisystem predilection are an added risk not necessarily because of incapacitation, but because of partial disability that could impede the performance of routine cockpit chores.

Consequently the aeromedical disposition of patients with SLE can be difficult. For example, arthralgias might impede proper rudder or yoke control, altered mentation and neuropathies could impair judgment and increase reaction time respectively, and inflammation of lung tissue may adversely affect oxygen diffusion; these are only a few undesirable effects that may compromise aviation safety. Others include constitutional symptoms and lack of a feeling of well-being. Another theoretical disadvantage to ponder is the exposure to excessive sunlight in the cockpit which is well known to exacerbate symptoms.

Certainly individuals with permanent or apparent long-term remission should be able to fly safely. Also a more liberal policy could be extended to aviators who are in the early stages of the illness. Another exception could be the patient who develops a lupus-like syndrome after taking medications (procainamide, hydralazine, and isoniazid are prime examples) known to cause this syndrome as a manifestation of drug reaction. Once the drug is discontinued, the lupus-like syndrome will spontaneously remit without further sequelae. In any case, if a decision is made to qualify an individual with SLE, very close following by the AME/FS would be mandatory.

Duodenal Ulcer Disease

Duodenal ulcer classically causes midepigastric pain or burning 30-60 minutes after meals and is usually relieved by food, milk, or antacids. One would expect duodenal ulcer to be a common illness among aviators in that its highest incidence is in individuals 30-50 years of age. The diagnosis is usually made by history, UGI series, or duodenoscopy. Although the etiology may be multifactorial, more than 90% of cases of duodenal ulcer are caused by *Helicobacter pylori*, a gram-negative flagellated spirochete that can be detected by gastric biopsy or serology.[6]

Treatment modalities for duodenal ulcer include antacids, H_2 receptor antagonists, sucralfate, and proton pump inhibitors (PPI). In general, these medications are benign although not completely free of side effects. Antacids can cause diarrhea or constipation depending on which preparation is used. Because sucralfate is not absorbed, there are no known systemic effects. H_2 receptor antagonists are very safe but may cause occasional headaches. Care must also be taken because they interact with warfarin, phenytoin, and theophylline. Omeprazole, a PPI, may cause headache and gastrointestinal symptoms in some patients.

For patients with *H pylori*, eradication therapy is strongly recommended because it reduces the ulcer recurrence rate to less than 5%.[7] There are several regimens although 14 days of triple therapy with bismuth, metronidazole, and either amoxicillin or tetracycline produces a 90% eradication rate.[6]

For aviators with uncomplicated duodenal ulcer, temporary restriction from flying is advisable when symptoms are present. In addition, healing may be facilitated by avoiding a stressful workplace and the irregular timing of meals sometimes necessitated by the aviator's schedule. In most cases a prescribed therapeutic regimen brings remission within 4-8 weeks. Unfortunately, ulcer disease has a high recurrence rate (70%-80%), particularly if *H pylori* infection has not been eradicated.[7] For those with *H pylori*–associated duodenal ulcer, the very low recurrence rate once the organism is removed gives added confidence for a favorable aeromedical disposition. In any event, aviators must understand that the risk of recurrence can be reduced by therapeutic compliance and avoidance of tobacco and alcohol. The final aeromedical disposition decision for uncomplicated duodenal ulcer depends upon the presence of symptoms, the requirement for medication, and the rate of recurrence.

Fifteen to twenty percent of patients with peptic ulcer disease will have a bleeding complication.[8] If this occurs following treatment what is the risk of an episode of rebleeding? This question is of particular concern to the AME/FS because of possible inflight incapacitation. Because it has been reported that 20% of patients presented with melena, 30% with hematemesis, and 50% with both,[9] some were probably incapacitated to some degree.

The risk of rebleeding depends very much on the treatment method used. For those who undergo *H pylori* eradication, the risk for rebleeding is small. In one study, only 1 of 23 of such patients had a recurrence by 48 months.[8] Other studies in the literature are consistent with these results. Maintenance H_2 receptor antagonist therapy is another option, although the findings are inconsistent, with some studies reporting a significant reduction in rebleeding and others reporting no improvement.[10,11]

In general, the risk for rebleeding is less after a surgical procedure than with medical treatment. However, there is a tradeoff because some patients develop long-term postoperative complications such as dumping syndrome (with its attendant symptoms of postprandial tachycardia, diaphoresis, hypotension, and abdominal pain) and diarrhea.

There are 3 major surgical procedures used to treat ulcer disease: parietal cell or highly selective vagotomy, vagotomy-antrectomy, and vagotomy and drainage (pyloroplasty).[12] For parietal cell vagotomy, the recurrence rate ranges from 5%-30% (depending on the center) and 6% for the dumping syndrome; for vagotomy-antrectomy it is 2% and 25% respectively; and for vagotomy-drainage, 0%-17% and 12% respectively.

With the variety of available medical and surgical therapeutic options for bleeding duodenal ulcer disease, the aeromedical disposition decision can be a difficult one. Other variables found in published studies can further cloud the issue, including the skill of the surgeon, the varying periods of patient follow-up, the loss of patients to follow-up, and patient compliance with prescribed treatment. Furthermore, studies may include hospitalized patients from a heterogeneous population, making it tenuous to apply data from these studies to a well-defined population of otherwise reasonably healthy aviators.

Nevertheless, we can arrive at some generalizations regarding the aeromedical disposition of aviators with bleeding duodenal ulcer disease:

- Gastrointestinal bleeding can pose an additional threat to flying safety.
- Once a patient has a bleeding ulcer, there are no prognostic risk factors to reliably predict which patients will rebleed.
- Those with *H pylori* infection who undergo eradication therapy have a low recurrence rate (5%).
- Of the surgical procedures available today, vagotomy-antrectomy has the lowest recurrence rate (2%).

- The incidence of dumping syndrome and its severity should be taken into account.
- If a waiver is granted, postoperative recovery must be complete with very close follow-up to ensure that a second bleeding episode has not occurred.

Gastric Ulcer

Gastric ulcers are much less common than duodenal ulcers. Incidence is highest in those 40-55 years old, and approximately 4% are malignant. Furthermore, gastric ulcers have a significant recurrence rate within 5 years. Otherwise, aeromedical disposition for gastric ulcer is similar to that of duodenal ulcer. Once malignancy has been ruled out by UGI series, gastroscopy, or cytology studies, the aviator should be temporarily restricted from flying until medical (or surgical) management is concluded and the ulcer has healed.

Gastroesophageal Reflux Disease (GERD)

With gastroesophageal reflux disease (GERD), there is lower esophageal sphincter (LES) relaxation and reflux of gastric contents that can eventually cause esophagitis with its attendant symptoms of substernal pain (heartburn), cramping, and vomiting. A more serious sequela of long-term esophagitis is occult upper gastrointestinal bleeding and anemia. The diagnosis of GERD can be made by esophagogastroduodenoscopy, esophageal pH probe, and manometry. Current therapeutic modalities include antacids, histamine H_2 receptor antagonists, prokinetic agents, cytoprotective agents, and proton pump inhibitors (PPI).[13]

H_2 blockers (cimetidine, ranitidine) reduce gastric acid secretion and rarely cause significant side effects. Long-term maintenance therapy may be necessary in many patients. Prokinetic agents such as bethanechol, metoclopramide, and cisapride act by increasing the LES pressure and accelerating gastric emptying. The former 2 medications are of questionable efficacy and have cholinergic effects (ie, miosis, bronchorrhea, bradycardia, hyperperistalsis). Metoclopramide may also cause mental depression and Parkinsonian-like symptoms. Cisapride was taken off the market because it causes heart rhythm abnormalities as this book went to press. Sucralfate protects the mucosal lining and is nonabsorbable causing no systemic effects. At worst it sometimes causes mild constipation. Gastric acid secretion can be suppressed by PPIs such as omeprazole, which are well tolerated with minimal side effects.

Besides pharmacological treatment, patients may also benefit from weight reduction, smoking cessation, and avoidance of alcohol. Dietary modification with avoidance of foods that decrease LES pressure such as fatty foods, chocolate, and coffee is also advisable. For patients with severe disease or disease refractory to medical treatment, fundoplication is an option.

Unfortunately, GERD has a high recurrence rate depending on the medication or combination of medications prescribed.[13] The aeromedical disposition consequently must be individualized according to the frequency and intensity of the episodes as well as the presence of complications such as bleeding. In general, the medications prescribed for GERD are benign but special consideration must be given if bethanechol or metoclopramide are prescribed as they may have side effects as described above that may be significant in the cockpit. And finally, the lifestyle modifications demanded by this illness, particularly dietary ones, may be impractical in some types of flying operations.

Inflammatory Bowel Disease

Inflammatory bowel disease includes Crohn's disease and ulcerative colitis. Crohn's disease or regional ileitis is a serious gastrointestinal disorder usually involving the ileum but which may also involve the stomach, the entire small intestine, or colon. It usually occurs in a relatively young population and has an unpredictable course of remissions and exacerbations. The inflammatory-like lesions of regional ileitis can cause episodic fever, abdominal pain, and diarrhea as well as a host of complications including abscess and fistula formation, obstruction, perforation, bleeding, and malabsorption. There is also evidence that these patients have a higher incidence of small and large bowel cancer than the general population.[14] Although an occasional patient with this disease will suffer only a single acute episode or enjoy a long respite, perhaps measured in years, the majority of patients will progress to chronicity, the interval between attacks becoming shorter and shorter, with eventual development of one or more of the complications almost a certainty.

The medical treatment of Crohn's disease is only supportive. It includes dietary therapy, 5-aminosalicylic acid compounds, antibiotics, corticosteroids, and immunosuppressants, all of which offer amelioration and transient remission of symptoms at best.[15] Although the 5-aminosalicylic acid compounds (sulfasalazine, mesalamine) and antibiotics sometimes prescribed (metronidazole, ciprofloxacin) have few side effects, this is not necessarily true for the corticosteroids and immunosuppressants. The former can cause mood changes, adrenal insufficiency, and cataract formation while the latter (azathioprine, mercaptopurine, cyclosporine) can cause leukopenia, pancreatitis, lymphoma, and leukemia. Hence, close monitoring is required. Surgical treatment (resection, permanent ileostomy, etc) also leaves much to be desired in that there is a 75% or higher recurrence rate of the disease postsurgery; furthermore, of those patients requiring surgery, as many as 50% will need another operation within 10 years.[16,17]

In one study, 592 patients with Crohn's disease were followed for an average of 13 years.[14] Of these patients, 438 or approximately ⅔ required surgical intervention sometime during the course of the disease. Although survival rates of the surgically and medically treated groups were high, symptoms continued sporadically for over half the patients, resulting in decreased quality of life for many years regardless of treatment. Recurrence of the disease after surgery was a major problem with 42% of the patients relapsing within 15 years, the great majority within 8 years.

Because Crohn's disease is characterized by remissions and exacerbations, serious complications, and in many cases refractoriness to treatment, prognosis for a full career in aviation is guarded. The AME/FS must take special care if long-term corticosteroids or immunosuppressants are prescribed because of their significant side effects. Exceptions might be made for those with infrequent symptoms who do not require long-term therapy.

Ulcerative colitis, although an entirely different entity, does have some clinical and diagnostic similarities to Crohn's disease; hence the aeromedical disposition lends itself to the same reasoning. Ulcerative colitis is an inflammatory disease of the colon causing abdominal pain, bloody diarrhea, and weight loss varying from mild to severe. The course of the illness is usually one of remissions and exacerbations with a number of patients developing complications such as anemia, arthritis, fistulas, ocular lesions, and colonic strictures; there is also a high incidence of colonic carcinoma. There are a number of treatment modalities similar to those for Crohn's disease including surgery (total colectomy with permanent ileostomy or an ileoproctostomy).

Ulcerative colitis appears to be less severe than Crohn's disease. Even though a majority of patients may have few or no symptoms after the first episode, as many as 27% will require surgery within 5 years of diagnosis.[18] Twenty to thirty percent of patients with ulcerative colitis will require surgery and 7%-15% will have recurrences.[19] And for those with colectomy and permanent ileostomy, the need for an ileostomy bag may be incompatible for certain types of flying, particularly in aircraft that require the wear of extensive life support equipment or impose high G forces. For patients with an ileoproctostomy, this may not be a consideration, but those who have this procedure can be inconvenienced by a large number of stools per day. The rationale of aeromedical disposition for patients with ulcerative colitis would be the same as for those with Crohn's disease.

Irritable Bowel Syndrome

Irritable bowel syndrome (IBS) is a disease of many names: irritable or spastic colon, nervous colon, nervous diarrhea—all of which aptly describe its manifestations. It is an extremely common disorder most often afflicting young and middle-aged adults. In some cases, it is a chronic, lifelong disorder. Although the etiology is unknown, there is considerable evidence of an association with stress, in particular domestic, financial, and occupational stressors. In addition to stress, there is also evidence that some patients develop symptoms related to sensitivity to certain foods. In any event, patients complain of abdominal pain or bloating, constipation, and diarrhea of varying severity and frequency without objective evidence of organic cause (barium enema and sigmoidoscopy may reveal only nonspecific changes). The gastrointestinal tract appears to be the target organ system with hypermotility and an increased sensitivity to stimulation.

Treatment is mainly supportive with dietary modification, antidiarrheals and anticonstipation agents frequently prescribed; psychotropic agents may also be helpful.[20] If food sensitivity is suspected, various elimination diets must also be tried. In any event, close follow-up with frequent and regular return visits to the managing physician will go a long way in helping the patient.

The psychological aspects of IBS deserve further emphasis as many patients have a rigid personality type with some degree of depression, hysteria, or other neurotic symptoms. Common complaints include fatigue, insomnia, depression, anorexia, and weeping. Therefore, treatment is often prolonged requiring frequent office visits, at least early in the course of the disease, and the active psychological support of the managing physician. Although the course of the disease varies from patient to patient, chronicity is the rule especially if there is concomitant psychiatric illness.

Flying status for individuals with IBS comes into question not necessarily because of potential incapacitation, but rather because of its chronicity. The frequency of symptoms, whether mild or severe, the need for dietary modification, and the need for close patient following with strong psychological support may be difficult to overcome in a flight operation. Furthermore, some drugs prescribed for this condition have side effects which preclude safe operation of an aircraft. For example, anticholinergics interfere with normal vision by causing mydriasis and by impairing the muscles of accommodation. Antidepressants and anxiolytics can cause drowsiness and a host of other side effects. Likewise, the tricyclic antidepressants may cause anticholinergic effects, hypotension, and disorientation, among other adverse reactions. And finally, if dietary therapy is necessary, the nature of the flying mission may make it extremely inconvenient if not impossible. In patients who do not have severe and frequent symptoms and do not require regular use of psychotropic medication or anticholinergics, a more liberal policy is in order.

Pancreatitis

Pancreatitis is a serious disease which, if not treated vigorously, has a significant fatality rate. The disease has a legion of underlying causes although the majority are related to gallstones, alcohol intake, or an idiopathic process. Patients frequently have severe abdominal pain, shock, and systemic symptoms. The onset of symptoms may be sudden, resulting in some degree of incapacitation. The treatment of pancreatitis is medical or surgical depending on the circumstances of the illness. In many cases the patient responds well to therapy with swift and permanent recovery within days; however, other patients will have recurrent acute attacks and progress to the chronic state.

The disease is of aeromedical significance because of the potential for sudden incapacitation and risk of recurrence. If an aviator develops acute pancreatitis, an underlying cause must be sought. Following successful treatment of gallbladder disease or alcoholism there would be reasonable assurance that another attack will not occur. In this case a request for a medical waiver for acute pancreatitis would be appropriate. However, if there is no apparent underlying cause, the probability of a relapse or progression to a chronic form of the disease cannot be predicted. Therefore it is advisable to observe the patient for 12-18 months before requesting a waiver.

Cholecystitis

Acute or chronic cholecystitis is associated with gallstones in over 90% of cases. Patients will complain of severe right upper quadrant pain, nausea, vomiting, and fever; occasionally there is also jaundice. Diagnosis is usually made by ultrasound study. The preferred therapeutic modalities are open cholecystectomy and laparoscopic cholecystectomy, and which is chosen depends on a number of variables. The latter is often preferred because there is less postoperative pain, an earlier discharge (6 hours to 3 days postsurgery), and an earlier return to normal activities (7-16 days postsurgery) compared to open cholecystectomy.[21,22] Without surgery, recurrence of symptoms is common and there is an increased risk of empyema and perforation. Attacks may be unheralded, causing frequent periods of discomfort lasting hours at a time. Although cholecystectomy is curative in most cases, some patients may develop the postcholecystectomy syndrome, a constellation of symptoms including flatulence, abdominal pain, and fatty food intolerance, the cause of which is not well defined.

Other therapeutic modalities include gallstone dissolution with chenodeoxycholic and ursodeoxycholic acid. Although this appears to be an attractive alternative to surgery, there are drawbacks in that these medications must be taken for several years and are only effective for small stones. Furthermore, there is a 50% failure rate and a 25%-50% recurrence rate.[23] For some patients extracorporeal shock wave lithotripsy is preferred, but it too is effective only for small stones and has a 5-year 15%-50% recurrence rate.[23]

In some cases, gallstones found fortuitously remain silent causing no symptoms. Some have advocated cholecystectomy to avoid future episodes of cholecystitis, bile duct obstruction, infection, and a host of other complications. However, studies today indicate that it is prudent not to treat a patient with asymptomatic gallstones. One study of military pilots and navigators indicated that about 10% will develop symptoms within 5 years, suggesting that watchful waiting is the most prudent course of action.[24]

For aviators with asymptomatic cholelithiasis, there should be little risk because most will not have symptoms and for those that do, the chances of an acute, incapacitating attack of cholecystitis in the cockpit is very small. If an aviator has a surgical procedure, cure can be expected in the great majority of cases. Caution is advised, however, if the unfortunate aviator develops the postcholecystectomy syndrome with severe and frequent attacks. Likewise, for those undergoing gallstone dissolution with bile salts or lithotripsy, the failure and recurrence rates are very high, increasing the probability of unwanted symptoms of gallbladder disease in the cockpit.

Diverticular Disease of the Colon

Diverticulosis is characterized by saccular outpouchings of the large bowel, usually in the sigmoid colon. The great majority of patients have no symptoms although some will complain of abdominal discomfort, constipation, or diarrhea; occasionally there will also be rectal bleeding. The treatment for symptomatic diverticulosis includes dietary therapy (fiber) and supportive care. Medical waivers can usually be granted for individuals who are asymptomatic or who have symptoms requiring only occasional medication.

Diverticulitis is a complication of diverticulosis in which there is a superimposed inflammatory process. It has been thought that this occurs when undigested food or fecal matter becomes trapped in the outpouchings. In any event, patients can become quite uncomfortable with abdominal pain and fever. Furthermore, they are prone to develop many other complications such as abscesses, perforation, fistulae, bleeding, or obstruction. The medical treatment for uncomplicated diverticulitis includes diet, broad-spectrum antibiotics (ciprofloxacin, metronidazole), and symptomatic care. If complications occur (eg, obstruction, perforation, or refractoriness), surgery may be necessary with resection of the diseased portion of the colon.

Whether treated medically or surgically, persistent or recurrent symptoms are common. In one study of 297 cases of diverticulitis, 26% of patients treated medically needed further care.[25] In another study of patients who underwent surgery, 27% had recurrences.[26]

Most patients with diverticulitis should be able to return to the cockpit once they are asymptomatic. A more cautious approach is necessary for those with frequently recurring symptoms, particularly if symptomatic treatment includes sedatives, anticholinergics, or analgesics.

Pilonidal Disease

Pilonidal sinus is of particular importance in military aviation. During World War II, U.S. Army hospitals treated over 80,000 cases with an average hospital stay of 55 days; in other studies hospital stays ranged from 4-50 days with recurrence rates a significant 10%-30%.[27]

Pilonidal sinuses are most frequently found in hirsute men and are usually located over the sacrococcygeal area. There are currently two schools of thought regarding etiology: one advocates that the sinus tract results from a congenital defect; the other contends that the tract is acquired by an ingrowth of hair which forms a nidus of infection in the subcutaneous tissue. Regardless of etiology, the condition is aggravated by poor hygiene and trauma. (It was called "the Jeep Disease" in World War II.) However, regardless of which theory one favors, an abscess or draining sinus forms, causing the patient some discomfort.

Treatment may be conservative (ie, incision and drainage with sitz baths) or surgical. There are several procedures in use including complete excision or marsupialization. Whatever mode of therapy is indicated, most patients can expect fairly lengthy follow-up care including packing and the inconvenience of daily sitz baths.

Because to some degree dirt, sweat, and trauma are causal factors of pilonidal sinus disease, it is no wonder that jeep drivers and helicopter crews are often afflicted. Some rotary wing pilots who develop pilonidal sinus may be lost to duty for weeks to months because of long-term treatment and/or recurrences. A return to a helicopter cockpit—well known for its propensity for vibration and buffeting—before adequate healing will certainly provoke a recurrence. Although cockpits of fixed wing aircraft are not as traumatic as those of rotary wing aircraft, there still exists a lesser degree of unfavorable conditions for patients with pilonidal sinus. Therefore, flying status must be determined by the extent of the disease and the degree of disability. Prevention in the form of scrupulous hygiene in the anal and sacrococcygeal areas is highly recommended, particularly for those at high risk for this benign yet terribly annoying condition.

Sarcoidosis

Sarcoidosis most commonly occurs during the third and fourth decades of life. The etiology of this disease, which causes characteristic noncaseating granulomatous lesions of multiple organ systems, is uncertain. Most frequently it affects the hilar nodes and the lungs, causing lymphadenopathy and a fibrous infiltration leading to abnormal pulmonary function and oxygen diffusing capacity. Patients may complain of fever, fatigue, cough, and diarrhea. Although its pulmonary manifestations are most common, sarcoidosis is a multiorgan disease that can affect the heart, eyes, skin, liver, kidney, and nervous system, causing significant dysfunction and impairment.

Cardiac involvement occurs in 3%-5% of patients as determined by autopsy, and it may cause bradyarrhythmias, tachyarrhythmias, cardiomyopathy, and congestive heart failure, as well as sudden death in up to 25% of patients.[28,29] Therefore, AMEs and flight surgeons should be fully cognizant of the effects of myocardial sarcoid, of its uniformly poor prognosis, and of its propensity to cause incapacitation and sudden death.

To illustrate, in a series of 250 patients followed for a number of years, there were a large number of reported complications: complete heart block (49), premature ventricular contractions and ventricular tachycardia (48), myocardial disease (43), sudden death (37), bundle branch block (33), supraventricular arrhythmia (23), valvular lesions (21), simulated myocardial infarction (15), and pericarditis (6). Furthermore, it was noted that cardiac problems could be the initial manifestation of sarcoid or could occur years after the original pulmonary manifestations had cleared. Sudden death was noted at all ages with a spike between 35 and 44 years of age.[30]

Therefore, it appears that the granulomatous lesions of sarcoidosis, should they occur in the myocardium, frequently cause dysrhythmias (PVCs and ventricular tachycardia most commonly), serious conduction disturbances such as complete heart block, and myocardial damage. It is not surprising then that such patients have a high incidence of sudden death. It is extremely important, therefore, that myocardial involvement be considered in any patient who has sarcoidosis.

Other protean manifestations of sarcoid include erythema nodosum, uveitis causing blurred vision and photophobia, and hypercalcemia/hypercalciuria with possible nephrocalcinosis and renal failure. In addition, lesions can occur in bone, liver, and the central nervous system causing cranial nerve neuropathies, encephalopathy, and seizures.

Although there are no definitive blood tests with which to diagnose sarcoid, many patients will have an increased angiotensin converting enzyme level, increased sedimentation rate, hypergammaglobulinemia, hypercalcemia, and hyperuricemia. The diagnosis is best made by tissue biopsy, gallium scan, thallium scintigraphy, and chest x-ray. The latter characteristically shows bilateral hilar adenopathy and is occasionally first detected in asymptomatic individuals. Pulmonary disease is of particular significance because it can cause abnormal diffusion and a lowered arterial pO_2.

The course of sarcoid is extremely variable. In many cases, the patient may develop only hilar adenopathy remaining entirely asymptomatic with spontaneous remission of the radiologic abnormality at a later date. Seventy to seventy-five percent will clear within 2 years.[29] In other cases, the disease may be progressive causing pulmonary symptoms, cough, hemoptysis, and shortness of breath, as well as symptoms referable to other organ involvement. There are 2 recognized forms of sarcoidosis, acute and chronic, which can be a useful differentiation for the AME/FS because each has its own course and prognosis. The acute form is of sudden onset, is often responsive to therapy or remits spontaneously, and in general has a favorable prognosis with most patients enjoying complete resolution of the disease process. The chronic form, on the other hand, has an insidious onset, is progressive, and offers little hope for complete recovery.

There is no known cure for sarcoid, with corticosteroids the mainstay of therapy benefitting those with pulmonary, eye, and skin involvement. Medication may be necessary for as long as 1 year, mandating particular vigilance for steroid side effects. Another medication with questionable efficacy is methotrexate. In some cases, supportive care such as antiarrhythmics, pacemakers, or implantable cardioverters-defibrillators may be necessary.

In general, the prognosis for patients with sarcoid is good, particularly if there is only pulmonary involvement. However, because of the potential for multiorgan disease, especially cardiac, a thorough evaluation is of utmost importance. Every effort should be made to rule out cardiac sarcoid because of its potential for incapacitation and sudden death.

In summary, the aeromedical disposition of aviators with sarcoidosis is as follows:

- The patient should have a complete evaluation, including the lungs, heart, eyes, kidneys, liver, skin, and central nervous system. Cardiac involvement should be carefully explored.
- If the patient only has active pulmonary disease as evidenced by symptoms, chest film, or abnormal pulmonary function tests, revocation of flight status is advisable with a return to duty once the patient is asymptomatic, off all medication (particularly steroids), and all studies are normal.
- If there is evidence of myocardial sarcoid, the poor prognosis demands permanent restriction.
- If other organ systems are affected by the disease process, a return to the cockpit would be in order as long as the patient is in remission and has no permanent sequelae that threaten flying safety.
- In all cases, close follow-up is essential.

Asthma

Asthma is a respiratory disease characterized by recurring acute attacks of wheezing, coughing, and shortness of breath. Airway inflammation is the primary problem. Between attacks the patient is asymptomatic and may enjoy perfectly normal pulmonary function. The asthmatic episodes can be triggered by a host of factors such as allergens, infection, exercise, emotional distress, and irritants. Diagnosis can be made by history, physical examination during an attack, and pulmonary function tests (a decreased FEV at 1 second improved with a bronchodilator). A number of drugs including antiinflammatory agents, beta agonists, anticholinergics, and xanthines are available to physicians for treatment as well as prophylaxis of this disease.[31]

Asthmatic attacks are to some extent incapacitating and are clearly unwelcome in the cockpit. Although current therapy almost always reverses airway obstruction and aborts the acute attack, there may be a need for maintenance medication for those with a more severe form of disease.

Antiinflammatory agents that may be prescribed include cromolyn, nedocromil, and corticosteroids. The former two are used to prevent attacks triggered, for example, by exercise, and cause no significant side effects. Inhaled corticosteroids such as beclomethasone are not absorbed to any great extent, thereby sparing the patient the side effects of oral corticosteroid therapy. The frequently prescribed beta ago-

nists, usually delivered by inhaler, may cause tremulousness, dizziness, and disturbances of cardiac rhythm. Ipratropium can have anticholinergic side effects.
Theophyllines can cause gastrointestinal symptoms, central nervous system dysfunction (dizziness, vertigo, nervousness, seizures) and cardiac arrhythmias (tachycardia and ectopy).

The aeromedical disposition of aviators with bronchial asthma is controversial.
Some reason that if a pilot with asthma is asymptomatic between attacks and
requires no maintenance medication, he or she can continue flying as long as the
asthmatic episodes occur infrequently and require only short courses of medication.
Occasional temporary restriction may be necessary when symptomatic and on medication. Contrary to this point of view, others are of the opinion that asthma, because
it is potentially incapacitating and because recurring attacks are unpredictable,
should be disqualifying. Furthermore, the need for only short-term therapy following an asthmatic attack cannot be guaranteed; many patients will require maintenance medication.

The aeromedical disposition of trained aviators who develop asthma will
depend on the frequency and severity of attacks as well as the need for multiple or
high-dose maintenance medication. Because asthmatic attacks are potentially incapacitating, policy should ensure that the risk is kept to a minimum. If maintenance
medication is necessary, this might be an indication that attacks are frequent.
Furthermore, the type of medications prescribed as well as their side effects must be
given careful consideration, long-term oral corticosteroids being one example. In
general, aviators with infrequent attacks well controlled with short-term therapy
could be given favorable consideration. For others, aeromedical disposition would
be more guarded.

Spontaneous Pneumothorax

Spontaneous pneumothorax is an entity in which air, often secondary to a ruptured
bleb, accumulates in the pleural sac. The mechanism is unclear in that it can occur in
normal as well as diseased lungs. Because spontaneous pneumothorax is most common in young healthy males between 20 and 29 years old, it can be expected to
occur in a number of aviators.

Spontaneous pneumothorax is probably diagnosed most frequently by the
patient's symptoms of sudden chest pain with shortness of breath and possibly a
cough. However, some patients may have no symptoms whatsoever. The symptoms
depend on the extent and size of the pneumothorax and therefore may encompass a
broad spectrum from no symptoms to a life-threatening situation. Of course, once

spontaneous pneumothorax is suspected, diagnosis can usually be confirmed by chest x-ray.

Therapy may be conservative or surgical. For a smaller pneumothorax, the managing physician may prescribe only bedrest because many lesions spontaneously remit in a short period of time. Other conservative treatment modalities include needle aspiration or negative pressure closed-tube thoracostomy with the negative pressure causing expansion of the lung by reabsorption of the air in the pleural sac. Unfortunately, there are significant first, second, and third recurrence rates with conservative therapy of 10%-60%, 17%-80%, and 80%-100% of cases respectively.[32-34]

There are several surgical options: chemical or mechanical pleurodesis by which scarification of the pleura is done causing obliteration of the pleural space, pleurectomy by open thoracotomy, resection of blebs, and pleurodesis by thoroscopy. For pleurodesis the recurrence rate is up to 30% and for pleurectomy it is 1%.[32] The choice of therapy depends, among other things, on the size of the pneumothorax, the severity of symptoms, and history of recurrence.

Because a pneumothorax can cause incapacitating symptoms, the recurrence rate is of particular significance for the AME/FS. As seen in published studies, recurrences are the rule rather than the exception for conservative therapy and pleurodesis. Although pleurectomy by open thoracotomy is a far more extensive procedure with a longer period of recuperation, the risk of another episode of spontaneous pneumothorax is reduced to a comfortable 1%. For patients who do have a second spontaneous pneumothorax, the majority will occur within 1 year of the initial event and ⅔ within 2 years. However, some patients may have another event even years later.

Pneumothorax is a condition of aeromedical concern not only because of severe symptoms (ie, chest pain, dyspnea, and shortness of breath), but also because of the possibility of gas expansion at altitude. In accordance with Boyle's law, the trapped gas could expand causing a mediastinal shift and serious respiratory distress. This is a potential threat not only inflight, but also in an altitude chamber, where it is not uncommon for some aviators to be taken to altitudes as high as 10,670 m (35,000 ft).

Although one could postulate that aviators are at increased risk of developing spontaneous pneumothorax because of the aviation environment, lowered barometric pressure, positive pressure breathing, rapid decompression, and acceleration, in reality, few cases have been reported inflight (one was recently reported in a F-16 pilot)[32] or in an altitude chamber. Fuchs reports that the occurrence of spontaneous pneumothorax in a decreased ambient pressure environment is extremely rare.[35] In a review of the literature, he has found only a handful of sporadic cases and even these were questionable. Furthermore, several studies encompassed thousands of subjects who had undergone altitude chamber indoctrination. Again, even in those studies the occurrence of spontaneous pneumothorax was rare. Therefore, it was concluded that exposure of aviators to decreased ambient pressure in aircraft or in an altitude chamber did not increase the risk of developing spontaneous pneumothorax.

Nevertheless, there are a multitude of factors which must be considered when determining the aeromedical disposition of anyone who has had a spontaneous pneumothorax. Among these are the high recurrence rate, the potential for incapacitation, and the mode of treatment.

The following criteria are suggested requirements for medical waivers for idiopathic spontaneous pneumothorax:

- There has been a single episode.
- There has been complete recovery with full expansion of the lung.
- Pulmonary function tests are normal.
- There is no demonstrable underlying pathology that would predispose the individual to recurrence.
- One year has elapsed, since most recurrences are within 12 months. (A few months' wait should suffice for patients having pleurectomy because of its low recurrence rate.)

If there is a recurrence in spite of therapy, the risk of subsequent episodes becomes even higher, so even more stringent criteria for a waiver would be advisable. For example, a pleurectomy might be recommended. In addition, military operations might opt to evaluate the pilot in an altitude chamber to ensure that lowered ambient pressure and rapid decompression could be withstood. In any event, precautions should be taken to minimize the risk of a recurring spontaneous pneumothorax.

Pulmonary Blebs and Bullae

A pulmonary bleb is a collection of air located between the visceral pleura and lung substance; a pulmonary bulla is a collection of air within the lung substance itself. Most individuals with blebs or bullae are asymptomatic with the abnormality usually first noted incidentally on chest x-ray. Although blebs and bullae may remain asymptomatic, they do pose a potential threat to individuals who are exposed to lowered barometric pressures. As the ambient pressure decreases, a bleb or bulla may slowly enlarge resulting in compression of adjacent structures, bleeding, or formation of a pneumothorax or pneumomediastinum. These untoward complications are particularly likely if the bleb or bulla is not in communication with the respiratory tree, or if the communication is partial or intermittent. However, with good communication the pressure can readily equalize as the aircraft ascends.

Although the aeromedical implications of these defects appear ominous, there is some evidence to suggest that at least in selected cases there is no added hazard to flying safety. Tomashefski and colleagues studied 6 individuals with chronic lung disease and blebs or bullae.[36] The subjects were taken to 5472 m (18,000 ft) in an altitude chamber with chest x-rays taken at various altitudes. It was found that the blebs and bullae had not increased in size as seen on films made at sea level, intermediary altitudes, and 5472 m. The most plausible explanation for failure of the blebs and bullae to enlarge when subjected to lower barometric pressure is the presence of good communication with the respiratory tree.

Thus there should be no hazard if the patient has no other disqualifying pulmonary pathology and there is reasonable confidence that the blebs or bullae communicate with the airway. (The gold standard for proof should be a chest x-ray in an inflight altitude chamber with no demonstrable enlargement of the blebs or bullae when the aviator is subjected to lower barometric pressure.)

Coccidioidomycosis and Histoplasmosis

Coccidioidomycosis is a fungal infection caused by *Coccidioides immitis*, an organism endemic in the southwestern part of the United States. The disease, which is contracted by inhalation of spores found in the soil, may involve multiple organ systems although pulmonary infection is its most common manifestation. Diagnosis of coccidioidomycosis can be made by chest x-ray, skin test, culture, and serology. Sixty percent of patients infected may be asymptomatic or develop a flu-like syndrome with full remission requiring no treatment.[37] However, some patients who develop extensive pulmonary infiltrates, cavitation, or disseminated disease may require therapy with amphotericin B, azole therapy, or surgery.

Histoplasmosis is a fungal disease caused by *Histoplasma capsulatum*, an organism found chiefly in the eastern and midwestern United States. Like coccidioidomycosis, it is primarily a pulmonary disease contracted by inhalation of spores from the soil. It is most frequently a benign self-limiting illness, although occasional patients become seriously ill with extensive pulmonary or extrapulmonary involvement. In such cases the treatment of choice is similar to that for coccidioidomycosis.

Since most cases of either fungal infection are self-limiting, aviators need be disqualified only temporarily from flying duty until the disease has run its course. However, for those with more serious forms of the disease requiring therapy for several months, disqualification is the prudent course because of potential side effects of the medications. For example, amphotericin B may cause nausea, fever, myalgia, and is nephrotoxic. The azoles can cause gastrointestinal symptoms and hepatotoxicity. Furthermore, there is a 75% relapse rate of coccidioidomycosis.[37] Once treatment is discontinued and the patient is asymptomatic with a normal or stabilized chest x-ray, a return to flying would be in order.

Chronic Obstructive Pulmonary Disease (COPD)

Any disease involving the lung is of compelling aeromedical interest because compromise of its normal function will decrease its ability to withstand physiological stresses such as decreased barometric pressure, a hypoxic environment, and accelerative forces. COPD is an excellent example illustrating the incompatibilities of a diseased lung and flight. The pathologic process affects the airways causing an inflammatory obliteration, fibrosis, and rupture of the alveolar sacs, eventually leading to abnormal ventilation/perfusion and an impaired diffusing capacity. Because of inadequate oxygen delivery and underperfusion or underventilation of the alveoli, the patient develops shunts by which poorly oxygenated blood reaches the systemic circulation.

In its early stages the disease process may cause no symptoms, but eventually the patient will complain of productive cough, wheezing, and dyspnea. As more and more lung tissue is destroyed over the years, the diffusion inward of oxygen and outward of carbon dioxide will become increasingly impaired, and hypoxemia and then hypercapnia will develop. Other late complications include bullae formation, pulmonary hypertension, cor pulmonale, and heart failure.

COPD can be easily diagnosed once it has reached its later stages. A patient with a smoking history, barrel chest, abnormal pulmonary function tests, and depressed diaphragm with hyperinflated lungs seen on chest x-ray is no diagnostic enigma. However, in the early stages when the patient is either asymptomatic or has mild symptoms without telltale laboratory or radiologic signs, detection and diagnosis is far more difficult. It is desirable to detect COPD in its early stages not only because treatment improves the prognosis, but also for aeromedical purposes. One way to accomplish this is by spirometry, which is employed by some medical departments as part of the regular periodic physical examination. Useful pulmonary function tests include FEV_1, FEV_1:FVC ratio, and the more sensitive maximum midexpiratory flow (MMEF) rate, all of which will be abnormal in obstructive airway disease. (Other tests purportedly useful in detection of early disease include flow volume curves, closing volume, and diffusion tests. However, these are controversial and often require special equipment.) Additionally, alpha$_1$-antitrypsin deficiency is a known risk factor for COPD and could be assessed in questionable cases. Although the above pulmonary function tests (FEV$_1$, FVC, and MMEF rate) may detect early disease, studies have shown no correlation with the degree of airway obstruction.

Although various modes of therapy including beta agonists, corticosteroids, and antibiotics are commonly prescribed, their efficacy for slowing or halting the disease process is highly questionable. Cessation of smoking is critical since this will bring symptomatic improvement. One study demonstrated that cigarette smokers will show improvement of their pulmonary function tests within 6-14 weeks of abstinence.[38] Thus there appears to be some degree of reversibility of the disease process, particularly if the diagnosis is made early and appropriate therapy instituted.

Regarding the aeromedical disposition of aviators with COPD, disqualification from the cockpit need not be predicated on the diagnosis per se, but rather on the extent of the disease process and degree of pulmonary insufficiency. AMEs and flight surgeons would probably have no disagreement over patients with advanced or even moderate disease. Such patients would pose an added risk to flight safety not only because of symptoms and the need to use medication, but also because of hypoxemia. In most cases, arterial pO$_2$, even at sea level would be lower than normal, and would get even lower at altitude. Thus an aviator at sea level might have an arterial pO$_2$ equivalent to that of a normal individual at 1520-2128 m (5000-7000 feet).

For aerobatics and high-performance aircraft pilots, ventilation/perfusion defects can be further aggravated by accelerative forces, depending on which portions of the lung are diseased, causing even more unoxygenated blood to be shunted into the systemic circulation.

Bullae formation occasionally found in patients with COPD is another consideration. If the bullae communicate with the airway, there is much less immediate danger. However, if the bullae do not communicate, there is the possibility that they will expand as the barometric pressure decreases with altitude or during a rapid decompression. Besides the danger of rupture, the expanding bullae can compress adjacent normal lung tissue, further depriving the patient of remaining functioning alveoli.

Another consideration is pulmonary hypertension. It is well known that hypoxia is the single strongest stimulus to cause increased pressure of the pulmonary vasculature. Most patients with COPD already have some degree of pulmonary hypertension which is aggravated at altitude due to the decreased barometric pressure. Serious sequelae of pulmonary hypertension which may eventually develop are cor pulmonale, congestive heart failure, and syncope.

Finally, patients with moderate or advanced COPD will undoubtedly be on some treatment regimen. Drugs normally prescribed are generally the same as those used to treat asthma. As discussed in the section on asthma, they do have side effects which can be undesirable in the cockpit.

Thus most patients with moderate or advanced COPD are not suited for the cockpit because of a decreased tolerance to a hypoxic environment, the possibility of bullae formation, the danger of pulmonary hypertension and its sequelae, and the need to take medication with undesirable side effects.

As for the aviator with a normal chest x-ray who is asymptomatic or with mild symptoms and shown to have abnormal pulmonary function tests on physical examination, the outlook for continued flying need not be so bleak. This is particularly true if the patient stops smoking and demonstrates some improvement in pulmonary function testing. Also consider arterial blood gas studies to determine the pO_2 at sea level. (The military services can sometimes also obtain blood gas studies in aircraft as well as in decompression chambers at various altitudes.) Therefore, a patient with early COPD could qualify for flying with some organizations as long as he or she is reasonably physically fit, does not have significant shunting of unoxygenated blood, has a normal chest x-ray, and stops smoking.

Tuberculosis

Although tuberculosis has become a relatively uncommon disease in the United States, the incidence has been increasing in recent years in part because of its association with HIV infection. Aviators with active disease should be temporarily disqualified from the cockpit for at least the early part of their therapy because of symptoms, side effects associated with treatment, and the need for close follow-up. Possible major adverse effects of first-line antituberculosis drugs are as follows[39]:

- Isoniazid: hepatitis, peripheral neuropathy
- Rifampin: gastrointestinal upset, hepatitis, skin eruptions
- Ethambutol: retrobulbar neuritis, blurred vision, scotomata
- Pyrazinamide: hepatitis, hyperuricemia
- Streptomycin: ototoxicity with vertigo and hearing loss

Other factors to consider are close and continuous contact of the cockpit crew and the undesirability of sharing equipment such as headsets, microphones, or oxygen masks with a fellow aviator who is still contagious. Awareness of these effects and proper patient follow-up should ensure a timely and safe return to the cockpit, perhaps at some time during the maintenance phase of treatment.

For the occasional case when thoracic surgery is necessary to extirpate the disease process, a waiver could be requested once the patient is fully recovered from the operation, has reasonably normal pulmonary function tests and exercise tolerance, and is cured.

Regarding chemoprophylaxis, isoniazid is most commonly prescribed because of contact with a household member with active tuberculosis, or because of recent TB skin test conversion. Isoniazid is a relatively innocuous drug although there is the occasional individual who will develop hepatitis, rash, gastrointestinal symptoms, or peripheral neuropathy.[40] However, aviators taking prophylactic isoniazid may continue flying without compromising flight safety because the untoward effects of isoniazid are quite uncommon and in no way cause an acute, incapacitating reaction when they do occur.

Shub and his group followed 58 military airmen who were prescribed isoniazid prophylaxis, 300 mg qd, for 1 year because they were skin-test converters.[41] Only 2 of the subjects had to discontinue the drug because of its side effects: one airman with rising transaminase and hepatomegaly and another with arthralgias. In both cases there was remission of the signs and symptoms once the isoniazid was discontinued. None of the 58 subjects experienced an acute crisis of any kind.

In another study of 13,838 patients on isoniazid prophylaxis, the incidence of hepatitis was directly related to age: 0.3% at 20-34 years of age; 1.2% at 35-49; and 2.3% at 50-64. It was also uncommon to develop peripheral neuropathy with conventional dosages.[42] Interestingly, even if a patient develops abnormal liver function tests, icterus, and dark urine, in most cases remission will take place even if the drug is continued. It is advisable to follow all patients on prophylaxis clinically, ordering laboratory studies when indicated.

Anemia

It is well beyond the scope of this book to discuss the many types of anemia. Only pernicious anemia, hereditary spherocytosis, hemoglobinopathies (including thalassemia and sickle cell trait), and G6PD deficiency will serve as examples. In general, the decision to grant flight certification depends on the type of anemia and its severity and the therapeutic regimen chosen. It should be remembered that an anemic condition, besides causing symptoms, can lower tolerance to hypoxia and acceleration. Furthermore, although anemic patients may have a normal hemoglobin saturation, the total hemoglobin pool is less than normal and consequently the total amount of available oxygen will be reduced, thereby resulting in the added burden of a compensatory increase in the cardiac output. Regarding aeromedical disposition, aviators who have curable anemia need be disqualified only temporarily and can return to flight status after treatment. The anemia of infection, of blood loss, or of dietary deficiency are examples of types that can be effectively treated with appropriate therapy.

Pernicious Anemia

Pernicious anemia is a megaloblastic anemia caused by the absence of intrinsic factor necessary for the absorption of vitamin B_{12}. If untreated its course is progressive, causing gastrointestinal, hematologic, and neurologic symptoms. The patient may complain of weakness, fatigue, paresthesias, incoordination, and altered cerebral function. The diagnosis can be confirmed by the presence of megaloblastic bone marrow, achylia gastrica, a positive Schilling test, and a response to a therapeutic trial of parenteral vitamin B_{12}. The treatment of choice for pernicious anemia is lifelong administration of parenteral vitamin B_{12} which may arrest the symptoms or even bring about complete remission.

Depending on the nature of operations some aviators can continue flying if they are asymptomatic, compliance with treatment is assured, and there is close following by the AME/FS. However, cogent reasons may exist for disqualifying some aviators with pernicious anemia from flying. The disease process and its symptoms are often irreversible even after therapy is initiated; it has a known association with carcinoma of the stomach; and for military personnel, therapy may become unavailable in the event of long-term deployment under field conditions or in cases of captivity. Once treatment is interrupted, the pathologic process recommences shortly thereafter. (Many airmen were in prison camps in North Vietnam for as long as 9 years.)

Hereditary Spherocytosis

Hereditary spherocytosis is a hematologic condition in which red blood cells have a shortened life span due to increased osmotic fragility. As a result, patients have a chronic hemolytic process with a decreased red blood cell count and a commensurate degree of anemia. Although the anemia may be mild to severe, it has a propensity to markedly worsen under certain stressful conditions such as infection, trauma, or hemorrhage. Other complications of hereditary spherocytosis include gallstones and leg ulcers. At this time there is no effective medical treatment for the disease. However, splenectomy has been curative in many cases with restoration of a normal red blood cell life span and correction of the anemia.

Patients with hereditary spherocytosis with significant anemia who are untreated should, in most cases, be disqualified from flying. In addition, the possibility of a further deterioration of red blood cells because of infection would pose an added risk. If the anemia is mild or if splenectomy is performed and there is a normal postoperative course as well as correction of the disease process, a return to the cockpit could be given favorable consideration.

Hemoglobinopathies

The hemoglobinopathies are those conditions in which the hemoglobin (Hb) molecule is abnormal due either to a structural abnormality or a reduced synthesis of portions of the polypeptide chains. These defects, which are genetically determined, can cause a hemolytic process of varying degree from mild to severe, and are therefore of concern to the AME/FS, as is any disorder affecting the body's oxygen transport system. Although a large number of hemoglobinopathies have been reported, most of them are quite rare with only 3 or 4 likely to be encountered by the AME/FS. In order to better understand these entities, a brief review of the hemoglobin molecule will serve as an introduction.

The hemoglobin molecule is a conjugated protein consisting of a heme portion and a globin portion and has a molecular weight of 64,500. The globin is made up of 2 pairs of polypeptide chains with one heme group, which is a complex of iron and a porphyrin, attached to each chain. There are 4 types of normal polypeptide chains designated α, β, γ, and δ, differing in composition or sequence of the amino acids constituting the chain. It is changes in these chains, either qualitative (ie, a different amino acid sequence) or quantitative (ie, a failure to synthesize enough of one of the amino acids) that cause the various types of hemoglobinopathies.

Normal hemoglobin types found in adults are HbA (which has 2 α and 2 β chains), HbA_2 (2 α and 2 δ chains), and HbF (2 α and 2 γ chains), with the entire hemoglobin pool consisting of approximately 96%-98% HbA, 2%-3% HbA_2, and <1% HbF. The normal as well as abnormal hemoglobins can be differentiated by electrophoresis and chromatography.

One of the more common hemoglobinopathies is sickle cell trait (SCT) which is found in individuals who are heterozygous for HbS. In previous years, SCT was a controversial condition in regard to aeromedical disposition, with diverse opinions ranging from the very conservative (who felt that no aviator with SCT should be certified to fly) to the very liberal (who felt that there should be no restrictions on these aviators' flight status). Some considered SCT to be an entirely benign condition without significance, at least to aviators flying at moderate altitudes, while those of a more conservative orientation considered SCT a serious enough threat that flying should be precluded for all individuals with the disorder.

By way of background, individuals with SCT have an abnormal hemoglobin, called hemoglobin S, which comprises 22%-45% of the total amount, the remaining portion being normal hemoglobin A. Although SCT has been historically associated with African Americans (7%-9% of them have SCT), it has now been recognized that this disorder is also found rather frequently among individuals from the Mediterranean area, particularly those of Greek lineage. The diagnosis can be made by sickle cell preparation and hemoglobin electrophoresis. Notwithstanding this abnormality, individuals with SCT usually have normal hematological studies including hemoglobin-hematocrit, indices and RBC and reticulocyte counts.

If red blood cells containing hemoglobin S are exposed to low enough oxygen tension, there is a propensity for them to become sickled and to obstruct blood vessels. This has been demonstrated in vivo as well as in vitro at altitudes even below 3048 m (10,000 ft).[43] Therefore there is the possibility of suffering cerebral, splenic, and visceral infarction with their attendant symptoms including severe pain and incapacitation. It is this fact that those who favored disqualification from flight status used to defend their position.

Although the literature was divided on the issue, many flight operations opted to allow aviators with SCT to continue flying, albeit in some cases with certain operational restrictions. Consequently, over the past 20 years a large number of aviators with SCT have not only flown all types of military and civilian aircraft, but also have taken altitude chamber flights to altitudes as high as 7620-10,670 m (25,000-35,000 ft). To the author's knowledge, there have been no untoward reactions reported inflight or in an altitude chamber in the military or civilian sectors. One might conclude that in spite of the theoretical risks of exposing individuals with abnormal amounts of HbS to hypobaric environments, the risk of sickling, at least in those healthy enough to pass a flight physical examination without serious sequelae, is practically nil.

Nevertheless, the AME/FS must be mindful of reports in the literature of sickling with incapacitating events such as splenic or vasoocclusive crises as well as sudden death occurring on mountaintops as low as 2743 m (9000 ft) or with extreme exertion.[44,45] Notwithstanding these reports, a liberal policy is clearly defensible based on 2 decades of experience. However, it is prudent to keep the risk minimal by subjecting such aviators to a thorough flight physical examination and proper acclimatization prior to strenuous exercise, as well as adequate conditioning and hydration.

Another hemoglobin, HbC, is formed by substituting lysine for glutamic acid in position 6 of the β-chain. Individuals who are heterozygous (HbAC) have hemoglobin C trait while those who are homozygous (CC) have hemoglobin C disease.

Although the peripheral smear of a heterozygote may show target cells, patients do not have hemolysis, anemia, or any other symptoms whatsoever, so there is no need to disqualify any aviator with this trait from flight status. Hemoglobin C disease, on the other hand, while not necessarily a severe disorder, is more serious than the trait in that patients will have hemolysis with an anemia, although it is usually mild, commensurate with the degree of red blood cell destruction. Furthermore, patients may be intermittently symptomatic with arthralgias, abdominal pain, and jaundice. The aeromedical disposition of aviators with HbC disease must be based on the degree of anemia, the frequency and severity of symptoms, and the nature of the mission. Obviously, for patients who are more than mildly anemic or who have frequent symptomatic episodes, restriction from the cockpit is advisable.

Another hemoglobinopathy variant is any condition in which 2 abnormal hemoglobins are inherited; HbS-C is an outstanding example. In such cases, the disorder is more serious than if the trait form of either HbS or HbC is inherited alone. Most patients with HbS-C have multisystem involvement of varying severity including pain of the muscles, bones, joints, and abdomen, hematuria, jaundice, vascular occlusions of the retina, splenic infarct, and constitutional symptoms. There is also a chronic anemia with many patients having hemoglobin levels 70% of normal. Therefore, it appears that 2 abnormal hemoglobins are pathologically synergistic. It would seem most prudent to disqualify individuals with S-C disease not only because of the disability it can cause, but also because of the added hazards of possible sickling at altitude.

Thalassemia is a quantitative hemoglobinopathy in which there is a reduced synthesis of hemoglobin causing a hypochromic microcytic anemia. There are 4 recognized forms, alpha and beta thalassemia (depending on which globin chain is deficient) each with a homozygous and heterozygous expression, the clinical manifestations of which are quite different in degree. The symptoms of both homozygous forms are usually so severe (few patients survive into adulthood because of severe anemia and cardiopulmonary complications) that flying is clearly contraindicated. On the other hand, heterozygous thalassemia, sometimes referred to as thalassemia minor or trait, usually causes only a slight anemia with hemoglobin levels never going below 9 g/dL. Furthermore, most patients have no symptoms whatsoever and live normal life spans. The differentiation of the thalassemia types can be made clinically and by hemoglobin electrophoresis. Treatment is usually not required of this benign hematologic disorder. Medical waivers for the minor form can be given favorable consideration as long as the anemia is minimal and the patient is symptom free. Most individuals with thalassemia minor require no medication and live normal lives suffering no ill effects or restrictions.

Glucose-6-Phosphate Dehydrogenase (G6PD) Deficiency

G6PD deficiency is a sex-linked disorder found in many ethnic groups, particularly African Americans, Asians, and people of Mediterranean stock. Individuals who have a G6PD enzyme deficiency may develop red blood cell hemolysis if challenged by a number of medications and/or infection. Although it is difficult to predict exactly which drugs will cause hemolysis, it has been clearly associated with nitrofurantoin, primaquine, and sulfas.[46] With a provocative drug, hemolysis begins in 2-4 days with continuous destruction of red blood cells for 7-12 days. As many as 30%-50% of RBCs can be destroyed. There is also evidence that hemolytic episodes can be triggered by bacterial and viral infections, hepatitis in particular.

In general, there are several variants of G6PD deficiency. Some serious forms will cause a chronic anemia due to a continuous hemolytic process. In the more mild variants, patients with the enzyme deficiency are asymptomatic with normal red blood cell count, morphology, and indices unless challenged. If challenged by an offending agent, a mild or severe hemolytic episode may ensue with hemoglobinuria and acute renal shutdown. The severity of the reaction is apparently dependent on which of the variants of G6PD deficiency the patient has and possibly the extent of enzyme deficiency. In general, most hemolytic episodes are mild with complete remission once the medication is stopped. In fact, it has even been demonstrated that hemolysis will discontinue and the hemoglobin level will soon return to normal even if the patient continues to take the offending medication. There is no known treatment for the disorder other than to avoid the inciting agent.

A retrospective study of 129 patients with G6PD deficiency was conducted in order to learn something about the natural history of the illness.[47] The study covered a 20-year period during which the patients were challenged 756 times with oxidant medications. There were only 25 reported cases of overt hemolytic episodes: 14 due to favism and 11 due to drugs (nitrofurantoin, 3; aspirin, 2; aminopyrine, 2; chloramphenicol, 1; sulfa, 1; streptomycin, 1; dipyrone, 1). Therefore, less than 1% of the patients had hemolysis secondary to drug ingestion, and some subjects had a second challenge with the same drug and still showed absolutely no hemolytic activity. Although the literature has few long-term studies on the natural history and prognosis of patients with G6PD deficiency, this particular study indicates that in the great majority of cases the disease is not particularly significant.

Regarding aeromedical disposition of aviator applicants, some medical departments may require a G6PD screening test as part of the initial physical examination and if the results are positive it is considered grounds for disqualification. This policy can be defended based on what we know of the enzyme-deficiency state as well as the nature of and requirements of the flight mission of that organization. However, the aeromedical disposition of an aviator who has inadvertently been found to have G6PD deficiency, perhaps 5-6 years after flight training, becomes much more difficult and controversial. Because of the great clinical variability of the disorder, it would not be efficacious to establish a rigid policy to apply to all cases regardless of circumstances. It seems much more reasonable to judge each case on its own merits taking into consideration the patient's hemoglobin level when unchallenged, and past history of hemolytic episodes, including the nature of the precipitant and the severity of symptoms. Certainly some patients may have a mild variant of the disorder and a history of an episode of mild hemolysis followed by total remission after taking a known oxidant-type medication. This individual should be able to continue cockpit duties with most flight operations if there is reasonable assurance that the known precipitant will be avoided. Of course, if a patient has chronic hemolysis or symptoms that are unpredictable and associated with a variety of medications as well as infectious disease, a more conservative policy would be in order. The AME/FS must therefore evaluate each case and recommend sensible aeromedical disposition based on the clinical circumstances.

Polycythemia

Occasionally, asymptomatic aviators will be found to have an elevated hematocrit during a periodic physical examination. Possible causes for this include polycythemia rubra vera (primary polycythemia), secondary polycythemia, and relative polycythemia (Gaisbock's syndrome). It is important to differentiate these 3 entities to determine appropriate therapy as well as aeromedical disposition.

Polycythemia rubra vera (or primary polycythemia) is a disease of unknown etiology in which there is not only an increase in red blood cell volume, but also increases in marrow cellularity, white blood cells, and platelets. These hematologic aberrations can cause a variety of symptoms and complications including shortness of breath, edema, dizziness, angina, myocardial infarction, and intracranial or gastrointestinal hemorrhage.

The most compelling problem is an abnormally high hematocrit (over 53% with some cases as high as 87%) that causes increased blood viscosity predisposing the patient to arterial and/or venous thrombotic events that may result in stroke, TIA, myocardial infarction, or deep venous thrombosis. As the hematocrit approaches 50%-60%, the blood viscosity increases sharply thereby increasing the risk. In one study, the overall rate of thrombotic events was 3.4 per 100 patients per year.[48] Treatment, which is not curative, consists of periodic phlebotomy and myelosuppressive agents. Whatever therapy is used, life expectancy is 11-15 years and many patients develop leukemia.[49]

Unlike polycythemia rubra vera, in secondary polycythemia there is an underlying pathologic process causing decreased arterial oxygen tension that is sensed by the marrow, resulting in increased red blood cell mass. So it is basically the body's response to a hypoxic state. For example, it may develop in individuals living at high altitude, those with chronic lung disease such as emphysema, or patients with congenital heart disease and right-to-left shunts. For reasons not well understood, there may also be an increased red blood cell mass associated with a variety of tumors, renal carcinoma being the outstanding example. Treatment must be focused on the underlying disease; temporary symptomatic relief may be attained with periodic phlebotomy.

Polycythemia rubra vera can be differentiated from secondary polycythemia by a number of laboratory tests. The former has normal arterial oxygen saturation and frequent leukocytosis and thrombocytosis; secondary polycythemia, however, has a lowered arterial oxygen saturation and usually normal levels of platelets and white blood cells.

In Gaisbock's syndrome, there is an increased hematocrit not necessarily due to a real increase in red blood cell mass, but due instead to decreased plasma volume. This would seem to put it in contradistinction to an absolute polycythemia. This condition is seen on regular periodic physical examination in individuals who have a slightly elevated hematocrit without other clinical or laboratory indications of secondary polycythemia or polycythemia rubra vera. It is most frequently found in hard-working, aggressive individuals who are anxious and tense. Although the exact mechanism causing stress polycythemia is not known, it is considered clinically insignificant and in no way compromises flight safety. A medical waiver request for this condition should be given favorable consideration.

There are multiple factors to consider in the aeromedical disposition of flight personnel with polycythemia. For those with the secondary type, the most important consideration is the underlying illness and its seriousness. For example, mild emphysema may pose no hazard in some air operations whereas advanced pulmonary disease would. In any event, regardless of the underlying process of secondary polycythemia, the AME/FS should remember that the arterial oxygen saturation is characteristically lower than normal. Because of this physiological aberration and because secondary polycythemia is merely a manifestation of a serious underlying disease, afflicted individuals may be unsuitable for flight duty.

Regarding polycythemia rubra vera, patients with this diagnosis should probably not be in the cockpit. The increased blood viscosity and thrombocytosis predispose the patient to potentially incapacitating sequelae. Furthermore, patients commonly complain of headaches, dizziness, lassitude, and weakness which would undoubtedly cause inflight performance decrement. Added to this is the chronic course of the disease and the absence of a definitive form of therapy. And finally, polycythemia rubra vera, for reasons not entirely clear, often coexists with other disease processes such as gout, peptic ulcer, hypertension, and chronic myelocytic leukemia.

Human Immunodeficiency Virus (HIV) Infection

HIV infection exhibits an extremely variable course, from an asymptomatic stage to multisystem disease including opportunistic infections, various cancers, and ultimately severe incapacitation and death. Because of the seriousness of this disease some flight organizations screen aviators with ELISA and Western blot testing. There is no evidence that HIV is prevalent in the aviator population, probably attributable to the fact that flight organizations screen out those who engage in high-risk behavior and test for the virus before hiring. Nevertheless, aeromedical disposition for the HIV+ aviator is an issue that occasionally comes up for consideration by aviation medicine authorities around the world.

Although an HIV+ patient can remain asymptomatic and normal for a long time, possibly as long as 10 years, eventually the virus will cause systemic symptoms, compromise the immune system, and the patient will convert from being HIV+ to fulfilling the criteria for full blown acquired immunodeficiency syndrome (AIDS). Along the way opportunistic infections such as *Pneumocystis carinii, Mycobacterium tuberculosis* or *M avium, Toxoplasma gondii,* cytomegalovirus, *Candida,* and *Cryptococcus* among others can occur, as well as cancers such as Kaposi's sarcoma and lymphoma.

The medical authority determining aeromedical disposition of the HIV+ aviator must take into consideration a number of factors, including the patient's symptoms, the presence of opportunistic infection or cancer, and the prescribed treatment.

For the asymptomatic HIV+ aviator not on medication the aeromedical disposition is controversial. One school advocates disqualification based on the fact that the virus penetrates the central nervous system and a number of patients develop neuropsychiatric symptoms including disturbed mentation, forgetfulness, and impairment of memory early in the course of illness.[50-52] Furthermore, studies indicate that 40% of asymptomatic HIV+ patients have encephalopathy with 25% presenting with neurological dysfunction.[53] Proponents argue that even subtle neurological changes can to some degree impair pilot performance and pose a threat to flying safety.

Others believe there is no need for disqualification as long as the pilot remains asymptomatic and is followed carefully by an AME/FS. Many patients will be perfectly normal for years, therefore disqualification is wasteful and unnecessary. As part of follow-up, clinical evaluation should include CD4 counts and viral load quantitation to confirm the patient's stage of illness. Viral load predicts rate of progression of the disease process and is a strong predictor for AIDS.[54] There are also tests for psychomotor and cognitive function including information processing, reaction time, memory, attention, spatial processing, and arithmetic skills that could be administered.[55]

Another factor to consider is the patient's emotional reaction to his or her diagnosis of HIV. Distraction, preoccupation, and depression are not unusual even if the patient is asymptomatic. It may be wise to temporarily disqualify the HIV+ aviator until the AME/FS is sure the patient is emotionally stable.

Another dimension to the aeromedical disposition decision of the HIV+ aviator is the implementation of medical treatment. Although controversial, the initiation of treatment is usually correlated with the CD4 count and serum viral load. There are 3 types of medications: nucleoside analog reverse transcriptase inhibitors (NAIs), nonnucleoside reverse transcriptase inhibitors (NNIs), and protease inhibitors (PIs).[56] In general, side effects of these medications are surprisingly benign and would become apparent well before they could cause problems in the cockpit. NAIs may cause peripheral neuropathy, anemia, neutropenia, gastrointestinal symptoms, myopathy, and pancreatitis. The most common side effect of NNIs is a rash and PIs can cause gastrointestinal upset with one of them, indinavir, associated with nephrolithiasis. Special caution is advisable when the patient is on indinavir.

For HIV+ aviators who are symptomatic, have opportunistic infection or cancer, or who have developed AIDS, the aeromedical disposition would be unfavorable in most cases. Given the associated symptoms and downhill course, flight safety would be compromised. In addition, many of these patients are prescribed not only antiretroviral medication, but also prophylaxis and treatment for opportunistic infections and cancer. Although many of the drugs commonly prescribed (*P carinii*—trimethoprim-sulfamethoxazole; tuberculosis—isoniazid; toxoplasmosis—trimethoprim-sulfamethoxazole; *M avium*—clarithromycin; *Candida*—fluconazole; *Cryptococcus*—fluconazole; cytomegalovirus—ganciclovir) may be innocuous alone, the additive effects of the disease process itself and polypharmacy leave the issue of aeromedical disposition in doubt.[57]

Alcoholism

Because of the ubiquity and frequent use of alcohol in our society, the AME/FS must be particularly aware of the signs and symptoms of alcohol abuse and their potential threat to flight safety. Although alcohol has rarely been implicated as a cause of a major commercial or military aircraft accident, the same cannot be said for general aviation. For several decades, the rate of alcohol-associated fatal general aviation accidents has been relatively stable at 15%.[58,59]

Several studies have clearly demonstrated that even small amounts of alcohol cause a performance decrement and have a synergistic effect with the physiologic stresses of flight. In an early study, a performance decline in a Link trainer was demonstrated in experienced pilots with blood alcohol levels ranging from 20-70 mg %.[60] Furthermore, target-tracking performance during G maneuvers was significantly degraded after drinking only 3 ounces of alcohol.[61] A number of other investigators have reported that tolerance to hypoxia is reduced as manifested by changes in auditory acuity, impaired neuromuscular control, delayed decision and reaction times, and abnormal nystagmic reactions.[62] In another interesting study, pilots with blood alcohol of 40, 80, and 120 mg % were allowed to fly with observer pilots who assessed their performance.[63] Procedural errors were significantly increased and there was frequent loss of control of the aircraft. The literature is also replete with evidence that drinkers can be compromised inflight by alcohol-induced hypoglycemia, postalcohol impairment, and positional alcohol nystagmus.[64] In a more recent study, a blood alcohol level of .04% (40 mg/dL) or more was found in 8% of pilots fatally injured between 1989 and 1993.[65] Wherever one turns in the literature, there is abundant and consistent evidence of the negative effects of alcohol on the skills necessary for safe flight operations.

Aviation medicine practitioners can view the effects of alcohol from 3 perspectives: acute, chronic, and subclinical. Clearly, anyone drinking such that there are manifestations of acute intoxication on duty are not fit to fly in any cockpit. Besides the immediate effects of intoxication (drowsiness, ataxia, dysarthria, emotional lability), the long-term effects such as cirrhosis, peripheral neuropathy, and various forms of encephalopathy are well known. The aeromedical disposition of patients with obvious signs of intoxication is not problematic; rather, flying safety is most threatened by the subclinical drinker, the aviator who has had enough alcohol to affect performance, but not enough to cause overt drunkenness.

Alcohol is readily absorbed in the stomach and small intestine with peak blood levels reached 60 to 90 minutes after a single dose. It is metabolized at a rate of about

10 mL/hour (equivalent to about 4 ounces of whiskey in 5 to 6 hours) by an oxidative process in the liver. Even relatively low blood alcohol levels of 30-100 mg % such as might be incurred by social drinking can cause undesirable effects such as euphoria, decreased inhibitions, impaired attentiveness and judgment, and increased reaction time. Interestingly, in responses from 835 anonymous questionnaires sent to pilots, approximately 50% of the respondents felt it was perfectly safe to fly within 4 hours of drinking.[66]

In spite of these sobering data, rehabilitation programs for alcoholic aviators have met with considerable success, allowing many to be requalified for the cockpit. This is largely due to changing attitudes in the medical community regarding alcoholism, the availability of excellent rehabilitation programs, the compliance of aviators with these programs, and possibly the deterrent effects of urine screening. Illustrative of this was a report on 600 pilots granted a special issuance after treatment for alcoholism. The rate of successful rehabilitation was 85%.[67] If rehabilitation has been successful and no end organ disease is present, and there is reasonable hope that the patient will not resume drinking, a medical waiver with a proviso for close patient following should be considered. A major airline has described its rehabilitation program as a multidisciplinary approach, including participation by the flight surgeon, family and colleagues of the patient, recovered alcoholic pilots, and Alcoholics Anonymous; 25 aviators of that airline were successfully treated and recertified for flying status.[68] Likewise, in our experience there are some military airmen who successfully completed rehabilitation programs and have subsequently enjoyed successful and productive flying assignments. Therefore, alcohol abuse should be viewed as any other disease in that effective treatment is available, and if successful, a return to the cockpit should be considered.

Pyelonephritis

Acute pyelonephritis is most commonly caused by gram-negative bacilli. Although it sometimes afflicts individuals in good health, there appears to be an association with other pathologic processes, such as obstruction of the urinary tract, vesicoureteral reflux, and diabetes. Patients frequently experience sudden fever, chills, and tenderness in the flanks or costovertebral areas. The diagnosis is highly likely when a patient has these symptoms along with leukocytosis and white blood cells and bacteria in the urine. Treatment consists of prescribing the appropriate antibiotic and addressing any other underlying pathology. In patients with no underlying cause, complete recovery can be expected shortly after antibiotic therapy has begun. Aviators must be temporarily restricted from flying during the treatment period, but once cured a medical waiver can be issued. Exceptions to this might be aviators who have frequent episodes of acute pyelonephritis, the chronic form of the disease, or an underlying pathologic condition that remains uncorrected.

Glomerulonephritis

Glomerulonephritis is a disease seen in adults of all ages characterized by an inflammatory process of the glomeruli. There are several types, among them poststreptococcal (following a group A beta-hemolytic streptococcus pharyngitis or cellulitis), IgA nephropathy (Berger's disease), and membranoproliferative. The diagnosis can be made by urinalysis (hematuria, proteinuria, RBC/WBC casts), creatinine clearance, BUN, ultrasound, and renal biopsy if necessary. Individuals with the acute form of the disease may be asymptomatic with only proteinuria and microscopic hematuria or, at the other extreme, may have severe constitutional symptoms, such as edema, hypertension, and congestive heart failure. Some will develop the chronic form of the disease and progress to renal failure and death. There is no known specific treatment for glomerulonephritis other than supportive care. In some cases disease progression can be slowed by ACE inhibitors, low protein diet, and good control of blood pressure.

The prognosis for patients with glomerulonephritis is variable in that some patients with the acute form will succumb rapidly, others will have spontaneous permanent remission, and yet others will develop the chronic form of the disease. For patients with the acute form, the majority will resolve spontaneously with some developing the chronic form. Of those with the chronic form 35% will go on to end-stage renal disease.[69]

For aviators with acute glomerulonephritis, a return to flying would be in order once the disease is in remission. For those who develop the chronic form, most could probably continue flying at least for a time, because the disease process is a slowly progressive one with significant symptoms becoming manifest long before any degree of incapacitation takes place. Furthermore, the use of an ACE inhibitor such as lisinopril has very few if any side effects. Patients granted a waiver or special issuance would require close following by the AME/FS.

Thyroid Disease

Because thyroid disease—its pathogenesis, diagnosis, and treatment—is a broad and complex subject not without controversy, a complete discussion will not be attempted. Only a few remarks of a general nature follow in order to lend some guidance to the AME/FS.

Graves' Disease

Patients with Graves' disease have a diffuse enlargement of the thyroid gland with an excess production of thyroid hormone leading to signs and symptoms of thyrotoxicosis. Heat intolerance, sweating, irritability, emotional lability, palpitations, and weight loss despite increased food intake are common complaints. The diagnosis is not difficult in the presence of such symptoms and several diagnostic laboratory tests including the T4 index and the T3 resin uptake.

The 3 conventional therapeutic modalities are surgery, radioactive iodine ablation, and antithyroid medication.[70] Partial thyroidectomy is currently rarely performed unless the diffuse goiter is cosmetically unattractive or is causing interference with the vital structures of the neck. Even though many patients become euthyroid postsurgery, up to 50% will develop hypothyroidism. Radioactive iodine is preferable treatment because it is convenient and safe with few side effects. If antithyroid medication (propylthiouracil and methimazole) is the chosen therapy, most patients will become euthyroid in about 2 months. Adverse effects include fever, rash, arthralgias, myalgias, and gastrointestinal disturbances. Agranulocytosis is another serious albeit rare side effect. Interestingly, in a number of cases, Graves' disease will go into permanent or temporary remission if the medication is discontinued after 1 to 2 years of treatment.

Regarding aeromedical disposition, the symptoms of Graves' disease necessitate restriction from flying at least until treatment is completed and the patient is euthyroid. In general, regardless of the treatment modality, waivers for flying could be granted once the patient is euthyroid and there are no ill effects from therapy. For those undergoing partial thyroidectomy, there is a risk of laryngeal palsy, hypothyroidism, and hypoparathyroidism secondary to inadvertent removal of the parathyroid glands. If propylthiouracil or methimazole is prescribed, the AME/FS must be mindful of their possible adverse effects. For aviators granted a waiver, close followup would be mandatory to ensure a continued euthyroid state and freedom from adverse side effects of therapy.

Hypothyroidism

Although there are many causes of hypothyroidism, the chief categories include those which are idiopathic, those secondary to antithyroid medications or thyroid surgery, and those which are inflammatory (Hashimoto's disease and Reidel's thyroiditis). Regardless of the etiology, the symptoms of hypothyroidism, including weakness, lethargy, and fatigue, preclude flight safety. However, in most cases patients can be restored to a euthyroid state and lead perfectly normal lives with any one of the many forms of thyroid medications on the market. Because thyroid is a relatively innocuous drug, a request for a medical waiver can usually be given favorable consideration as long as the patient is followed at reasonable intervals to ensure medication compliance and a continued euthyroid state.

Diabetes Mellitus

Diabetes is occasionally diagnosed in aviators after appearance of symptoms (polyuria, polydipsia, polyphagia, weight loss) or from hyperglycemia or glucosuria noted on a routine physical examination. The diagnosis will be Type II NIDDM in 90%-95% of cases.[71] In any event, the cornerstone of therapy is diet and exercise. If glycemic control cannot be attained, medication must be prescribed. Oral hypoglycemics include sulfonylureas (eg, tolbutamide, chlorpropamide, glyburide, glipizide), metformin, alpha-glucosidase inhibitors, rosiglitazone, and repaglinide. Insulin is required in juvenile diabetes and eventually in up to 50% of those on oral medication.[72] Because of the availability of reliable equipment for self-monitoring of blood glucose, tight control is achievable in most patients who are in compliance with their therapeutic regimen. Most aviators with diabetes can be well controlled because they are a disciplined population that understands the illness and the dangers of poor control or a hypoglycemic event inflight.

The aeromedical disposition of individuals with diabetes mellitus can be difficult and in some cases controversial. Diabetics who are poorly controlled and symptomatic are clearly unsuitable for any cockpit. Only with good control and no significant long-term complications should consideration be given for qualification. The use of hypoglycemic agents must be taken into account as well.

For those fortunate aviators who can be controlled by diet and exercise alone, a medical waiver can be granted with confidence as long as the patient is closely followed clinically. However, the course of action is not so clear for patients requiring oral hypoglycemic agents such as the sulfonylureas because of the risk of hypoglycemia. Hypoglycemia is unwelcome in any cockpit because it can cause dizziness, fatigue, tremulousness, seizures, and coma. However, hypoglycemia is reported to be rare and when it does occur, very mild.[73] Consequently, a liberal policy is acceptable for an aviator who is well controlled on these medications, has no significant side effects, has no history of a hypoglycemic event, and is followed closely by his or her physician. (Military aviation is a possible exception to this because of erratic schedules, unforeseen deployments, irregular meals, and other stressors not normally imposed upon civilian aviators.)

Other oral hypoglycemics include metformin and alpha-glucosidase inhibitors (acarbase) both of which can cause mild gastrointestinal symptoms but neither of which cause hypoglycemic reactions. Although metformin can cause lactic acidosis, this reaction is extremely rare. Therefore, both of these medications pose little if any threat to flight safety.

Regarding patients requiring insulin, the risk of a hypoglycemic reaction is of great concern not only because of the possibility of loss of consciousness, but also because of subtle deficits in nervous system function that could degrade cockpit performance. Although the exact incidence of such reactions is not known, they do occur, particularly if there is poor compliance with prescribed therapy or added stress such as an infection.

The Diabetes Control and Complications Trial (DCCT) clearly demonstrated that tight glycemic control to keep the blood sugar level as close to normal as possible will significantly delay the progression of the long-term complications of diabetes. It was shown that the microvascular complications of nephropathy, neuropathy, and retinopathy were reduced a substantial 35%-70%.[74] The study also suggested that macrovascular complications including coronary artery disease, peripheral vascular disease, and stroke might also be reduced by intensive therapy. However, there is a price for the salutary effects of tight control: a 3-fold increase in hypoglycemic events. Nevertheless, the DCCT found that the risk of hypoglycemia with intensive therapy is outweighed by the reduction in microvascular changes.

In considering qualifications of a diabetic aviator, even one well controlled with insulin, there is a dichotomy in that good medical treatment calls for tight control which increases the risk of a hypoglycemic event. On the other hand, if tight control is not maintained for whatever reason, there is a significantly higher likelihood of serious long-term complications.

There are 2 schools of thought on the aeromedical disposition of aviators who are insulin dependent. One school argues that selected individuals may be given favorable consideration as long as these provisions are met:

- There have been no episodes of hypoglycemia.
- There are no microvascular or macrovascular complications.
- The blood sugar is well controlled.
- There is a full understanding of the disease and the effects of poor control and hypoglycemia.

- Frequent clinical following is assured.
- There will be periodic self-monitoring of blood glucose (including pre-flight and inflight) and that guidelines will be provided on taking snacks should the blood sugar become too low.
- There are reasonable guarantees of full compliance with the therapeutic regimen.

Interestingly, there is a Canadian helicopter pilot on insulin who has met similar criteria and has flown safely with a medical aviator waiver for a number of years.[71] Those who oppose a liberal policy argue that the risk of hypoglycemia is too great and that this poses an unacceptable risk to flight safety. They also argue that some aviators might intentionally maintain a degree of hyperglycemia in order to minimize the occurrence of a hypoglycemic event. This would not be good medicine because the DCCT recommended tight control to minimize the risk of long-term complications. And finally, many believe it is unrealistic to expect pilots to monitor their blood sugar preflight and inflight. For these reasons the recommendation of this school is to disqualify all aviators who are on insulin.

The debate on the question of flight certification for diabetic aviators will undoubtedly rage for some time before it is resolved. In the meanwhile, regulatory agencies must make their own policies.

References

1. Larson RH, Lofren EP, Myers TT, et al. Long-term results after vein surgery. *Mayo Clin Proc.* 1974;49:114-117.

2. Pinals RS. Rheumatoid arthritis: A pharmacological overview. *AFP.* 1988;37(3):145-152.

3. Calabro JJ. The seronegative spondyloarthropathies. *Postgrad Med.* 1988;80(2):173-188.

4. Emerson BT. The management of gout. *N Engl J Med.* 1996;334(7):445-451.

5. Dudley JS, Lawler J. Systemic lupus erythematosus in a naval aviator. *Aviat Space Environ Med.* 1998;69:788-792.

6. Domianos AJ, McGarrity TJ. Treatment strategies for *Helicobacter pylori* infection. *AFP.* 1997;55(8):2765-2774.

7. Lang KA, Pickard JS. Peptic ulcer disease in the military aviator: A management approach. *Aviat Space Environ Med.* 1998;69:1100-1103.

8. Macri G, Malani S, Surrenti E, et al. Eradication of *Helicobacter pylori* reduces the rate of duodenal ulcer rebleeding: A long term follow-up study. *Am J Gastroenterol.* 1998;93: 925-927.

9. Laine L, Peterson EL. Bleeding peptic ulcer. *N Engl J Med.* 1994;331:717-727.

10. Vaira D, Menegatti M, Miglioli M. What is the role of *Helicobacter pylori* in complicated ulcer disease? *Gastroenterol*. 1997;113:578-584.

11. Jensen DM, Cheng S, Kovacs TOG, et al. A controlled study of ranitidine for the prevention of recurrent hemorrhage from duodenal ulcer. *N Engl J Med*. 1994;330:382-386.

12. Pappas TN. The stomach and duodenum. In: Sabiston DC, Lyerly HK, eds. *Textbook of Surgery*. 15th ed. Philadelphia: Saunders; 1997:859-861.

13. Fass R, Hixson LJ, Ciccolo ML, et al. Contemporary medical therapy for gastroesophageal reflux disease. *AFP*. 1997;55(1):205-212.

14. Farmer RG, Whelan G, Faxio VM. Long term follow-up of patients with Crohn's disease. *Gastroenterol*. 1985;88:1818-1825.

15. Botoman VA, Bonner GF, Botoman DA. Management of inflammatory bowel disease. *AFP*. 1998;57(1):57-68.

16. Stenson WF. Inflammatory bowel disease. In: Goldman L, Bennett JC, eds. *Cecil Textbook of Medicine*. Vol. 1. 21st ed. Philadelphia: Saunders; 2000:78.

17. Glotzer DJ. Surgical therapy for Crohn's disease. *Gastroenterol Clin North Am*. 1995;24(3):571-596.

18. Sales DJ, Kirsner JB. The prognosis of inflammatory bowel disease. *Arch Int Med*. 1983;143:294-299.

19. Weiss EG, Wagner SD. Surgical therapy for ulcerative colitis. *Gastroenterol Clin North Am*. 1995;24(3):559-575.

20. Bonis PAL, Norton RA. The challenge of irritable bowel syndrome. *AFP*. 1996;55(4):1229-1236.

21. Hobbs KEF. Laparoscopic cholecystectomy. *Gut*. 1995;36:161-165.

22. Rappaport WD, Gordon P, Warneke J, et al. Contraindications and complications of laparoscopic cholecystectomy. *AFP*. 1994;50(8):1707-1711.

23. Tait N, Little JM. The treatment of gall stones. *BMJ*. 1995;311:99-105.

24. Saboe GB, Slauson JW, Johnson R, et al. The aeromedical risk associated with asymptomatic cholelithiasis in USAF pilots and navigators. *Aviat Space Environ Med*. 1995;66:1086-1088.

25. Schoetz DJ. Uncomplicated diverticulitis. *Surg Clin North Am*. 1993;73(5):965-974.

26. Ferzoco LB, Raptopoulos V, Silen W. Acute diverticulitis. *N Engl J Med*. 1998;338(21):1521-1526.

27. Jordan MH, Meinecke HM. Ambulatory surgery for pilonidal disease. *Am Surg*. 1979;45(6):360-363.

28. Rose CS, Maier LA. Sarcoidosis. *N Engl J Med*. 1997;336:1224-1234.

29. Belfer MH, Stevens RW. Sarcoidosis: A primary care review. *AFP*. 1998;58(9):2041-2050.

30. Fleming HA, Bailey SM. The prognosis of sarcoid heart disease in the United Kingdom. *Ann NY Acad Sci*. 1986;465:543-550.

31. Gross KM, Ponte CD. New strategies in the medical management of asthma. *AFP*. 1998;58(1):89-100.

32. Robb DJ. Aerospace medicine residents teaching file. *Aviat Space Environ Med.* 1994;65(2):170-172.

33. Voge VM, Antracite R. Spontaneous pneumothorax in the USAF aircrew population. *Aviat Space Environ Med.* 1986;57:939-949.

34. North JH. Thoracoscopic management of spontaneous pneumothorax allows prompt return to aviation duties. *Aviat Space Environ Med.* 1994;65(12):1128-1129.

35. Fuchs HS. Incidence of spontaneous pneumothorax in apparently healthy aircrews. *Aerospace Med.* 1967;38:1286-1288.

36. Tomashefski JF, Freeley DR, Shillito FH. Effects of altitude on emphysematous blebs and bullae. *Aerospace Med.* 1966;37:1158-1162.

37. Stevens DA. Coccidioidomycosis. *N Engl J Med.* 1995;332:1077-1082.

38. Bode FR, Dosman J, Martin RR, et al. Reversibility of pulmonary function abnormalities in smokers. *Am J Med.* 1975;59:43-52.

39. McColloster P, Neff NE. Outpatient management of tuberculosis. *AFP.* 1996;53(5):1579-1586.

40. Pickwell SM. Positive PPD and chemoprophylaxis for tuberculosis infection. *AFP.* 1995;51(8):1929-1934.

41. Shub C, Salmonsen PC, Jordan JE, et al. Safety of INH chemoprophylaxis in aviation personnel. *Aerospace Med.* 1971;42:1325-1335.

42. Treatment of tuberculosis and tuberculosis infection in adults and children. Joint statement of the American Thoracic Society and Centers for Disease Control. No author cited. *Am Rev Respir Dis.* 1986;134:355-363.

43. Diggs LW. The sickle cell trait in relation to the training and assignment of duties in the Armed Forces: I—Policies, observations, and studies. *Aviat Space Environ Med.* 1984;55(3):180-185.

44. Tiernan CJ. Splenic crisis at high altitude in 2 white men with sickle cell trait. *Ann Emerg Med.* 1999;33:230-233.

45. Kerle KK, Nishimura KD. Exertional collapse and sudden death associated with sickle cell trait. *AFP.* 1996;54(1):237-240.

46. Beuther E. G6PD deficiency. *Blood.* 1994;84(11):3613-3636.

47. Herman J, Ben-Meir S. Overt hemolysis in patients with glucose-6-phosphate dehydrogenase deficiency. *Israel J Med Sci.* 1975;11(4):340-344.

48. Grupo Italiano Studio Policitemia. Polycythemia vera: The natural history of 1213 patients followed for 20 years. *Ann Int Med.* 1995;123:656-664.

49. Linker CA. Polycythemia vera. In: Tierney LM, McPhee SJ, Papadakis MA, eds. *Current Medical Diagnosis and Treatment.* 37th ed. Stamford, Conn: Appleton & Lange; 1998:501.

50. Clifford DB. AIDS and the brain. *AFP.* 1987;36(6):101-106.

51. Berger JR. Neurologic complications of the human immunodeficiency virus infection. *Postgrad Med.* 1987;81(1):72-79.

52. Searight HR, McLaren AL. Behavioral and psychiatric aspects of HIV infection. *AFP.* 1997;55(4):1277-1237.

53. Patt HOL, Pagano MA, Garau MA. HIV encephalopathy: Should we await a catastrophe before screening? *Aviat Space Environ Med*. 1994;65:70-73.

54. Chesbro MJ, Everett D. Understanding the guidelines for treating HIV disease. *AFP*. 1998;57(2):315-322.

55. Damos DL, John RS, Parker ES, Levine AM. Anti-retroviral therapy and cognitive function. *Aviat Space Environ Med*. 1997;68:900-906.

56. Maenza J, Flexner C. Combination antiretroviral therapy for HIV infection. *AFP*. 1998;57(11):2789-2798.

57. Montauk SL, Gebhardt B. Opportunistic infections and psychosocial stress in HIV. *AFP*. 1997;56(1):87-96.

58. Ryan LC, Mohler SR. Current role of alcohol as a factor in civil aircraft accidents. *Aviat Space Environ Med*. 1979;49:275-279.

59. Mohler SR. Civil aviation medicine. In: DeHart RL, ed. *Fundamentals of Aerospace Medicine*. 2nd ed. Baltimore: Williams & Wilkins; 1996:755.

60. Aksnes EG. Effects of small doses of alcohol upon performance in a link trainer. *J Aviat Med*. 1954;25:680-693.

61. Burton RR, Jaggars JL. Influence of ethyl alcohol ingestion on a target task during sustained $+G_z$ centrifugation. *Aerospace Med*. 1974;45(3):290-296.

62. Bishop JA. *Alcohol and Aviation. Review 3-75*. USAF School of Aerospace Medicine, Brooks AFB, Texas: 1975.

63. Billings CE, Wick RL, Gerke RJ, et al. Effects of ethyl alcohol on pilot performance. *Aerospace Med*. 1973;44(4):379-382.

64. Gibbons HL. Alcohol, aviation, and safety revisited: A historical review and a suggestion. *Aviat Space Environ Med*. 1988;59:657-660.

65. Canfield D, Fleming J, Hordinsky J, Birky M. *Drugs and Alcohol Found in Fatal Civil Aviation Accidents Between 1989 and 1993*. DOT/FAA/AM – 95/28. Federal Aviation Administration, Office of Aviation Medicine, Washington, DC: November 1995.

66. Damkot DK, Osga GA. Survey of pilots' attitudes and opinions about drinking and flying. *Aviat Space Environ Med*. 1978;49(2):390-394.

67. Russell JC, Davis AW. *Alcohol Rehabilitation of Airline Pilots*. DOT/FAA-AM-85-12. Civil Aeromedical Institute. Federal Aviation Administration, Oklahoma City: October 1985.

68. Schwartz FR, Kidera GJ. Method of rehabilitation of the alcohol-addicted pilot in a commercial airline. *Aviat Space Environ Med*. 1978;49(5):729-731.

69. Michaud VJ. Chronic glomerulonephritis: Medical and aeromedical disposition. *Aviat Space Environ Med*. 1997;68:225-227.

70. Hennessey JV. Diagnosis and management of thyrotoxicosis. *AFP*. 1996;54(4):1315-1324.

71. Gray GW, Dupre J. Diabetes mellitus in aircrew—type I diabetes in a pilot. *Aviat Space Environ Med*. 1995;66:449-452.

72. Lipsky MS, Zimmerman BR. Diagnosis and management of type II diabetes mellitus. *AFP*. Monograph 1, 1999:13.

73. Baliga BS, Fonseca VA. Recent advances in the treatment of type II diabetes mellitus. *AFP.* 1997;55(3):817-824.

74. The Diabetes Control and Complications Trial Research Group. The effect of intensive treatment of diabetes on the development and progression of long term complications in insulin-dependent diabetes mellitus. *N Engl J Med.* 1993;329:977-986.

Chapter 3
Orthopedics

Orthopedic pathology accounts for a significant number of waivers in many flying organizations. This is explained in part by the fact that many of the pathologic conditions are caused by trauma—we live in an accident-prone society. Injury to the musculoskeletal system can cause a wide variety of fractures, dislocations, sprains, tears, or amputations, each requiring some form of orthopedic care, be it open or closed reduction; casting; internal fixation with screws, pins, and plates; or soft tissue repair. Due to space limitations, it is not possible to describe the multitude of injuries and treatment methods in this chapter. However, regardless of the extent of injury or nature of treatment, the final judgment on aeromedical disposition is largely dependent on the degree of residual functional impairment once the lesion or injury has healed and treatment and rehabilitation are completed. Clearly, the AME/FS must render judgment as to whether residual limitation of motion, loss of strength, or functional impairment is great enough that safe operation of the aircraft is compromised. If so, disqualification from flying status is mandatory. Exceptions are made for minimal disabilities that in the opinion of the AME/FS would not interfere with the safe performance of all cockpit duties.

One of the most common complaints is low back pain. In most cases, the cause is probably lumbar-sacral muscle spasm or strain, which is self-limiting and causes the patient only temporary disability, after which normal activity can be resumed without further difficulty. However, in other cases there may be a more serious underlying etiology making aeromedical disposition more problematic. A discussion follows of several such disorders causing low back pain that the AME/FS may occasionally encounter.

Herniated Nucleus Pulposus (HNP)

Herniated nucleus pulposus (HNP), a sequela of degenerative disk disease or trauma, occurs most commonly in young adult to middle aged persons. In HNP, the nucleus pulposus herniates posteriorly putting pressure on the spinal cord or nerve root, causing pain and/or neurologic dysfunction. Although this pathologic process can occur at any vertebral level, it is most common between L4-L5 and L5-S1.[1] Therefore, patients usually complain of severe low back pain with radiation down one leg in the distribution of the affected nerve root. In 50% of cases, there is a history of trauma, straining, or lifting heavy weights, causing the application of sudden compressive forces along the vertebral column. The diagnosis can be made by history and physical examination: decreased knee or ankle reflexes, decreased range of motion of the spine, decreased dorsal flexion strength of the ankle, and limited straight leg raising are some common signs. Confirmation of the diagnosis can be made with CT or MRI scan, lumbar diskography, electromyography, and myelography.

The treatment of HNP is either medical or surgical. Conventional medical treatment is supportive and includes bedrest on a hard surface, heat, analgesics, and muscle relaxants. Selected patients may also be treated with chymopapain which, when injected into the disk space, causes lysis of the nucleus pulposus. A common surgical procedure is laminectomy with diskectomy. Surgery is usually performed when conservative measures fail and the patient experiences recurrent symptoms, intractable pain, or neurologic deficit. However, surgery is not always curative and a number of patients will continue to complain of discomfort after operation. In studies of cases undergoing surgery, 80%-95% had good to excellent relief of pain with 2% having neural damage.[2]

Flying status would be in doubt if the aviator did not respond to conservative therapy or if after surgery he or she was among the 5%-20% of patients with recurrent pain requiring frequent bedrest and use of analgesics. For military aviators flying ejection seat–equipped aircraft and for helicopter pilots, the potential for reinjury caused by high G forces, excessive vibration, and ejection must be taken into account. Interestingly, a number of reports have indicated that HNP or low back pain occurs relatively frequently in these populations.[3,4] Although there are no precise data, it would stand to reason that there is an added risk of symptom recurrence should an aviator be exposed to high G forces, particularly if they are abrupt as is the case when ejecting. If surgery is performed, it is advisable to wait 3-4 months before returning to the cockpit to ensure that healing is complete.

Spondylolysis

Spondylolysis is a defect in the neural arch of the lower lumbar vertebrae. The etiology of this entity is unknown, although there is evidence that it might be congenital or caused by a stress fracture. Although 10% of adults will demonstrate spondylolysis on x-ray,[5] few individuals complain of low back pain. Treatment for symptomatic individuals is supportive and includes the use of a back brace and analgesics.

The lesion is of aeromedical significance not only because it can cause occasional low back pain, but also because it involves the portion of the spine most vulnerable to accelerative stresses. Symptomatic aviators who need to take medication frequently should probably not be on flight status. This is particularly true for military and aerobatic aviators because exposure to G forces may aggravate the condition.

Spondylolisthesis

Spondylolisthesis is a condition in which there is slipping forward of a vertebra, most commonly the fifth lumbar vertebra. The cause of this defect may be congenital or it may be secondary to degenerative disk disease or spondylolysis. In any event, patients complain of low back pain as well as sciatica if there is nerve root compression. The diagnosis of spondylolisthesis can usually be confirmed radiologically. Medical treatment consists of bedrest, analgesics, and bracing. If symptoms are unremitting or frequent and severe enough to require regular use of analgesics, flight certification would be unadvisable. It is also possible that continued exposure to vibration and accelerative forces could aggravate the condition by causing further vertebral slippage. However, this hypothesis is conjectural, and was contradicted in a study examining fighter pilots with spondylolisthesis; all of them had a benign course.[6] If conservative therapy is ineffective and the patient has frequent, severe low back pain, various surgical procedures including spinal fusion are available.[7] A waiver request would be in order 4-6 months postsurgery to ensure full healing.

Compression Fracture

Aviators who eject from high-performance aircraft are at risk of sustaining compression fracture of the vertebral column. Any portion of the vertebral column can be injured depending on the characteristics of the ejection seat system. Such injuries are quite common, with incidence rates of 10%-30% reported in some types of aircraft.[8] Treatment for compression fractures is bedrest and analgesics for several weeks to months. In the RAF patients are admitted to the hospital for a minimum of 3 weeks. Symptomatic treatment is prescribed with physiotherapy commencing once the pain is in remission. After 3 months, the aviator may be returned to flying if she or he is asymptomatic and there is full range of motion of the spine.[9]

However, there are differences of opinion as to when it is most appropriate to return an aviator to the cockpit because of the possibility of a second ejection, which may cause more severe injury to the previously injured vertebral column. Smelsey reported on 6 USAF crewmen who each ejected twice during an interval ranging from 2 months to 8 years.[10] None of them sustained injury of the vertebral column from the second ejection despite the fact that each of the 6 aviators had sustained a compression fracture on the first ejection. It is probably prudent, however, to wait 3-6 months postejection before requesting a medical waiver. Although this recommendation is empirical, enough time would have elapsed to provide healing sufficient to withstand high G forces should a second ejection become necessary. Probably the most important guide for the flight surgeon deciding when to request the waiver is the presence or absence of symptoms, ie, back pain.

Another consideration is the long-term effect of ejection on the vertebral column. It has been shown that aviators who have normal spine x-rays immediately postejection may develop radiologic abnormalities as long as 10 years later. In one study of 70 such crewmen, 30 developed radiologic evidence of compression fractures months to years later, despite a normal x-ray of the spine made immediately postejection.[11] Another study by the USAF Armstrong Aerospace Medical Research Laboratory also admonishes flight surgeons about the possible occurrence of these delayed x-ray changes and low back pain.[12] Therefore, it is advisable to follow all aviators who have ejected and to obtain repeat spine films at a later date.

References

1. Schlesinger EB. Intervertebral discs. In: Rowland LP, ed. *Merritt's Textbook of Neurology*. 8th ed. Philadelphia: Lea & Febiger; 1989.

2. Laminectomy and microlaminectomy for treatment of lumbar disk herniation. No author cited. In: Cole HM, ed. *JAMA*. 1990;264(11):1469-1472.

3. Mason KT, Harper JP, Shannon SG. Herniated nucleus pulposus: Rates and outcomes among US Army aviators. *Aviat Space Environ Med*. 1996;67(4):338-340.

4. Thomas MK, Porteous JE, Brock JR, et al. Back pain in Australian military helicopter pilots: A study. *Aviat Space Environ Med*. 1998;69:468-473.

5. Salter RB. *Textbook of Disorders and Injuries of the Musculoskeletal System*. 2nd ed. Baltimore: Williams & Wilkins; 1983.

6. Froom P, Ribak J, Tendler Y, et al. Spondylolisthesis in pilots: A follow-up study. *Aviat Space Environ Med*. 1987;58:588-589.

7. Gaines RW, Humphrey WG. Spondylolisthesis. In: Chapman MW, ed. *Operative Orthopaedics*. 2nd ed. Philadelphia: Lippincott; 1993.

8. Osborne RG, Cook AA. Vertebral fracture after aircraft ejection during Operation Desert Storm. *Aviat Space Environ Med*. 1997;68:337-341.

9. Ward MW. *Orthopedics*. In: Ernsting J, Nicholson AN, Rainford DJ, eds. *Aviation Medicine*. 3nd ed. Oxford: Butterworth-Heinemann; 1999:362.

10. Smelsey SO. Study of pilots who have made multiple ejections. *Aerospace Med.* 1970;41(5):563-566.

11. Crooks M. Long term effects of ejecting from aircraft. *Aerospace Med.* 1970;41(7):803-804.

12. Kazarian LE. F/FB-111 Escape Injury Mechanism Assessment. AMRL-TR-77-60. Aerospace Medical Research Laboratory, Wright-Pattersen AFB OH. 1977.

Chapter 4
Neurology

In both civil and military aviation experience, neurologic disease ranks second only to cardiovascular disease among medical conditions that threaten an aviator's fitness to fly. Many neurologic disorders including epilepsy, stroke with severe deficit, and dementing neurologic illnesses are clearly incompatible with aviation safety, but fortunately many other neurologic disorders are not. If the condition is cured, arrested, static, or characterized by a predictable course, aeromedical certification may be possible. The ability to accurately monitor the illness is another important determinant in a certification decision. With slowly progressive neurologic disorders, monitoring allows identification of the point beyond which aviation safety might be compromised necessitating disqualification. Parkinson's disease is an example of such a condition. Also infrequent or fully controlled migraine, benign vasovagal syncope, mild neuropathy or myopathy, treated radiculopathies, and mild traumatic brain injury without residua need not bar aeromedical certification in many instances. This chapter addresses a number of neurologic disorders that are encountered in aviators and discusses aeromedical disposition.

Aviation activities include military operations, scheduled air carrier services, commercial operations (including charter, corporate, air taxi, and agricultural activities), aerobatic flying, and private pilot operations. An existing neurologic condition might compromise aviation safety in military activities, where full fitness and readiness for worldwide deployment is essential, and yet pose no threat to private pilot activities. In this chapter general principles important in considering aeromedical certification of individuals with neurologic disorders will be presented. The principles set forth are intended only as guidelines to provide the reader with important factors in the decision-making process, without attempting to provide a rigid framework or strict algorithm for the certification process.

Birth and Developmental Abnormalities

Cerebral Palsy

Cerebral palsy is a general term encompassing neurologic disorders of diverse etiology and of either developmental or acquired origin. The term refers to a static, nonprogressive encephalopathic motor disorder with varied manifestations including spasticity, ataxia, dyskinesia (chorea, athetosis, dystonia), and hypotonia.[1] In addition, seizures and cognitive changes may accompany the motor deficit (oligophrenic triad), though cognition is often normal. Intrauterine stroke, developmental anomalies and intraparenchymal hemorrhage in premature infants are among the etiologic considerations in this illness.

Diagnosis of cerebral palsy is often made by history taking and standard neurologic examination, and abnormalities are usually evident in early life. For example, the aviator may describe a static motor deficit present since birth, with delayed developmental milestones. In mild cases poor coordination when participating in school sports activities (minor motor disability) may be reported.[1] Signs may range from mild incoordination without significant functional impairment to severe motor disability, spasticity, and contracture. In addition, involuntary movements or ataxia may be present. Neuroimaging studies, such as computed tomography (CT) or magnetic resonance imaging (MRI) may reveal developmental or acquired pathologic changes, such as infarction, atrophy, porencephaly, and developmental abnormalities.

Management of cerebral palsy is symptomatic and often directed at relief of spasticity. Muscle relaxants such as baclofen are used to treat spasticity, and physical therapy is often employed. Several muscle relaxants, including baclofen, may cause sedation. Anticonvulsants are used to treat seizures, and tailored education programs have proven useful.

Aeromedical disposition is based on individual assessment of the degree of neurologic impairment and extent to which motor disability precludes safe operation of an aircraft. Many persons with cerebral palsy have minimal neurologic impairment and no significant functional disability. For example, mild spasticity of one or more limbs characterized by hypertonia, slightly impaired rapidly alternating movements, hyperreflexia, and perhaps a Babinski sign, may only impair running, leaving other motor functions intact. Consideration of aeromedical certification for most aviation activities would be acceptable. However, severe motor deficit, ataxia, involuntary movements, speech and cognitive impairment, and the presence of seizures preclude aeromedical certification. The use of potentially sedating medications may also disallow certification. These include the muscle relaxants baclofen and cyclobenzaprine, and the benzodiazepines.

Attention Deficit-Hyperactivity Disorder (ADHD)

The term *attention deficit-hyperactivity disorder* refers to a behavioral disorder characterized by a variety of symptoms that may include incoordination, distractibility, inattention, hyperactivity, impulsiveness, labile affect, and restlessness.[2] There may be motor incoordination and a learning disability, though most individuals with ADHD possess normal intelligence.[2] The condition is static, though hyperactivity may improve with maturation. ADHD is characteristically seen in children (prevalence, 4%), though in recent years its presence in adolescents and adults has been emphasized. Male prevalence is two- to threefold that in females.

The history will disclose childhood symptoms including inattention, distractibility, hyperactivity, impetuous or explosive behavior, impulsivity, impatience, disorganization, and inability to follow instructions. There may be a family history of similar difficulties. Subtle neurologic findings may be present, including incoordination, clumsiness, and minor reflex abnormalities. Although hyperactivity and inattention can occur independently, they are more commonly seen in combination. Affected adolescents may exhibit immaturity and argumentative or explosive behavior. Neurological examination is often normal, though restlessness, inattention, and distractibility may be grossly evident. Laboratory studies are normal, although neuropsychological testing may disclose an underlying learning disability.

Medications used to treat hyperactivity include the stimulants methylphenidate, dextroamphetamine, and pemoline. Common side effects include insomnia, anorexia, weight loss, and nervousness. Dizziness, irritability, and tachycardia may also occur. In some cases antidepressants including imipramine and nortriptyline may be prescribed. Frequently-encountered side effects include drowsiness, dizziness, dry mouth, headache, and lightheadedness. Medication may be discontinued if hyperactivity subsides with maturation.

A history of ADHD does not preclude certification if symptoms are mild and unacceptable medication has not been prescribed. The potential sedating or mind-altering effects of stimulants and antidepressants generally precludes certification. In many cases the major symptoms improve over time, and implementation of adaptive strategies may eliminate the need for medication, allowing consideration of aeromedical certification.

ADHD has been recognized with increasing frequency in adults. History might disclose symptoms of difficulty focusing attention, distractibility, and restlessness. As in children with ADHD, there are no characteristic neurologic findings. Family history may be positive, and diagnosis in a parent is often made when an affected child is brought to medical attention. Laboratory studies are normal. Because diagnostic criteria have not been strict or uniform, diagnosis of this illness in adults can be confusing, although available psychological test batteries are sometimes useful in identifying ADHD.

A history or current diagnosis of ADHD in adults is not invariably disqualifying, since mild forms may not compromise aviation safety. As mentioned above, a major barrier to aeromedical certification relates to the use of disqualifying medications, including stimulants and antidepressants. If medication is discontinued and symptoms are not functionally disabling, certification may be possible following a period of observation of perhaps a year or more.

Structural Malformations

Structural malformations include developmental abnormalities of the skull and spine.[3] Congenital fusion of cervical vertebrae (Klippel-Feil syndrome) is one example that characteristically causes no functional impairment or neurologic deficit. On the other hand, basilar impression, a condition in which the skull base is flattened with the odontoid process extending upward into the posterior fossa, can cause distortion of brainstem structures and induce spasticity, ataxia, cranial nerve palsies, and hydrocephalus. In Arnold-Chiari malformation the brainstem is lengthened and, along with lower cerebellar structures, descends into the upper cervical spinal canal, causing symptoms similar to those occurring in basilar impression.

History will disclose a problem present since birth or discovered after development of a neurologic deficit. Neurologic findings may include ataxia, spasticity, and cranial nerve palsies. Neuroimaging studies (conventional radiographs, CT, MRI) often demonstrate the abnormality. Structural abnormalities producing no neurologic deficit, such as Klippel-Feil syndrome, may require no treatment, while symptomatic basilar impression and Arnold-Chiari malformation (depending on degree of severity) may necessitate surgical decompression of the posterior fossa, effecting cure.

Aeromedical disposition should address the nature and degree of neurologic deficit, presence or absence of hydrocephalus, and temporal profile of the illness (stability versus progression). If surgery has been performed, a symptom-free and neurologically stable period of observation of 6-12 months should be observed before considering medical certification. The underlying condition may render an individual unsuitable for military operations while presenting no problem with civil aircraft operations.

Infections of the Nervous System

General Principles

Infectious agents capable of producing neurologic disease include bacteria, viruses, fungi and yeasts, spirochetes, and parasites. Prion particle disorders such as Creutzfeldt-Jakob disease might also be included here because the causative prion particle, like a virus, is transmissible, although it contains no detectable nucleic acid. Central nervous system infection may lead to leptomeningitis, encephalitis, cerebritis, subdural or epidural empyema, and brain abscess.[4] In general, aeromedical concerns relate to the possibility of residual neurologic impairment from prior CNS infection. Complications of such infections include seizures, cognitive deficits, behavioral abnormalities, cranial nerve palsies, motor deficits, and possibly hydrocephalus, all of which are of aeromedical significance.

Office interview and review of pertinent records will document the infectious exposure. Gait abnormalities (spasticity, ataxia), cranial nerve palsies, behavioral changes, and cognitive impairment may be evident to the examiner. Neuroimaging studies may reveal hydrocephalus or focal atrophy, and electroencephalography (EEG) may demonstrate potentially epileptiform changes. If chronic infection persists, cerebrospinal fluid examination may reveal pleocytosis, elevated protein, and depressed glucose, depending on the infectious agent. In some cases the organism can be identified by appropriate studies.

The aviation medical examiner/flight surgeon (AME/FS) will likely encounter the aviator when the infection is remote and treatment has been completed. However, in some cases medications might be prescribed beyond those needed to eradicate infection, such as anticonvulsants, muscle relaxants, hypnotics, and minor or major tranquilizers. If this is the case, potential side effects of sedation, cognitive impairment, and mood alteration might present a barrier to aeromedical certification. Once medication is discontinued, return to flight status is feasible if there are no significant neurologic sequelae from the initial infection.

Human Immunodeficiency Virus (HIV)

Because of the singular importance of human immunodeficiency virus (HIV) infection, it will be discussed in some detail. Acquired immune deficiency syndrome (AIDS) was initially recognized in 1981, and the causative agent, the retrovirus HIV-1, was isolated in 1983. After a latency of several years, HIV infection can lead to opportunistic infection, neoplasia, a chronic wasting syndrome, and neurologic syndromes. Acute infection may mimic aseptic meningitis, while chronic infection may lead to cognitive changes, psychiatric abnormalities, vascular (stroke-like) symptoms, ataxia, seizures, myelopathy, polyradiculopathy, peripheral neuropathy, and myopathy.[5]

The epidemiology of HIV infection is changing. The 1986 CDC (Centers for Disease Control and Prevention) classification of HIV infection was based on clinical criteria, but it was modified in 1987, when dementia and myelopathy were added as AIDS-defining illnesses. In a further 1993 revision, the CDC included laboratory-based categories (CD4+ lymphocyte cell counts) and additional clinical categories.[6] Asymptomatic HIV-positive individuals were now reportable as AIDS cases if the CD4+ count fell below 200 cells/mL.[6] (The World Health Organization did not adopt this classification.)

Ongoing development of new antiretroviral agents has expanded treatment options, and improved assessment of viral activity and treatment response is now possible through HIV-1 RNA assay (viral load). Because early treatment has gained favor and is now advised for individuals with CD4+ lymphocyte counts below 500/mL, an increasing number of asymptomatic HIV+ individuals are under treatment, often with multiple agents. Highly active antiretroviral therapy (HAART) is in wide use.

Though the risk of dementia being the presenting illness in an otherwise asymptomatic HIV+ individual is small, it is not absent. Consequently, medical certification of asymptomatic HIV+ individuals, with or without treatment, is a controversial issue. If vigorous treatment of these persons based on cytologic criteria is begun, side effects from the medical regimen also become an issue.

In chronic HIV infection a major aeromedical concern is the possibility of HIV dementia beginning with subtle incapacitation. When an AIDS-defining illness occurs, the risk of AIDS dementia increases dramatically, and aeromedical certification is generally precluded.

The AME/FS may be involved in initial certification of an aviator with HIV infection. Several variables affect a certification decision, including national policy, military versus civil aviation activity, access to state-of-the-art treatment, and ability to monitor individuals with the disease. If an HIV+ aviator, treated or untreated, is granted aeromedical certification, regular monitoring is necessary because of the concern for HIV-related dementia.[7] Periodic neuropsychological testing can be employed to monitor cognitive function. Standard neuropsychological instruments, including the Halstead-Reitan test battery and other more comprehensive test instruments, are subject to practice effect with repeated use. Computerized test batteries such as COGSCREEN have been used to monitor cognitive changes, and test material can be varied to minimize practice effect. In addition to the neurologic deficits potentially affecting HIV+ individuals, psychological reactions to the diagnosis (anger, depression, reckless thought) also merit serious consideration in a certification decision.

Aeromedical certification of HIV-infected aviators is likely to remain a controversial issue despite advances in treatment and ability to monitor the infection, and recent research only complicates the issue. Despite the use of HAART, smoldering low-level replication of the virus can be demonstrated in peripheral blood mononuclear cells. Cell-free virion RNA may also be found in peripheral plasma.[7] Long-term follow-up of individuals being treated with HAART will undoubtedly shed further light on the course of the disease in these individuals.

Traumatic Brain Injury

General Principles

Although traumatic brain injury is a major cause of neurologic disability in the adult population, **head** injury may not necessarily be accompanied by **brain** injury. Disturbance of or loss of consciousness, focal neurologic deficit, or abnormalities on brain imaging studies indicate brain injury has occurred. When evaluating an aviator with a recent or remote history of head injury, one must seek to determine whether brain injury occurred and its extent. The Glasgow Coma Scale (GCS) and duration of posttraumatic amnesia (PTA) are useful indicators in assessing severity of traumatic brain injury.[8] The Glasgow Coma Scale has a range of 3-15 points based on 3 basic clinical parameters (see Table 4-1). Another measure of severity of brain injury is duration of posttraumatic amnesia (PTA), defined as the amount of time between injury and the return of continuous memory (see Table 4-2). Patients with a GCS score of 9 or less and/or PTA of greater 24 hours duration, have a significant risk of permanent neurologic sequelae. The majority of civilian head injuries are closed head injuries, in which there is no violation of the cranial vault. Individuals with penetrating head injuries involving dural or parenchymal laceration with subsequent scar formation (the meningocerebral cicatrix described by Penfield) are at high risk for posttraumatic epilepsy. Injury to certain cortical areas, such as the central sulcus, are also associated with a greater risk of seizures.

The AME/FS is likely to encounter an aviator seeking aeromedical certification after recovery from acute injury. Along with the history and neurologic examination, records will be helpful in assessing the severity of residual deficit. Determination of the presence of persistent or permanent sequelae then becomes the overriding concern in the aeromedical disposition decision. Significant sequelae of traumatic brain injury are *postconcussion syndrome*, *focal neurologic deficit*, *posttraumatic epilepsy*, and *posttraumatic neuropsychological impairment*.

Table 4-1. The Glasgow Coma Scale

Eye opening
Spontaneous	4
To sound	3
To pain	2
None	1

Best motor response
Follows commands	6
Localizes stimulus	5
Withdraws	4
Flexion posturing	3
Extension posturing	2
No movement	1

Verbal response
Oriented	5
Confused	4
Words	3
Sounds	2
None	1

Add scores from all 3 categories above to calculate total GCS.

Postconcussion syndrome is a condition that often follows a seemingly trivial head injury, and is characterized by a number of subjective symptoms including headache, nonspecific dizziness, insomnia, restlessness, irritability, poor concentration, and attentional problems.[9] Neurological examination, brain imaging studies (CT, MRI), and EEG are often normal, and neuropsychological testing reveals no persistent deficits. There is evidence that diffuse axonal injury (DAI) characterized by axonal shearing, axonal retraction bulbs, and petechial hemorrhages provide the pathologic substrate for postconcussion syndrome. Because secondary gain issues may complicate the picture, litigation confounds clinical assessment. Postconcussion syndrome usually improves and resolves with the passage of time (6 months

Table 4-2. Duration of Posttraumatic Amnesia (PTA)

Mild brain injury:	0-1 hour of posttraumatic amnesia
Moderate brain injury:	1-24 hours of posttraumatic amnesia
Severe brain injury:	1-7 days of posttraumatic amnesia
Very severe brain injury:	>7 days of posttraumatic amnesia

to 2 years). With resolution of symptoms and absence of use of disqualifying medications, aeromedical certification can be considered. Narcotic analgesics, sedative hypnotics, antidepressants, sedating muscle relaxants, and tranquilizers ordinarily preclude certification until they are discontinued, followed by a medication-free observation period.

Focal neurologic deficit resulting from traumatic brain injury is determined by the area of brain or nerve affected, with motor deficit a common finding. For example, trauma resulting in a left subdural hematoma is often associated with contusion of the underlying cortex, producing right hemiparesis and aphasia. This deficit may persist despite early and successful evacuation of the hematoma. Other deficits include cranial nerve palsies, visual field defects, and ataxia.

The most common mechanism of traumatic brain injury involves frontal deceleration. These forces may cause stretching of the olfactory filaments at the cribriform plate, resulting in anosmia. If sense of smell does not return within 6 months, the filaments are likely severed rather than stretched, producing permanent anosmia, and an aviator would lose the ability to detect fumes or odors in the cockpit. Much of what we interpret as taste involves the sense of smell. Anosmic patients often complain of loss of taste, though taste fibers to the tongue (cranial nerves VII and IX) are not injured. Nerves to the extraocular muscles may be traumatized in orbital blowout fractures or at the level of the brainstem if sufficient forces are applied. Hearing and facial nerve function may be affected by basilar skull fractures involving the temporal bone. Frontal deceleration may also expose the anterior surfaces of the frontal and temporal lobes to contusion, which may lead to changes in personality, behavior, intellect, and memory. The more posterior parietal and occipital regions are somewhat more cushioned and protected, though at times are affected by contrecoup injury.

Posttraumatic epilepsy (PTE) is far more common in penetrating (open) head injuries in which laceration of cerebral tissue has occurred, leaving a "meningocerebral cicatrix" (Penfield) that may give rise to posttraumatic seizures. With penetrating head injury, risk of epilepsy can range from 20%-57%. Civilian trauma more likely involves closed or blunt injury, in which the cranial vault is intact (although a linear nondepressed fracture may be present). The risk of PTE with closed head injury is approximately 5%, although certain factors may increase the risk. These include a history of febrile seizures, a sibling with epilepsy, occurrence of an intracranial hematoma, and injury to certain cortical areas such as the central sulcus, a highly epileptogenic zone.

Seizures may be partial elementary seizures, partial complex seizures, partial seizures with secondary generalization, or primarily generalized seizures (see section on epilepsy for clinical characteristics of each). A seizure occurring at the time of impact (impact seizure) may not have long-term significance, but seizures beginning weeks or months after injury suggest scar formation (gliosis) and persistent seizure potential. If seizures are going to occur, they will develop within 6 months in approximately 50% of individuals, within 1 year in 75%, and within 2 years in 85%-90%. Ninety-seven percent of susceptible individuals will have had their first seizure within 3 years of trauma.[8]

Posttraumatic neuropsychological impairment is often overlooked in the acute injury phase, being overshadowed by clearly evident disturbed consciousness and focal neurologic deficit. When alert wakefulness returns and focal deficit clears, neuropsychological deficits may surface. Cognitive deficit may not become evident until the individual attempts to resume normal activities, whereupon problems at home, at work, and in social settings appear.[10] Attention, concentration, information processing speed, mental flexibility, and frontal lobe executive functions may be disturbed. When traumatic brain injury is of significant severity, as measured by Glasgow coma score or length of posttraumatic amnesia, the AME/FS must inquire carefully about changes in personality, behavior, intellect, and memory. Observers such as family members, friends, and associates can provide valuable information, which may not be mentioned or recognized by the aviator. A high index of suspicion is warranted with increasing severity of trauma. Neuropsychological testing is employed to determine the nature and extent of posttraumatic cognitive deficit.

History from the patient (and observers when needed) along with careful review of adequate medical records will characterize the injury. Focal neurologic deficit will be evident on neurological examination. Brain imaging studies may indicate areas of posttraumatic encephalomalacia or focal atrophy, with MRI being more sensitive than CT imaging. EEG may also be useful in assessing posttraumatic seizures, though a normal EEG by no means excludes the possibility of epilepsy. Potentially epileptiform abnormalities (eg, a frontal or temporal spike focus) may be seen. Since activation of an epileptiform focus may occur only during sleep, a sleep-deprived wake and sleep EEG is appropriate when considering seizures.

The majority of neurologic recovery from traumatic brain injury will take place within the first 6-12 months following injury. Further recovery at a lesser rate may occur in the following 1-2 years, with younger age groups being favored.[8]

The AME/FS is faced with the difficult task of assessing severity of brain injury, determining the nature and extent of sequelae, and deciding whether or not sufficient time has passed to achieve maximal neuronal recovery. The declining risk of posttraumatic epilepsy with time is another parameter in deciding aeromedical disposition. Since each case deserves careful individual consideration of all variables, only general aeromedical disposition guidelines can be suggested.

In mild concussion with loss of consciousness lasting from seconds to minutes, upon complete recovery and freedom from symptoms, a 60-90 day period of observation might be sufficient before return to flight status. One must remain vigilant for delayed development of neurologic symptoms following seemingly minor head injury, which may indicate subdural hematoma. Symptoms may appear weeks or months later, and the inciting injury may be all but forgotten. Moderate to severe brain injuries require a longer period of observation. Individuals with cerebral contusion, manifested either clinically as focal neurologic deficit or appearing on neuroimaging studies, should be observed for a year or more before return to flight status is considered. In persons with an intracranial hematoma (epidural, subdural, intraparenchymal) a 1-3 year period of observation might be appropriate. Early evacuation of an epidural hematoma followed by rapid and complete recovery would allow earlier consideration of return to flight status (eg, 6-12 months), whereas an aviator with a large subdural hematoma, underlying cortical contusion, and slowly resolving hemiparesis might require 2-3 years of observation. Patients with severe brain injury might warrant 3 years of observation to ensure maximal neuronal recovery and lessening of seizure risk.

Intracranial Neoplasms

General Principles

Tumors involving the brain or its coverings may be primary or metastatic and benign or malignant. Benign tumors may involve cranial nerves (eg, acoustic neuroma), the meninges (eg, meningioma), and the pituitary gland (eg, adenoma). Likewise, certain parenchymal tumors (eg, low-grade astrocytoma) may follow a relatively benign, protracted course. The gliomas (astrocytoma, oligodendroglioma, glioblastoma multiforme) are the most common primary malignant intracranial neoplasms, representing 60% of intracranial tumors.[11] In general, tumor incidence rises markedly after age 65.

Tumors arising from structures outside the brain parenchyma tend to be benign, causing symptoms due to compression of adjacent brain tissue. Therefore, these tumors lend themselves to total removal and cure without significant residual neurologic deficit. However, certain benign neoplasms may be "malignant by position," meaning attempted total removal carries a high risk of severe deficit or death, this being particularly true of tumors involving the base of the brain (eg, craniopharyngioma).

Tumors arising within the brain parenchyma, whether primary or metastatic, commonly have malignant characteristics, with tumor cells often infiltrating normal parenchyma in finger-like fashion. Tumor spread typically extends beyond gross surgical margins, mingling with surrounding normal parenchyma. Though the tumor is debulked, neoplastic cells remain. Attempts at wider excision would remove normal parenchyma along with tumor, increasing the degree of postoperative neurologic deficit. Therefore, the gliomas and metastatic tumors are characterized by recurrence rather than cure, although there are some exceptions, such as cystic astrocytomas of the cerebellum with a mural tumor nodule and certain solitary well-defined metastatic lesions.

Craniopharyngiomas (Rathke's pouch tumor) are more common in childhood and adolescence. Though benign, these tumors commonly involve basal brain structures, prohibiting complete resection. Recurrence is the rule. Benign, functioning or nonfunctioning pituitary adenomas can often be resected, but larger adenomas may cause significant visual field defects and also involve the cavernous sinus and internal carotid arteries.

Recent-onset worsening headaches, partial or generalized tonic-clonic seizures, mental status changes, and cumulative neurologic deficit may indicate the presence of tumor. Tumors may also cause personality change that might be mistaken for an emotional disorder. Projectile vomiting is not uncommon. Unlike the sudden-onset neurologic deficit typical of stroke, tumors are characterized by a progressive temporal profile, and if located in a relatively silent area of the brain such as the cerebellum, frontal lobes, temporal lobes, or nondominant parietal lobe, they may reach appreciable size before discovery. Slowly growing tumors such as meningioma allow for compensatory changes in surrounding tissue, sometimes becoming quite large before causing symptoms.

Neurological examination might reveal papilledema secondary to increased intracranial pressure, and focal deficit including visual field defects, aphasia, hemiparesis, or mental status changes. Spinal cord tumors are far less frequently encountered and often present with a progressive myelopathy accompanied by spastic weakness, a sensory level, and bladder and bowel dysfunction.

Though computed tomography (CT) brain imaging studies are useful, magnetic resonance imaging (MRI) studies with and without gadolinium has become the gold standard for detection of brain tumor, since small lesions may escape detection with CT.

The treatment of brain tumors includes surgical removal, chemotherapy, and radiotherapy, depending upon tumor type, location, and clinical circumstances.

An aeromedical disposition decision will normally be considered when treatment is completed and recovery assured. Typically, a suitable period of observation (1 year or more) is appropriate before considering aeromedical certification when dealing with benign extraparenchymal tumors. The AME/FS must gather records including reports of imaging studies and operative and radiation oncology reports if applicable. In addition, pathology reports are essential and follow-up notes are useful in documenting deficit and recovery. Upon review, the appropriate licensing authority might consider certification if complete tumor resection has effected cure and residual deficit (if any) is not functionally significant. Seizures must be absent and there must be an appropriate period of observation. As noted earlier, tumors arising within the brain parenchyma generally recur and are unpredictable, usually precluding certification. Close follow-up is essential in all cases.

Hereditary, Degenerative, and Demyelinating Disorders

General Principles

The hereditary, degenerative, and demyelinating disorders represent a wide variety of neurologic disorders, some of which follow a static or predictable slowly progressive course. Ability to monitor the condition might allow special issuance certification until aviation safety is compromised. In this section the more common disorders causing aeromedical certification concerns will be addressed.

Multiple Sclerosis

Onset of multiple sclerosis occurs most commonly from age 20-40, with slight female preponderance. The disease is characterized by demyelinating plaques in the central nervous system with some axonal loss. A central scotoma due to optic neuritis may be a presenting symptom, although sensory symptoms, focal weakness, vertigo, diplopia, and ataxia are common complaints. In addition, bladder and bowel function may be impaired. Some patients note a tingling sensation radiating down the spine or into the extremities with head flexion (Lhermitte's phenomenon). Worsening symptoms following heat exposure or a hot shower may occur. In general, neurologic findings relate to the area of the central nervous system affected, with visual field defects, reflex asymmetries, focal weakness, sensory abnormalities, and pathologic reflexes often being present. Multiple sclerosis may follow a chronic progressive or relapsing and remitting course, with exacerbations lasting weeks or months.

MRI brain imaging studies have greatly facilitated confirmation of the diagnosis of multiple sclerosis, although in doubtful cases, adjunctive studies may be helpful, such as cerebrospinal fluid examination for oligoclonal bands and IgG synthesis. Visual, auditory, and somatosensory evoked potentials are sometimes also useful. Clinical diagnosis remains of utmost importance in multiple sclerosis.

Acute exacerbations of demyelinating disease are commonly managed with oral corticosteroids or intravenous methylprednisolone. In more severe cases that are unresponsive to corticosteroid treatment, immunosuppressive agents such as cyclophosphamide, methotrexate, and azathioprine may be employed. There is a growing trend to treat multiple sclerosis patients early with one of the interferons (beta-1a-interferon or beta-1b-interferon) or the copolymer glatirimer acetate in an effort to stem progression of the disease. A variety of muscle relaxants are used to treat spasticity. Other agents are used for symptomatic improvement of bladder function, some with anticholinergic properties. Fatigue has been treated with amantadine, pemoline, and more recently modafinil.

The AME/FS must address a number of important issues when considering certification of an aviator with multiple sclerosis. Age of onset, severity and frequency of exacerbations, degree of neurologic deficit, and rapidity of progression must all be taken into account. Duration of clinical stability is an important parameter, as is lesion location; for example, a pontine lesion might make the aviator susceptible to vertigo and diplopia. The possibility of cognitive deficit must also be addressed. Medication use is important, because sedative effects are common with muscle relaxants and anticholinergic agents used for bladder control. The well-known adverse effects of corticosteroids also merit consideration. Amantadine may be mind-altering, and flu-like symptoms or depression may accompany interferon injections.

An aviator with mild disease and no significant neurologic deficit might be considered for certification following an appropriate period of demonstrated stability (months to a year or more). Certification might have provisions including limited certificate duration, periodic follow-up visits, or operational limitations (eg, restriction to a multicrew cockpit). Certain operations (military, aerobatic, agricultural) might preclude special issuance.

Parkinson's Disease

Parkinson's disease is characterized by the symptom triad of tremor at rest, rigidity, and bradykinesia. In addition, a general attitude of flexion, freezing of gait, and loss of postural reflexes are often present. The usual age of onset is the mid-fifties, though the age range is wide. In Parkinson's disease dopamine metabolism in the basal ganglia is disturbed. Pure Parkinson's disease is idiopathic, but Parkinsonism refers to a Parkinson-like state with multiple causes, such as postinfection (encephalitis lethargica), drug exposure (metoclopramide, antipsychotic agents), metabolic derangement, toxic exposure (carbon monoxide, manganese), and vascular insult. Other degenerative disorders, of which Parkinsonism is one component, are sometimes called Parkinson-plus syndromes.[12] These disorders are accompanied by additional symptoms including cognitive changes, disorders of ocular motility, ataxia, and autonomic disturbances with orthostatic hypotension.

Rest tremor in the hands, especially pill rolling tremor involving the thumb and index finger, is a common presenting symptom. Other signs and symptoms include slow and shuffling gait, gait arrest or freezing, diminished or absent arm swing, flexed posture, paucity of facial expression, infrequent blinking, diminished vocal volume, and paucity of movement. Cogwheel rigidity and impaired rapidly alternating movements (eg, finger wiggle or foot tap) are additional characteristic clinical features.

At the time of initial diagnosis, an attempt should be made to classify the illness as idiopathic Parkinson's or a Parkinson-plus syndrome. One must also search for underlying correctable causes, such as medication-induced Parkinsonism. Structural disease as an etiology is excluded with cerebral imaging studies.

The majority of patients with Parkinson's disease are managed medically with dopamine precursors (levodopa, most commonly combined with carbidopa), dopamine agonists, and anticholinergic agents. A number of newer dopamine agonists have shown promise in relieving symptoms of the disease. Unfortunately patients commonly develop receptor sensitivity to dopamine precursors over 4-7 years. Furthermore, fluctuating effectiveness (on-off phenomenon) and involuntary movements then limit further use of these agents. Early use of dopamine agonists might allow lower doses or delayed institution of dopamine precursors, preserving their usefulness for later years. There has been widespread interest in surgical solutions including pallidotomy and deep brain stimulation. Tissue implants remain under study.

The AME/FS encountering an aviator with Parkinsonism must consider the accuracy of diagnosis (idiopathic versus secondary Parkinsonism), duration of illness, severity of impairment and medications being used. Fine motor coordination for performance of cockpit tasks warrants specific consideration. Dopamine precursors and agonists may cause hallucinations, and anticholinergic agents may cause sedation and confusion, precluding certification. Duration of treatment and freedom from side effects must be documented if certification is to be considered.

Parkinsonism is in most cases a progressive disorder leading to cumulative disability. Some patients progress slowly, respond well to medication, and remain free of side effects. Others respond to surgery. In many individuals certification may be considered with appropriate provisions for follow-up. When cumulative disability impacts aviation safety, certification can be withdrawn.

Familial Tremor/Essential Tremor

Familial tremor, the most common movement disorder, often begins in adulthood and usually progresses very slowly over many years, but may appear static for long periods of time. It usually involves the hands and is most pronounced with the arms outstretched (postural tremor). Head and voice tremor may occur, and less commonly trunk and limbs may be involved. Patients will complain of tremor with writing and eating (soup on a spoon, peas on a fork, carrying an empty cup on a saucer). Performing fine movements such as threading a needle or using a small screwdriver may be difficult. The term *essential tremor* is used when there is no family history of tremor, but the disorder is identical. Alcohol commonly lessens the symptoms, while stress will aggravate the condition. There are no laboratory findings to support the diagnosis.

Many individuals have little impairment from tremor and require no treatment. However, if the tremor becomes bothersome, propranolol or primidone are quite effective and other medications have been prescribed including diazepam, lorazepam, and meprobamate. Surgical procedures such as deep brain stimulation have been employed in severe cases.

Many persons have mild tremor that may be embarrassing but causes no functional impairment. It is not uncommon for a patient to decline treatment once relieved of the threat of Parkinson's disease. Others will use medication only in stressful circumstances such as when delivering a speech. Aeromedical certification can be considered in many individuals as long as appropriate provisions are made for periodic follow-up. Changes may be imperceptible for years, allowing ample time for assessment of significant impairment. Treatment with propranolol or another beta-blocker should not preclude consideration for aeromedical certification in most cases (though mild sedation may be a factor in some) provided an appropriate observation period for side effects has been established. Primidone, an older anticonvulsant, has sedative properties which could impact aviation safety. Benzodiazepine and meprobamate usage will bar certification due to potential sedative and cognitive side effects.

Cerebrovascular Disorders

General Principles

Our population is aging. Many aviators are flying beyond age 70, some beyond age 80, and a few beyond age 90. Risk of stroke and cardiac disease rises sharply with age, with stroke being the third leading cause of death in the U.S. following heart disease and cancer. The incidence of stroke has declined from 106.3/100,000/year in 1900 to 60.2/100,000/year in 1995. This is presumably due to risk factor modification, particularly the treatment of hypertension. This section will deal with cerebrovascular disease including transient ischemic attack (TIA), thrombotic stroke, embolic stroke, intracerebral hemorrhage, and subarachnoid hemorrhage. Table 4-3 shows a breakdown of the causes of stroke.

It is also useful to consider stroke in terms of anatomic localization, such as in the anterior circulation (internal carotid territory) or posterior circulation (vertebral-basilar territory). Clinical differentiation is important, because strokes in the posterior circulation are more likely to be of embolic origin. Furthermore, anterior circulation strokes or transient ischemic attacks might be caused by surgically-correctable carotid artery disease.

Of paramount importance in any discussion of stroke is the assessment of risk factors, and they are detailed in Table 4-4.

Hypertension is the single most important modifiable risk factor for stroke, and it may play a role in as many as 70% of all strokes, with both systolic and diastolic hypertension increasing the relative risk of stroke to 6 times that of the normal population. Longstanding hypertension also increases the risk of heart disease and accelerates arteriosclerosis. Most intracerebral hemorrhages are due to hypertension. Consequently, persistent elevation of blood pressure in an aviator merits attention.

Table 4-3. Type, Pathogenesis, and Frequency of Stroke

Ischemic infarction of brain	83%
Large vessel thrombotic	31%
Embolic	32%
Small vessel thrombotic	20%
Hemorrhagic stroke	17%
Intracerebral hemorrhage	10%
Hypertensive	5%
Amyloid angiopathy	3%
Other	2%
Subarachnoid hemorrhage	7%
Aneurysmal	3%
Vascular-malformation related	2%
Other	2%

Table 4-4. Risk Factors for Stroke

Nonmodifiable risk factors

Major
> Advancing age
> Male sex
> Diabetes mellitus
> Prior stroke or transient ischemic attack
> Positive family history of stroke
> Asymptomatic carotid bruit

Less well documented
> Socioeconomic status

Modifiable risk factors

Major
> Hypertension
> Heart disease
> Atrial fibrillation
> Transient ischemic attack
> Tobacco use

Secondary
> Cholesterol level
> Lack of exercise
> Obesity

Less well documented
> Alcohol intake
> Infection

Heart disease ranks second only to hypertension among major risk factors, followed by ischemic heart disease, valvular heart disease, congestive heart failure, and arrhythmia. Additional risk factors include diabetes mellitus and tobacco use. Recognition of risk factors and dedication to their modification are integral components of a certification decision, since each affects an aviator's risk of initial and recurrent stroke. Clearly, risk of sudden incapacitation from stroke is the prime consideration in aeromedical certification decisions.

Transient Ischemic Attack (TIA)

A transient ischemic attack (TIA) is a short-term focal disturbance of neurologic function due to ischemia that resolves within 24 hours, with most lasting only minutes. Symptoms depend on the arterial supply to the involved area of brain.

Transient ischemic attacks can be broadly divided into retinal, anterior circulation (carotid territory), and posterior circulation (vertebral-basilar territory) types. The risk of stroke following TIA is in the range of 5%-6% per year over five years.[13]

The classic retinal manifestation of an ischemic episode is amaurosis fugax (fleeting blindness), with the patient reporting sudden monocular visual loss, often described as if a descending (or ascending) shade or curtain was drawn over the eye. Complete blindness usually occurs briefly, though a partial defect may also occur. Vision returns within 30-60 seconds. Amaurosis fugax usually signifies disease of the carotid artery in older individuals, though benign occurrences have been rarely reported in the young. In some cases examination of the optic fundus during or following an episode may disclose embolic material at the branches of retinal arterioles (Hollenhorst plaques). One must always search for carotid disease in an individual with amaurosis fugax.

TIAs in the anterior circulation may produce contralateral weakness and sensory loss, aphasia when the dominant hemisphere is involved, and at times visual field defects. If a TIA is purely motor or purely sensory, small vessel disease involving deep penetrating arteries is suggested.

TIAs in the posterior circulation give rise to brainstem symptoms including varying combinations of vertigo, ataxia, diplopia, dysarthria, facial numbness, crossed numbness or weakness, and bilateral visual field defects. Bilateral symptoms always suggest posterior circulation disease.

Once the TIA has ended, there may be no neurologic findings, although with amaurosis fugax or an anterior circulation TIA, a bruit may be heard over the ipsilateral carotid artery. Though symptoms may clear completely and neurologic examination may be normal, sensitive brain imaging studies such as MRI may demonstrate an infarct in a location appropriate to the TIA, rendering the definition of TIA somewhat arbitrary.

A TIA may be a harbinger of stroke and, when due to carotid disease, myocardial infarction. Consequently, occurrence of one or more TIAs should prompt assessment of vascular risk factors, consideration of associated heart disease, and development of a treatment plan. CBC, chemistry panel, blood lipid profile, carotid ultrasound, brain imaging studies, and an echocardiogram may be indicated. In younger individuals and those without common risk factors, search for a hypercoagulable state and other causes of stroke in the young is warranted.

If carotid artery stenosis of greater than 70% is present, carotid endarterectomy is the treatment of choice, as demonstrated by several studies.[14] There is also a general consensus that stenosis of less than 30% should not be addressed surgically. Ongoing studies are underway to assess treatment of patients with 30%-70% stenosis. Medical management of TIA is addressed below in the section on atherothrombotic brain infarction.

When considering aeromedical certification for an aviator with a history of TIA, the AME/FS should consider a number of factors. These include the nature of the event, the thoroughness of the medical evaluation, assessment of nonmodifiable and modifiable risk factors, medication use (and potential side effects), and the observation period since the event(s) occurred. Lowering risk for recurrence through attention to modifiable risk factors should be considered in a certification decision. Because of the association between carotid disease and cardiac disease, consideration of comorbid cardiac disease is important.

Asymptomatic Carotid Bruit

The asymptomatic carotid bruit in the aviator is of concern because of the associated risk of stroke. Asymptomatic bruits in the neck occur in 4%-5% of the population aged 45-80 and in up to 90% of individuals with stenosis of 75% or greater.[15] A bruit does not necessarily indicate carotid stenosis, as there are alternative causes, such as the radiation of an aortic stenosis murmur or tortuous artery.

The risk of stroke in patients with asymptomatic carotid stenosis has been variably reported, although the presence of a bruit does not appear to be as critical as the degree of stenosis subsequently found. In general, longitudinal studies suggest the overall risk is below 1% per year, but the annual risk approaches 5% when stenosis is 75% or greater.[16] Surgical treatment of asymptomatic high-grade stenosis remains controversial.

Atherothrombotic Brain Infarction

Sudden onset of neurologic deficit is characteristic of thrombotic stroke, although stuttering and progressive neurologic deficit may occur at times, mimicking the temporal profile of a structural lesion (tumor or abscess). Neurologic deficit relates to the area of the brain supplied by the affected vessel. For example, dominant hemisphere middle cerebral artery thrombosis may produce hemiplegia and aphasia, anterior cerebral artery thrombosis will affect the contralateral leg, while posterior cerebral thrombosis may produce a contralateral homonymous hemianopsia. Posterior circulation infarcts may cause a variety of brainstem symptoms including vertigo, diplopia, ataxia, dysarthria, and visual field defects. CT or MRI brain imaging studies are useful in documenting location and extent of the infarction.

Acute management of stroke is directed at halting progression of neurologic deficit, idealizing systemic factors in support of recovery, preventing secondary neuronal injury from edema, and commencing rehabilitation efforts. Specific varieties of acute stroke may be treated with recombinant tissue plasminogen activator (rtPA) if given within 3 hours of stroke onset. Intravenous and intraarterial thrombolysis are undergoing further study, as is widening the interventional window beyond 3 hours.

Long-term medical management of TIA and stroke consists of aspirin, ticlopidine, clopidogrel, dipyridamole, or warfarin. Recommendations vary regarding the optimal dosage of aspirin, with 50-325 mg/day being the dosage range suggested by the American College of Chest Physicians.[17] Warfarin is used less commonly. A combination of low-dose aspirin and extended-release dipyridamole has recently been introduced. Along with medical treatment, vigorous attention to modifiable risk factors is essential to reduce risk of recurrent stroke.

The AME/FS becomes involved when the aviator seeks certification following stroke. At this point all pertinent records should be reviewed, including history and physical examination, consultations, laboratory and imaging studies, discharge summaries, records of treatment, and follow-up reports. Assessment for residual neurologic deficit is particularly important. Modifiable and nonmodifiable risk factors should be considered along with the aviator's resolve in attending to risk factors. Side effects of medication must also be considered. Aspirin may cause GI upset and bleeding, while ticlopidine, clopidogrel and dipyridamole may cause headache and dizziness. Finally, an adequate period of observation (eg, 2 years) for recovery and risk factor modification is appropriate. This may vary depending on stroke mechanism. Stroke related to surgically-repaired patent foramen ovale or carotid stenosis may warrant earlier consideration than primary atherothrombotic stroke, since recurrence risk is lowered by treatment.

At 1 year following stroke, recurrence risk ranges from 5%-25%, depending on stroke subtype and comorbidity; over 5 years the total risk is 20%-40%. Cumulative risk at 3 years is approximately 18%, with risk factor burden affecting recurrence potential.[18] Those with large-vessel atherosclerotic stroke have the greatest risk of recurrence at 3 years (approximately 21%), while those with lacunar stroke have the lowest risk (about 14% at 3 years). Advanced age, hypertension, coronary artery disease, atrial fibrillation, congestive heart failure (CHF), hyperglycemia, high-grade carotid stenosis, and prior TIA are all associated with increased risk of late recurrence.[18] If good recovery has been achieved and risk factors addressed, certification may be considered after observation as noted above. If carotid endarterectomy has been performed and significant cardiac disease has been excluded, certification is often possible.

Embolic Cerebral Infarction

Sources of cerebral emboli include proximal arteries (artery-to-artery embolus), the ascending aorta, cardiac valves and chambers (cardiac emboli), and the venous system when a sufficient cardiac right-to-left shunt exists (eg, patent foramen ovale). Embolic infarction is more common in the posterior circulation and more often hemorrhagic. Sudden onset of deficit followed by rapid clearing are characteristic of embolus. Multiple bilateral infarcts suggest the possibility of an embolic source, with neurologic findings similar to those seen in atherothrombotic stroke, as are laboratory and imaging studies. When embolic stroke is suspected, appropriate studies include carotid ultrasound, transthoracic echocardiography, and transesophageal echocardiogram when indicated (stroke in the young, known right-to-left shunt, few or absent risk factors). Contrast echocardiography with intravenous bubble infusion has become increasingly important in demonstrating significant intracardiac right-to-left shunts.

Guidelines for neurologic recovery from embolic stroke are the same as those for atherothrombotic stroke. One additional consideration, however, is the embolic source and its management. For example, in the treatment of valvular disease, tissue valves do not require anticoagulation with warfarin, though eventually valve replacement is necessary. On the other hand, anticoagulation must be employed with mechanical valves. If embolus via a patent foramen ovale (prevalence of 20% in the population) is suspect, surgical treatment becomes an option. However, the mere presence of patent foramen ovale in an aviator with stroke does not indicate causation.

If stroke recovery is complete or near-complete, elimination of significant risk of future emboli becomes the major factor in a certification decision. If carotid stenosis or ulcerated plaque has been surgically corrected following stroke or TIA, recertification is possible. Follow-up carotid ultrasound studies should be performed to determine the likelihood of restenosis, and the possibility of underlying cardiac disease deserves scrutiny. Good follow-up and a suitable observation period are essential in deciding aeromedical disposition.

Stroke in the Young

Approximately 5% of strokes of various causes occur in younger individuals aged 15-45. Hence, one can expect an occasional case in the aviator population. A partial list of causes is detailed in Table 4-5.

Arterial dissection is high on the list as a cause of stroke in the young, as it constitutes about 4% of strokes in this population.[19] Multiple vessels in the carotid and vertebral systems may be involved. In one Mayo Clinic study, 200 patients with cer-

Table 4-5. Causes of Stroke in the Younger Patient

Atherosclerotic stroke	26.9%	Sick sinus syndrome (brady-tachy syndrome)	
Nonatherosclerotic vasculopathy	23.1%	Intracardiac defects	
Migraine		Septal aneurysm	
Arterial dissection		Cardiomyopathy	
CNS angiitis		Myocardial infarction	
Periarteritis nodosa		Left ventricular aneurysm	
Drug abuse		Intracardiac tumors (eg, atrial myxoma)	
Sjögren's syndrome		Invasive cardiac procedures	
Giant cell arteritis		Patent foramen ovale (PFO)	
Beçhet's syndrome			
Wegener's granulomatosis		Hematologic	12.2%
Cardioembolic	21.7%	Arteritis	
Rheumatic disease		Antithrombin III deficiency	
Mitral valve prolapse		Protein C deficiency	
Prosthetic valve		Protein S deficiency	
Subacute bacterial endocarditis		Anticardiolipin antibodies	
Noninfectious (marantic) endocarditis		Antiphospholipid antibodies	
Liebman-Sacks endocarditis		Lupus anticoagulant	
Calcific valvular disease		Elevated homocysteine levels	
Congenital valvular defects		Oral contraceptive use	
Atrial fibrillation		Unknown	16.1%

vical arterial dissections over a 20-year period were identified. Long-term prognosis was good, with a recurrence beyond the first month of about 1% per year.[20] This may allow a shorter observation period before certification is considered (eg, 1 year).

Intracerebral Hemorrhage

Primary brain hemorrhage most commonly occurs in hypertensive individuals, with the basal ganglia, brainstem (pons), and cerebellum being the most common sites, though subcortical hemorrhages may also occur. Hypertensive hemorrhages commonly produce severe deficit, usually permanent, or coma and death. Structural lesions that may lead to hemorrhage include vascular malformations, aneurysms rupturing into the parenchyma, hemorrhagic infarcts, mycotic aneurysms, tumors (especially malignant melanoma), and hypocoagulable states (leukemia, thrombocytopenia, etc).

CT brain imaging studies readily identify significant parenchymal hemorrhage. If hypertension is not the obvious cause of bleeding, a search must be made for other sources such as congenital aneurysm, vascular malformation, or hypocoagulable state. Conventional transfemoral arteriography may be employed in the search for aneurysm and vascular malformation. MRI may demonstrate small vascular lesions such as cavernous angiomas that may escape detection on CT scan or conventional angiography. Magnetic resonance angiography (MRA) is gaining favor as a useful noninvasive technique for imaging major cervical extracranial vessels, as well as the circle of Willis and its major branches.

Deep supratentorial hematomas and pontine hemorrhages are managed medically, with hyperosmolar agents and treatment of hypertension. Because cerebellar hematomas may be life-threatening, emergent surgical removal is sometimes indicated. Surgical evacuation of small well-circumscribed subcortical hematomas is occasionally employed.

Evaluation of intracerebral hemorrhage follows the same principles employed for atherothrombotic or embolic infarction, with determination of the cause of the hemorrhage of primary concern. If the hemorrhage was caused by hypertension, treatment of blood pressure and idealization of other cerebrovascular risk factors is essential. Individuals suffering lesser hypertensive hemorrhages who recover and vigorously address high blood pressure and other risk factors might be considered for certification. On the other hand, structural lesions causing hemorrhage, including vascular malformations and aneurysms, must be isolated from the circulation through surgical intervention before certification is considered. For example, clipping of an aneurysm or complete resection of a malformation may be curative, allowing certification after a suitable period of observation. Other procedures, such as embolization of a malformation or placement of a coil in an aneurysm, may lessen the risk of recurrent hemorrhage, but may not cure the patient.

Subarachnoid Hemorrhage

Like intracerebral hemorrhage, subarachnoid hemorrhage may result from a ruptured aneurysm or vascular malformation, though at times no source of bleeding is found (idiopathic subarachnoid hemorrhage). The characteristic presentation of subarachnoid hemorrhage is sudden severe headache with or without altered consciousness, vomiting and prostration, and nuchal rigidity. Noncontrast CT imaging studies may demonstrate obvious blood in the ventricles or subarachnoid space over the convexities and in the basilar cisterns. In the proper clinical setting (sudden severe headache), spinal fluid examination should be carried out in search of blood that escapes detection on CT imaging studies. Conventional transfemoral angiography, magnetic resonance imaging (MRI), and magnetic resonance angiography (MRA) may be indicated to determine the source of bleeding. Due to acute vasospasm and possible clot within an aneurysm, initial conventional angiography may not demonstrate the lesion in approximately 13% of cases. A second (and perhaps a third) angiogram may be necessary to completely exclude aneurysm. In addition to aneurysms, vascular malformations and other structural lesions may also be demonstrated by these studies.

Acute medical management of subarachnoid hemorrhage is not within the purview of this discussion, since certification is not an issue in this setting. Surgical treatment ideally isolates an aneurysm by placement of a clip across its neck, effecting cure. However, clipping may be precluded by location of the aneurysm, broadness of its base, or fusiform shape. In such instances alternative methods are used to reduce the risk of rebleeding, including wrapping with muscle, application of glue, and angiographic introduction of a metallic coil within the dome of the aneurysm to induce thrombosis. As noted above, though these measures may reduce risk of rebleeding to a variable extent they often are not curative, so risk of rebleeding is lessened but not eliminated. Assessment of risk reduction must be individualized and based on specifics including the nature of the procedure, the degree of obliteration of circulation within the aneurysmal dome, and the remaining compromise of vascular integrity.

Though surgical resection of a vascular malformation may eliminate the risk of rebleeding, seizures arising from the surrounding altered neuronal bed may persist. In fact, vascular malformations more often present with seizures than with hemorrhage. The presence of seizures precludes aeromedical certification.

Assuming curative treatment of the lesion responsible for subarachnoid hemorrhage is successful, certification may be considered after recovery and an observation period of 1 year or longer. The aviator must be free of significant residual deficit, such as motor deficit, speech impairment, visual field defect, or cognitive changes.

Idiopathic subarachnoid hemorrhage has a good prognosis. If complete studies, including follow-up angiography (where initial studies revealed no hemorrhagic source) are unremarkable, certification may be considered after a 1-year period of observation. The long-term prognosis of subarachnoid hemorrhage of unknown origin is good.

Intracranial Hemorrhage in the Young

When considering nontraumatic intracranial hemorrhage in the young adult, causes other than hypertension must be considered. In one study of intracranial hemorrhage in 72 young adults from ages 15-45,[21] cause of hemorrhage was as detailed in Table 4-6. As in thrombotic stroke, intracranial hemorrhage in the young adult warrants a careful search for less-common mechanisms of stroke.

Table 4-6. Cause of Hemorrhage in a Study of 72 Young Adults*

Vascular malformation	29.1%
Hypertension	15.3%
Aneurysm	9.7%
Substance abuse	6.9%
Tumor	4.2%
Acute alcohol intake	2.8%
Preeclampsia, eclampsia	2.8%
Systemic lupus erythematosus	1.4%
Moyamoya disease	1.4%
Cryoglobulinemia	1.4%
Undetermined cause	23.6%

From Toffol GJ, Biller J, Adams H. Nontraumatic intracerebral hemorrhage in young adults. Arch Neurol. 1987;44:483-485.

Episodic Disorders

General Principles

Episodic disorders are conditions that cause intermittent neurologic symptoms. These include vertigo, migraine, cluster headache, transient global amnesia, syncope, and seizure disorder. The potential threat these conditions pose to aviation safety is self evident. Each will be addressed separately.

Vertigo

Dizziness is a nonspecific term. An individual complaining of dizziness should be asked exactly what the word means to him or her. Many patients will describe a lightheaded, woozy, floating or swimming sensation as dizziness. These descriptions do not have diagnostic value and may relate to metabolic, toxic, circulatory, degenerative, endocrine, and emotional factors. The term **vertigo** is reserved for conditions in which there is an element of rotation (of the person or the environment). Swaying or falling sensations may also be described. True vertigo of greater magnitude may be accompanied by staggering gait, pallor, nausea, vomiting, and diaphoresis.

It is important as well to distinguish dizziness and vertigo from dysequilibrium or ataxia. With ataxia there is no spinning sensation, and while sitting, lying, turning in bed, or performing other head or body movements the person is asymptomatic. With standing there is a sensation of unsteadiness, often with a need to grasp a nearby object for reassurance and stability. Stance and gait may be wide-based. The person will complain of unsteadiness and lack of balance, but will deny spinning or dizziness. This type of dysequilibrium suggests a central lesion affecting cerebellar pathways.

If true vertigo is present, one must determine if it is of central or peripheral origin. Central vertigo is of brainstem origin, involving the vestibular nuclei and their connections, while peripheral vertigo involves labyrinthine structures. True vertigo, if accompanied by nystagmus, nausea and vomiting, and exacerbation by body or head movement is more likely of peripheral origin, especially if paroxysmal and recurrent. The individual is often normal between episodes.

When vertigo is the sole symptom, distinguishing central from peripheral vertigo may be difficult. For example, it is known that vertigo may be the sole presenting symptom of vertebrobasilar ischemia and be indistinguishable from labyrinthitis in the emergent setting. Nevertheless, symptoms associated with the vertigo often provide helpful clues in differential diagnosis. Peripheral vestibular disorders causing vertigo may be accompanied by hearing loss, tinnitus, ear fullness, and ear pain, while central vertigo may be accompanied by other symptoms of brainstem dysfunction including diplopia, dysarthria, facial or extremity sensory symptoms, and unilateral or bilateral weakness of the extremities.

Vertigo may compromise aviation safety by abrupt onset in an asymptomatic individual, abrupt recurrence in an asymptomatic individual, or by causing a persistent vertiginous state of variable degree.[22] Clearly, vertigo regardless of etiology is unwelcome in the cockpit. A general discussion of peripheral and central vestibulopathies follows; for specific diseases associated with vertigo see Chapter 6 (otolaryngology).

Acute peripheral vestibulopathies include benign positional vertigo, acute labyrinthitis (an isolated episode of acute peripheral vertigo), acute recurrent peripheral vertigo, and Meniere's disease. Additionally, chronic peripheral vertigo may result from trauma, a nonfunctioning labyrinth, or medications such as gentamycin.

Central vestibulopathies causing vertigo are of diverse etiology, including demyelinating disease (multiple sclerosis) in young individuals, posterior fossa space-occupying lesions, brainstem ischemia in older individuals, and acoustic neuroma. Neuromas characteristically present with tinnitus and hearing loss rather than vertigo, although a complaint of unsteadiness (ataxia) is common.

Evaluation of vertigo is directed at investigation of central and peripheral structures, with studies tailored to the suspected origin as determined by careful neurologic history. Brain imaging (computed tomography, magnetic resonance imaging), MRA of intracranial and extracranial cervical arteries, vascular ultrasound studies, and conventional transfemoral angiography are used to assess intracranial structures and vascular anatomy. Vestibular studies including caloric testing and electronystagmography are useful in distinguishing central from peripheral vertigo and may lateralize a labyrinthine disorder.

Aside from symptomatic treatment with fluids, antivertiginous medications, and antiemetic agents, treatment of peripheral vertigo varies with the underlying cause: benign positional vertigo may respond to vestibular exercises; acute labyrinthitis is self-limited; surgery may be employed for repair of a perilymphatic fistula.

The reader is referred to Chapter 6 for discussion of aeromedical disposition in individuals with vertigo.

Migraine Headache

Migraine headache is common, affecting approximately 5%-15% of the population, with women more frequently affected than men. It can occur at any age, though onset is often in childhood or adolescence. A family history of migraine is present in 60%-90% of cases. Many migraine sufferers are conscientious, anxious, organized, self-critical, and perfectionistic individuals, often with a history of allergy and/or motion sickness. Headaches may last hours to days and may be separated by days, weeks, months, or years, sometimes subsiding in later life.

There are many purported precipitants of migraine including emotional stress and the way it is managed, sleep deprivation, hunger, sun exposure, anxiety, menses, alcohol use, strong odors such as perfumes, intense mental activity, and relaxation after sustained intense concentration (Saturday morning headache). Certain foods may precipitate migraine including milk, cheese, dairy products, chocolate, onions, garlic, almonds, and other foods. Nitrate- and tyramine-containing foods, food additives, and some medications including oral contraceptives, may also trigger migraine.

Migraine is diagnosed by history, since neurologic examination and diagnostic studies are characteristically normal. In making a diagnosis, the AME/FS should inquire about family history, age of onset, headache characteristics, precipitating factors, emotional factors, personality features, and response to treatment.

The three varieties of migraine that are generally encountered are ***common migraine***, ***classic migraine***, and ***migraine equivalent*** (acephalgic migraine, migraine variant).

In common migraine the headache may begin slowly or abruptly, is typically though not always unilateral, throbbing or pulsating, and without an aura. Peak intensity may be sustained for hours to a day, less often for 1-3 days. Nausea, vomiting, photophobia, and hyperacusis are common accompanying features. A measure of relief may be obtained with darkened surroundings and sleep. Following the headache, fatigue, exhaustion, and a drained feeling are common. Severe migraine may be completely incapacitating to some individuals, while others have milder symptoms during which they can tolerate the discomfort and continue to function in a relatively normal fashion.

Unlike common migraine, classic migraine headache is preceded by an aura, which may be motor or sensory, but is most commonly visual in nature. For 15-30 minutes preceding the attack, the patient might see flashing sparklers, colored lights, geometric patterns, zig-zag or lightning bolt–shaped patterns, shapes resembling battlements of a fort or castle (fortification scotoma), or less commonly, visual field defects. Some patients have described colorful circles or globes appearing centrally and moving toward the periphery. Marching sensory symptoms, such as numbness beginning in the face and spreading to the arm and hand may also occur. The patient may also complain of difficulty with thinking and mental processing. After 15-30 minutes the aura begins to subside and the headache begins, though aura and headache quite often overlap. Headache characteristics are the same as those of common migraine. In some patients aura is the predominant feature, the headache being mild and barely remembered.

Migraine equivalent (migraine variant, acephalgic migraine) refers to a condition in which a migrainous aura, most commonly visual, is not followed by headache, and this entity may cause diagnostic confusion with TIA in older individuals. Other features such as history of childhood migraine, family history, and widely scattered episodes over many years may assist in diagnosis. Migraine equivalents with visual aura are common after age 50.

The diagnosis of migraine must be made by history, although testing may be necessary to rule out other more serious illness. Helpful diagnostic studies include CT and MRI of the brain; MRA to visualize the great neck vessels, circle of Willis and major intracranial vessels; and at times conventional transfemoral arteriography when aneurysm, usually at the circle of Willis, is suspected. EEG may demonstrate dramatic changes during the acute phase of migraine, causing concern for a structural lesion. However, the tracing returns to normal within a few days to a week following the migraine.

Milder forms of migraine may be treated without pharmacologic agents by avoidance of known precipitating factors, altering lifestyle, modifying habits, and recognizing stress factors and management choices that might trigger migraine. If migraines are infrequent, treatment is directed at the individual headache. To treat acute attacks, common analgesics including aspirin, acetaminophen, and NSAIDs may be effective. Other treatment modalities include sumitriptan and other activators of serotonin receptors, and ergotamine preparations may also be useful.

When migraines are frequent, prophylactic treatment might be warranted. Propranolol, other beta-blockers, and calcium channel blockers such as verapamil may be useful, as are amitryptiline, the selective serotonin reuptake inhibitor (SSRI) antidepressants including sertraline, methysergide, and valproic acid.

There are a number of parameters the AME/FS should consider when determining certification of an aviator with migraine. These include identification of precipitating factors, the nature of the aura, and degree of neurologic compromise from the aura. Headache frequency, rapidity of onset (time to peak), severity, and degree of incapacitation are also important parameters. The nature and success of treatment must be considered, since some medications might affect pilot performance. In general, a number of medications including aspirin, acetaminophen, and NSAIDs are acceptable. Beta-blockers and calcium channel blockers warrant individual consideration and observation for side effects. Others, including anticonvulsants and antidepressants, often preclude certification due to their potential cognitive or sedative effects. In some patients, avoidance of precipitating factors and lifestyle changes might allow reduction in dosage or even discontinuation of prohibitive medications, after which certification might be considered. Consequently, many migraine sufferers can be managed with treatment regimens compatible with certification, although more restrictive policies might be necessary in specific aviation operations, such as military operations where immediate worldwide deployment availability is an important issue.

Cluster Headache

Cluster headache (histamine headache, Horton's headache) is characterized by "clusters" of recurrent headache, lasting weeks to several months and separated by periods of quiescence lasting months to many years.

Individual headaches are characteristically abrupt in onset, reach peak intensity rapidly, are severe and usually of short duration (30-60 minutes), and may occur with remarkable regularity during a cluster. They are unilateral, located in, behind, or about the eye, and may be accompanied by ipsilateral nasal stuffiness, conjunctival injection, and Horner's syndrome (ptosis, miosis, anhydrosis). With recurrent episodes Horner's syndrome may become permanent. Neurologic examination is normal unless Horner's syndrome is present. Otherwise, diagnostic studies are unrevealing.

Individual headaches are commonly managed by analgesics, although oxygen, a potent vasoconstrictor, may abort the headache. Other treatment modalities for use during a cluster include beta-blockers, calcium channel blockers, ergot alkaloids, and corticosteroids. Histamine desensitization has also been employed with some success.

Cluster headaches are often excruciating, requiring narcotic analgesia, making grounding imperative during an attack. Certification may be possible once recovery has occurred, with provisions for grounding if symptoms recur. Certification parameters to consider include previous history of clusters, frequency of episodes, and response to treatment. Frequent clusters or chronic cluster headache might preclude certification.

Transient Global Amnesia

Transient global amnesia (TGA) refers to a global amnesic state with preserved personal identity, level of consciousness, and self awareness that resolves within 24 hours. Mean duration of attacks is 4-6 hours. Retrograde amnesia ranging from several months to 40 years is initially present, later shrinking to a permanent retrograde gap of 15 minutes to 10 hours. There are strict diagnostic criteria for true TGA, including presence of a capable witness for most of the attack, clear anterograde amnesia, absent clouding of consciousness, normal cognition outside of memory, absent focal symptoms and relevant focal signs, and resolution of symptoms within 24 hours. There can be no history of recent traumatic brain injury or active epilepsy. Incidence of TGA is about 10/100,000/year, with an age range of 5-92, though 90% of cases occur from ages 50-79.

TGA is a unique entity, clearly distinct from confusional states and other states of altered mentation. A brief case history best captures the essence of TGA.

A 48-year-old captain for a major air carrier was working vigorously in his yard in midsummer. The temperature approached 100° and the humidity was 94%. He spent 7 hours digging post holes in the rocky ground, then setting the posts in concrete. After finishing his work in late afternoon he showered. His wife returned home to find him standing near the closet in his robe. He look perplexed. Upon seeing his wife, he said "Something is wrong. What am I supposed to be doing? I can't remember." His wife replied that he was to pick up their daughter for a shopping trip. He had no recollection of such plans and could not explain how he spent the day. His wife instructed him to dress himself for a trip to the hospital. He appeared befuddled, but complied. He repeatedly asked his wife where they were going despite her consistent replies. En route to the hospital he was able to give his wife rather complex instructions for detouring around a highway construction site. In the emergency room he was alert. He complained of a mild headache and gave a history of childhood migraine. He had no memory for the preceding 4 months, including his daughter's college graduation. Physical and neurological examinations were normal except for memory loss. CT scan and laboratory studies were normal. Around 10:00 P.M. his memory began to return. By the following morning his memory had returned up to the time he dug his second post hole. He had no further episodes in 8 years of follow up.

Precipitating factors associated with onset of TGA include cold or hot water immersion (2%), sexual intercourse (3%), painful experience (2%-4%), physical exertion (18%), medical procedures (5%), and emotional stress (14%-44%). A history of migraine is present in 25%-33% of cases.

At onset of TGA there is often a brief flash of insight, the person sensing that something is amiss. There is a bewildered, perplexed appearance, with disorientation for time (90%) and for place (90%). Repetitive questioning is characteristic (92%), and headache is common (39%-58%). During the attack, complex motor acts can be performed flawlessly (flying a plane, making a cabinet, assembling a bicycle).

There are no focal neurologic findings in TGA. Brain imaging studies are normal, as is the electroencephalogram (EEG) during the attack. The pathology of TGA is thought to relate to a disturbance of the limbic system. An experimental condition, the spreading depression of Leao, characterized by slowly spreading cortical depolarization and changes in cerebral blood flow, has been a proposed mechanism for TGA and migraine aura as well. In pure TGA, there is no scientific evidence to support a vascular or epileptic etiology.

TGA must be distinguished from *transient ischemic amnesia*, which might superficially mimic TGA. In this condition, a variety of vertebrobasilar transient ischemic attack, focal signs and symptoms of brainstem dysfunction will accompany the amnestic state. Also to be considered is *transient epileptic amnesia*, characterized by unusually short attacks of amnesia lasting less than 10 minutes.[23]

Although there is no specific treatment for TGA, avoidance of precipitants may reduce risk of recurrence, which is approximately 3% per year over 5 years.

TGA is benign, and the sole aeromedical concern is risk of recurrence. When considering aeromedical certification the AME/FS should take into account the presence or absence and nature of precipitating factors, as well as the setting in which the episode occurred and the likelihood of exposure to similar circumstances. Often the setting is unique and unlikely to be reproduced. Possible relationship to migraine should be considered. Finally, a suitable period of observation of a year or more is appropriate before considering certification because other conditions, such as transient epileptic amnesia or transient ischemic amnesia, will usually become evident within that time.

Syncope

Syncope is defined as loss of consciousness and postural tone due to global cerebral hypoperfusion, while "near syncope" or "presyncope" refers to a state in which the individual feels faint, but cerebral perfusion is sufficient to preserve consciousness. Syncope is common, occurring in 3% of the population. Other terms describing this condition include **vasodepressor syncope**, which refers to collapse of peripheral resistance, hypotension, and loss of consciousness without bradycardia. This is the most common variety of syncope. Another term, **vasovagal syncope**, refers to the dual elements of collapse of peripheral resistance and vagus-mediated bradycardia.[24] Asystole will cause presyncope in 2-3 seconds in an upright person and loss of consciousness in 4-8 seconds (12-15 seconds in recumbency), while generalized tonic-clonic seizures will occur in 20-25 seconds.

Syncope represents a disturbance of homeostasis, which is dependent upon regulation of cardiac output, blood pressure, and blood volume. The balance between cardiac output and peripheral arteriolar tone (peripheral resistance) maintains the stability of the cardiovascular system. Normal cerebral blood flow (approximately 55 cc/100 gm/min for brain tissue) is usually assured by autoregulation in the cerebrovascular bed and a number of peripheral vascular and cardiac compensatory mechanisms.

Neural influences on homeostasis are abundant.[25] For example, higher cortical centers in the alert brain respond to external stimuli with perception and imagination. The limbic system is integral to the affective and emotional components of syncope, and there is an intimate connection between syncope and the emotion of fear, sometimes referred to as the "limbic connection." Consequently, an individual's emotional state may determine whether or not syncope will occur in a given setting.

The hypothalamus regulates autonomic function, and vasopressor and vasodepressor centers in the brainstem respond to sensory input. The intermediolateral cell column in the spinal cord provides sympathetic efferent input to peripheral arterial smooth muscle, which regulates peripheral resistance, while baroreceptors, chemoreceptors, and volume receptors respond to intravascular stimuli. Finally, skeletal muscle tone and contraction supports venous return.

When a person stands, venous pressure in the dorsum of the foot is barely able to return blood to the right atrium. Five hundred milliliters of venous blood pools in the lower body; central venous pressure declines by 3-5 mm Hg, and there is lower ventricular preload. Consequently, stroke volume declines by 50% and cardiac output by 30%, leading to diminished baroreceptor stimulation, reduced vagal (parasympathetic) and enhanced sympathetic tone. To compensate, peripheral resistance is increased, and heart rate increases 10-15 beats per minute. Mean arterial pressure is therefore preserved, and syncope does not occur.

It takes little to upset the delicate balance of homeostasis. Sudden fear, anger, pain (limbic connection), or other influences may result in an abrupt increase in heart rate, pulse pressure, and blood pressure. Baroreceptors respond, leading to sympathetic inhibition, collapse of peripheral resistance, diminished venous return, hypotension, and syncope. Vagus-mediated bradycardia may also occur (vasovagal syncope). Syncope is imminent when mean arterial pressure approaches 70 mm Hg. This is not disease, but rather overwhelmed homeostatic mechanisms whose capabilities have been exceeded.

Syncope is a diagnosis largely dependent on history, since general physical examination, neurological examination, and laboratory studies are often normal. Therefore, careful history taking is essential. Description by a witness to the event can prove invaluable in distinguishing syncope from other conditions that alter consciousness. A major challenge is to differentiate syncope from seizure. The AME/FS should consider the ***postural setting***, ***presyncopal symptoms***, the ***syncopal episode***, and the ***syncopal setting***.

Postural Setting

Syncope nearly always occurs in the upright position, rarely occurring while sitting or recumbent. Recurrence of syncope with resumption of upright posture is diagnostic of postural cerebral hypoperfusion.

Presyncopal Symptoms

The prodrome of syncope is often prolonged, as long as 5 minutes, with a mean duration of 2.5 minutes. Prodromal symptoms may include nausea, queasiness or a hollow abdominal sensation, repetitive yawning, and deep breathing. Visual symptoms, caused by retinal ischemia, include constriction of visual fields, darkening of vision, and bleaching and alteration of color (eg, "like looking through a yellow filter"). Usually the skin becomes cool and clammy, and there may be abdominal cramps and an urge for bowel emptying. Other symptoms include a feeling of warmth, dryness of the mouth, and a yearning for fresh air or a glass of cold water. To an observer, the person appears pallid.

Syncopal Episode

The episode itself is characterized by a sudden, hypotonic, flaccid collapse, with a brief period of unconsciousness ranging from 5-20 seconds. Collapse and recumbency restores venous return and cerebral perfusion. Syncope may be prolonged if the patient is kept upright by concerned bystanders trying to prevent a fall or by physical restrictions to falling (slumping in a chair or booth). This could lead to convulsive accompaniments. Respirations are shallow or imperceptible. Finally there is rapid recovery with little or no confusion, but frequent complaints of nausea, headache, and urinary urgency.

Approximately 15% of patients with syncope have brief ***convulsive accompaniments***, but not a fully developed generalized tonic-clonic seizure. There may be brief twitching of the face and hands, tonic posturing, or several myoclonic jerks. This is not an epileptic phenomenon, but a functionally decerebrate state related to hypoperfusion. An EEG would show suppressed or absent activity rather than the excessive neuronal discharges seen in a seizure. Epilepsy is erroneously diagnosed in approximately one-third of these individuals. As noted above, convulsive accompaniments are more common if the individual is kept in an upright position. Urinary incontinence, occurring in 10% of persons with syncope, would also heighten concern for an epileptic event. An erroneous diagnosis of seizure is very detrimental to the aviator, since medical certification would be unlikely.

Syncopal Setting

The AME/FS should determine what contributory environmental factors were present. Were there unpleasant sights, smells, or sounds? Was there sudden unanticipated pain or sustained upright posture with little movement? Was there sudden standing after a period of recumbency or squatting? Was there fatigue, fasting, worry, fear, intense emotion, or other stimulus (limbic connection)? Were there dehydration, salt loss, fluid loss, alcohol consumption, or other factors affecting homeostasis? Was there antecedent exertion or bladder or bowel evacuation?

If a diagnosis of syncope is made, then the causative mechanism must be determined, which is possible in 65% or more of cases.[26] The mechanisms of syncope are detailed in Table 4-7.

History is the cornerstone of diagnosis in syncope, because it alone will identify the correct mechanism in about 50% of cases. Syncope is idiopathic in about 35% of cases. Physical examination and basic laboratory studies (CBC, sugar and electrolytes, ECG or rhythm strip) will increase the yield, but additional studies including EEG, Holter monitor, and cardiac electrophysiologic studies are often normal.

Recently there has been increased interest in ***tilt table*** studies in the diagnosis of neurally mediated syncope. Although these studies may be useful in evaluating individuals with syncope, caution must be advised in their interpretation. The tilt table is used in an attempt to reproduce syncope by sustained gravity-mediated orthostatic stress. Usually passive tilt is performed, followed by provocation with isoproterenol infusion in doses ranging from 1-8 μg/minute. Isoproterenol was introduced to increase the rate of positive responses and lessen the time needed for testing, and it was hoped that it would not reduce specificity of a positive response. Several factors may cause difficulty in tilt table study interpretation including:

Table 4-7. Mechanisms of Syncope

Benign vasovagal syncope
　　Other terms: neurocardiogenic or neurally mediated syncope, common faint
　　Settings: anxiety, fear, pain, medical procedure, emotional stress, exertion, etc

Impaired peripheral resistance
　　Autonomic neuropathy (amyloidosis, diabetes)
　　Orthostatic hypotension (prolonged recumbency, medication, illness)

Altered blood quantity
　　Blood loss, dehydration

Altered blood quality
　　Anemia
　　Hypoxia
　　Hypoglycemia

Mechanically impaired venous return
　　Valsalva-induced
　　Breath holding
　　Pregnancy
　　Micturition
　　Tussive syncope
　　Weightlifting
　　Atrial myxoma

Altered cardiac output
　　Valvular stenosis
　　Idiopathic hypertrophic subaortic stenosis
　　Pump failure (cardiomyopathy)

Altered cardiac rhythm
　　Arrhythmias
　　　　Bradycardias (sick sinus syndrome, etc)
　　　　Tachycardias
　　Heart block
　　　　Mobitz type II second-degree block
　　　　Third-degree heart block

Specific syncopal syndromes
　　Swallow syncope (nearly always pathologic, indicating esophageal
　　　or cardiac disease)
　　Glossopharyngeal neuralgia
　　Carotid sinus syncope (sinus rhythm most often uninvolved,
　　　with underlying heart disease being the primary problem)

Lack of standardization of tilt angles: Tilt angles of 45° are associated with significant false-negative responses, while angles of 80° or greater result in more false-positive results. It has been suggested that 60°-70° be chosen as a standard.[28]

Variable tilt duration: It has been proposed that 45-60 minutes should be the standard.

Positivity criteria: It has been proposed that only syncope or presyncope accompanied by objective changes in heart rate and/or blood pressure be accepted as a positive vasovagal response.[27]

False positive rates of 8.9% without isoproterenol provocation and 27% with isoproterenol infusion are significant, perhaps leading to an incorrect diagnosis and unnecessary treatment.[28]

Lack of day-to-day reproducibility: In one study of 36 patients with vasodepressor syncope who had positive responses to tilt table testing, only 11 (31%) had reproducible positive responses when tested the following day.[29]

For these reasons, the usefulness of tilt table testing as a screening tool or predictor of recurrent syncope is limited. Therefore, clinical diagnosis remains the gold standard in evaluation.

Fortunately vasovagal syncope is a rare and benign occurrence in most individuals. Patient recognition of syncopal settings, precipitating factors, and prodromal symptoms may allow the person to prevent its occurrence with avoidance strategies and lying down if necessary. Nevertheless others may faint unpredictably. The medications listed below have been employed in attempts to prevent recurrence of syncope.

- Beta-blockers: The action of beta-blockers is theoretically linked to lowered activation of afferent vagal C-fibers, stimulated by mechanoreceptors in a vigorously contracting myocardium (Bezold-Jarisch reflex), and perhaps opposing circulating epinephrine. Reports of efficacy in preventing tilt table–induced syncope vary widely (25%-100%).
- Disopyramide: This agent has anticholinergic properties that can lower parasympathetic vagal tone and ventricular contractility by exerting a negative inotropic effect.
- Scopolamine: Its anticholinergic properties counteract vagal cardio-inhibition.
- Alpha-agonists: These agents exert their effects by enhancing venous tone and reducing venous pooling, thereby avoiding vigorous contraction of a small ventricle and resultant mechanoreceptor stimulation. Ephedrine, pseudoephedrine, midodrine, and etilifrine have also been used.

If an aviator required these medications for prophylaxis, revocation of flight status would be prudent in some cases because of potential sedative or anticholinergic effects of certain agents. Other medications such as beta-blockers may be acceptable. For detailed discussion of pharmacologic agents used in the treatment of neurally mediated syncope, the reader is referred to the monograph edited by Blanc et al.[30]

Not all syncope is benign, as there are patients who suffer a "malignant" type of cardio-inhibitory vasovagal syncope.[31] As in cardiac asystole, onset of syncope may be sudden and without warning, causing fractures and other injuries. If the physical setting leads to a slumped upright or semi-upright position, hypoxic-ischemic brain injury may occur. Medications may not be effective, and permanent pacemaker placement may be necessary to counteract the cardioinhibitory response.[32]

Micturition syncope is usually benign in the otherwise healthy young aviator. Typically a young cadet goes to bed after an evening of drinking. When partially awakened by the urge to urinate 1-2 hours later, he initially resists. Finally succumbing to strong signals from his bladder, he rises and voids a large amount of urine. Syncope may occur at the beginning, during, upon completion, or immediately following urination. The condition is benign and does not portend risk of sudden incapacitation in the cockpit. One proposed mechanism is the dual influence of orthostatic hypotension and reflex-induced vagus-mediated bradycardia.

Micturition syncope occurring in older individuals is another matter, as it is often associated with underlying heart disease such as serious cardiac arrhythmia or high degree heart block.

A decision to certify an aviator with a history of syncope must be made carefully. The AME/FS must attempt to determine the mechanism of syncope and decide if the condition is benign. Careful consideration should be given to the setting in which the episode(s) occurred. An estimation of recurrence risk is essential, as is judgment regarding likelihood of recurrence in a cockpit setting. Features such as the postural setting and emotional state also deserve scrutiny. Fear of bodily invasion and loss of control (eg, venipuncture, ear or eye examination, vaccination, etc) is more likely to cause syncope than external fears (eg, flying near a thunderstorm or executing an instrument approach to minimums). Measures to reduce recurrence risk, such as avoidance of hypoglycemia, dehydration, and use of medication deserve attention. Finally, a period of observation might be warranted. Fortunately, syncope is most often of benign origin, allowing a favorable certification decision once potentially serious disease has been excluded.

Seizure Disorder

Seizures represent the clinical expression of excessive and/or hypersynchronous, usually self-limited, abnormal discharge of neurons in the cerebral cortex.[33] *Epilepsy* is characterized by *recurrent unprovoked seizures*. The terms *seizure disorder* and *convulsive disorder* are synonymous with epilepsy. All imply chronic seizure potential. The person with a *single* seizure should not be labeled epileptic, since 2 or more seizures must occur to justify the diagnosis.

One percent of the population will have epilepsy by age 20, rising to 3% by age 75.[34] Febrile seizures occur in 2%-5% of the population. As many as 2%-3% of the population will have a single seizure sometime during their life.

Although a detailed discussion of the classification of epilepsy would serve no purpose here, familiarity with certain descriptive terms is useful in understanding seizures. Acquired, or *symptomatic seizures* may be divided into 2 varieties. One is an *acute symptomatic seizure* caused by an acute neurologic insult. Examples include seizures caused by hyponatremia, hypoglycemia, acute cerebral embolus, acute head trauma (including impact seizure), and acute bacterial meningitis. An acute symptomatic seizure often does not indicate potential for chronic, recurrent seizures (epilepsy). A *remote symptomatic seizure* would relate to a variably distant neurologic insult such as prior head injury (posttraumatic epilepsy), birth injury, stroke, or infection. Chronic seizure potential is implied. With acute symptomatic and remote symptomatic seizures there is a causal relationship between the insult and the seizure(s).

Another important descriptive term is a *provoked seizure*. With provoked seizures, the relationship is not causal, as in acute and remote symptomatic seizures. A provoked seizure is precipitated by a factor that lowers seizure threshold. Each person has a constitutional or genetically determined threshold for seizures, a degree of resistance, beyond which a seizure may occur. Seizure threshold may be altered by a number of nonspecific precipitants, which can provoke a seizure. These include sleep deprivation, emotional stress, intercurrent illness, menses, time of day, and other precipitants. Alternatively, sleep deprivation can provoke seizures in an individual with posttraumatic epilepsy (remote symptomatic seizures caused by previous head injury). In contrast, an *unprovoked seizure* has no identifiable precipitant.

Causes of seizures include genetic influences, traumatic brain injury, stroke, infection (meningitis, encephalitis), degenerative and demyelinating diseases (multiple sclerosis, Alzheimer's disease), substance abuse, and withdrawal seizures (alcohol, benzodiazepines, meprobamate, hypnotics, barbiturates). Seizures are idio-pathic in about 70% of persons newly diagnosed with epilepsy.

For this discussion a very basic classification of seizures is appropriate. Seizures may be *generalized from the onset, simple partial, complex partial,* and *partial with secondary generalization.*

In generalized seizures clinical manifestations indicate simultaneous involvement of both cerebral hemispheres at onset. Impairment or loss of consciousness may be the initial clinical manifestation of the event. Motor manifestations and electroencephalographic changes are bilateral, presumably indicating widespread abnormal neuronal discharges involving both cerebral hemispheres. Generalized onset seizures include absence (petit mal) seizures, atypical absence (petit mal variant) seizures, myoclonic seizures, clonic seizures, tonic-clonic seizures and atonic seizures.

A generalized tonic-clonic seizure may begin with a sudden, eerie decrescendo cry (epileptic cry), caused by forced expiration against partially closed vocal cords. The victim may fall and suffer injury. There follows a tonic phase, accompanied by apnea and resultant cyanosis, then a clonic phase with repetitive contractions of the extremities. The eyes are open and rolled upwards, the hands clenched, and the legs extended. Respirations are rough, blowing, and noisy. Tongue biting may occur, and blood-tinged frothy saliva may come from the mouth. Urinary incontinence may occur. The seizure lasts from 60-90 seconds in most cases, after which the patient may fall into a deep, snoring sleep. Upon awakening there is characteristically a postictal state with confusion, sleepiness, headache, nausea, vomiting, and muscle soreness. These clinical characteristics, when present, leave little doubt that a generalized seizure has occurred.

Classic petit mal (absence) seizures are also generalized from the onset. These are characterized by brief lapses of awareness that come without warning and last only seconds. During the spell the individual may pause and stare blankly, and the eyelids may flutter. There is no postictal state, and normal activity and responsiveness are immediately resumed. Seizures may occur many times per day. If spells are very brief, the patient may not be aware of their occurrence. Classic petit mal epilepsy is a disease of childhood, and the characteristic EEG abnormality is 3-per-second spike and wave. In some cases generalized tonic-clonic seizures may also occur. In addition to classic petit mal epilepsy, there is a petit mal variant in which seizures may differ somewhat clinically. EEG in these individuals will demonstrate "atypical spike and wave" (eg, polyspike and wave) rather than the classic 3-per-second spike and wave discharge.

A partial (formerly known as focal) seizure arises from a discrete area of the cerebral cortex. With *simple partial seizures* there is no alteration of consciousness.

For example, focal twitching of one hand in an alert, awake individual might constitute a simple partial seizure. The event would imply an irritative lesion in the contralateral cerebral cortex. In addition to motor symptoms, somatosensory, special sensory, autonomic, and psychic symptoms may occur.

Complex partial seizures (formerly known as psychomotor or temporal lobe seizures) are accompanied by alteration of consciousness. Seizure content might include repetitive vegetative movements such as lip smacking or chewing, staring (automatisms), a dazed appearance, and unresponsiveness to voice or other stimuli. Such an event would suggest a seizure of temporal lobe origin. Unlike absence (petit mal) seizures, complex partial seizures are commonly followed by a postictal state of variable length characterized by fatigue, headache, or a period of confusion.

Any partial seizure may end spontaneously or progress to a generalized tonic-clonic seizure. This is described as a partial seizure with secondary generalization. A seizure with motor manifestations beginning in one hand might gradually progress up the extremity as adjacent areas of cortex are involved in the seizure, later involving the face and lower limb. This is sometimes referred to as the **Jacksonian march**. Secondary generalization might follow. Partial onset may be very brief and undetected by the patient and the examiner, although at times it is evident electrographically during EEG recording.

Distinguishing partial from generalized seizures is essential, since a partial seizure implies the presence of a focal cortical lesion. This lesion must be identified, and a progressive process, such as tumor, must be excluded. Risk of neoplasm with partial seizures is approximately 5% in childhood, rising to 20% in partial seizures of adult onset.

As in syncope, neurologic history is of utmost importance in the evaluation of seizure disorder. The AME/FS must inquire about a history of febrile seizures, family history of seizures, remote neurologic insult such as traumatic brain injury or CNS infection and use of medication and alcohol (and withdrawal from medication, substances of abuse, and alcohol). Inquiry should be made about the setting of the event (sleep deprivation and other potential provocative factors) and about any aura that may have been present. If at all possible, an observer who witnessed the event should be interviewed. This is often essential for diagnosis and may be far more valuable than extensive laboratory testing. Symptoms following the event should also be elicited. Antecedent and postictal symptoms might strongly support a diagnosis of seizure despite the absence of a witness.

When evaluating an applicant with a history of seizures, the AME/FS should inquire about risk factors that bear upon risk of recurrent seizures. These are:

- History of febrile seizures
- Family history of seizures in a first-degree relative
- History of remote neurologic insult
- Abnormal neurologic examination
- Abnormal EEG
- Abnormal cerebral imaging study
- Prior acute symptomatic seizure

Aside from basic laboratory studies, tools used in the investigation of seizure disorders include cerebral imaging studies and EEG. MRI has become the gold standard for the assessment of seizure disorders. Lesions, such as small cavernous angiomas or early gliomas, that escape detection with CT imaging may be demonstrated by MRI. Volumetric MRI studies for mesial temporal sclerosis, a common cause of complex partial seizures, may be helpful. Vascular imaging studies including MRA and conventional transfemoral arteriography may be useful in demonstrating vascular malformations and other vascular lesions associated with seizures.

The EEG is helpful in the evaluation of seizure disorder, but it is an imperfect tool since patients with epilepsy commonly have an initially normal EEG. Furthermore, 25% of persons with epilepsy have normal EEGs throughout life. In addition, specific epileptiform abnormalities may be present in persons without clinical seizures, causing further confusion. A small percentage of the population has mild to moderate nonspecific EEG abnormalities, but no specifically epileptiform discharges or clinical seizures. At times these nonspecific changes are incorrectly linked to an episode of simple syncope (particularly when there are convulsive accompaniments and/or urinary incontinence), leading to an erroneous diagnosis of seizure disorder, with tragic consequences for the aviator.

The EEG is useful when it demonstrates specifically epileptiform abnormalities or a normal pattern for exclusionary purposes. The AME/FS should remember that the EEG is a useful tool in the assessment of disorders of consciousness, but results must be correlated with the entire clinical picture. When seizure disorder is suspected, a sleep-deprived wake and sleep EEG should be obtained, because certain epileptiform discharges, such as spikes and sharp waves, may be activated only during sleep. A normal waking record alone is not sufficient when seizure disorder is strongly suspected. In difficult cases, sophisticated EEG techniques employing nasopharyngeal electrodes and/or prolonged EEG with video monitoring may be warranted.

Although some individuals may enjoy permanent remission from seizures without medication, this is the exception rather than the rule. Consequently, most patients require anticonvulsant therapy indefinitely, precluding aeromedical certification due to recurrence risk and the cognitive effects of medication. In refractory cases, epilepsy surgery (eg, anterior temporal lobectomy) is at times employed.

It is prudent for the AME/FS to recognize that seizures tend to recur, which is of aeromedical significance. With 2 or more seizures recurrence risk approaches 73%, and for this reason a thorough neurologic evaluation should precede a certification decision. In some cases evaluation at an epilepsy center may be necessary to differentiate seizure from other varieties of disturbed consciousness. It is noteworthy that a significant proportion of patients referred to an epilepsy center for surgery have nonepileptic seizures (pseudoseizures). A history of febrile seizures in infancy and early childhood does not preclude certification, although complex or complicated febrile seizures do carry an increased risk of recurrence. Persons with benign Rolandic epilepsy in adolescence characteristically enjoy permanent remission. Acute symptomatic seizures do not necessarily portend chronic seizure potential. Remote symptomatic seizures occurring months or years after a neurologic insult indicate persistent potential for recurrence. Years of seizure-free and medication-free observation are important when considering certification of an individual with a history of seizures.

With thorough history, assessment of risk factors, careful neurologic examination, cerebral imaging studies, and use of EEG one may arrive at a reasonable estimate of recurrence risk. Extreme caution is advised in the evaluation of applicants with a history of seizures. If the risk approaches that of the normal population, aeromedical certification may be possible. In general, a diagnosis of epilepsy is in itself disqualifying in all segments of aviation. Although good control may be achieved with anticonvulsants, risk for recurrence remains significantly higher than that of the normal population. In addition, all antiepileptic drugs (AEDs) have potential cognitive effects, which might further compromise aviation safety. At present, certification of individuals with epilepsy well controlled on medication is not recommended.

The Single Seizure

Many patients have had multiple seizures when they come to medical attention. However, some may suffer a single seizure, often generalized tonic-clonic, with no antecedent history of seizures. This problem is not uncommon in aeromedical certification and requires an assessment of recurrence risk. The isolated seizure is treated as a unique entity, since long-term prognosis for recurrence may be as low as 30% when risk factors are absent, as opposed to a 73% risk when seizures are multiple.[35]

When evaluating an individual with a single, adult-onset, generalized tonic-clonic seizure, the AME/FS should consider risk factors. These include a history of febrile seizures, family history of seizures in a first degree relative, history of an acute symptomatic seizure, history of a remote neurologic insult, abnormal neurologic examination, abnormal cerebral imaging study, and abnormal EEG, all of which increase seizure risk. If **all** risk factors are absent, risk for subsequent seizure is about 30% over 5 years.[36] If an individual without risk factors remains seizure free for 5 years without medication, certification could be considered because recurrence risk beyond that point is acceptably low. Treatment with anticonvulsants following a single seizure clouds the issue of recurrence risk because one cannot determine whether freedom from recurrence is due to medication. Thus, the decision to treat an isolated seizure has important implications for the aviator. Often neurologists elect not to treat an isolated seizure.

Unexplained Loss of Consciousness

In certain instances, identifying the cause of an episode of disturbed consciousness may be difficult. Differentiating syncope from seizure, transient ischemic attack from transient global amnesia, and a metabolic disturbance from a psychiatric disorder might be challenging. In such instances detailed history is essential for accurate diagnosis. The guidelines below can be useful in the investigation of disturbances of consciousness. The applicant, and a witness if possible, should describe the episode in detail, covering the following points:

- *Posture:* Did the event(s) occur standing, sitting or lying?
- *Symptoms preceding the event:* What feelings or warning symptoms occurred?
- *Description of the event:* What is the last recollection before the event and the first recollection after the event? Was there tongue-biting or loss of bowel or bladder control?
- *Symptoms following the event:* Was there headache, nausea, vomiting, confusion, or muscle soreness? Was alertness and awareness regained immediately, or was it delayed?
- *Setting of the event:* Was there fatigue, fasting, sleep deprivation, emotional upset, worry, fear, other illness, or dehydration that might have triggered the event?
- *Medication, alcohol, drugs:* List medications used, both prescribed and over-the-counter. List dosage and timing. Was there alcohol consumption or consumption of other substances? What were the amounts?
- *Past history:* Was there history of febrile seizures, developmental difficulties, fainting, migraine, dizziness, or serious illness earlier in life?

- *Family history:* Is there a family history of syncope, seizure, migraine, or other illness?
- *History from an observer:* Though not always obtainable, an observer's history may solidify the diagnosis.
- *What did the observer note before the event?* Was there staring, diaphoresis, pallor, or change in respiration?
- *What occurred during the event?* Were respirations rough and blowing, or shallow and imperceptible? Was breathing noisy? Was there convulsive movement or motionless flaccidity? Was there pallor, cyanosis, apnea, thrashing, shaking, or posturing? How long did the spell last?
- *What happened after the event?* Was there immediate return to alertness? Was there confusion, sleepiness, combativeness, vomiting, or other symptoms?
- *Take history from medical records:* Records from emergency medical services, paramedic flow sheets, and the emergency room might be very helpful in documenting clinical findings. Hospital records and physician records will provide further valuable information.

Miscellaneous Conditions

Tension Headache

Tension headache is the most common headache in humans. Unlike migraine, which often occurs infrequently, tension headache may be quite frequent, occurring several times per week or even daily (chronic daily headache). Tension headaches tend to be less severe than migraine, though they are annoying and frustrating. Often the patient will complain of tightness and stiffness in the neck. Although there may be tenderness at the occipital insertion of the paraspinal muscles, neurological examination and laboratory studies are normal, emphasizing the importance of a thorough history.

Tension headaches in themselves are not disabling, and for some, medication may not be necessary. Chronic or daily use of medications, some of which might have sedating or habit-forming qualities, might compromise aviation safety, thereby precluding aeromedical certification. If the problem is sufficiently severe, evaluation and treatment of emotional factors and strict control of acceptable medications might be necessary before considering aeromedical certification. Medication use and overuse is the major concern in certification of an aviator with tension headache.

Sleep Disorders

Sleep disorders comprise a broad spectrum of sleep disturbances bridging the specialties of internal medicine, psychiatry, otolaryngology, pulmonary medicine, pediatrics, and neurology. A sleep disorder is defined as a sleep disturbance that is harmful to the individual's health or well being. Clearly, excessive daytime sleepiness may compromise aviation safety, though at times only minor discomfort is the result (eg, jet lag). In the International Classification of Sleep Disorders, conditions are divided into four categories[37]:

1. Dyssomnias
    A. Intrinsic sleep disorders: Includes narcolepsy, obstructive sleep apnea, restless legs syndrome, psychophysiological insomnia.
    B. Extrinsic sleep disorders: Includes insufficient sleep syndrome, hypnotic-dependent sleep disorder.
    C. Circadian rhythm sleep disorders: Includes shift-work sleep disorder, delayed sleep-phase syndrome.
2. Parasomnias
    A. Arousal disorders: Sleepwalking, sleep terrors.
    B. Sleep-wake transition disorders: Rhythmic movement disorder (head banging).
    C. Parasomnias (usually associated with REM sleep): REM sleep behavior disorder, sleep paralysis.
    D. Other parasomnias: Nocturnal paroxysmal dystonia.
3. Medical/psychiatric sleep disorders.
    A. Associated with mood disorders: Depression, anxiety disorder, psychosis.
    B. Associated with neurological disorders: Sleep-related epilepsy, parkinsonism, electrical status epilepticus of sleep.
    C. Associated with other medical disorders: Sleep-related asthma, fibrositis, sleep-related gastroesophageal reflux.
4. Proposed sleep disorders: Sleep-related laryngospasm, short sleeper, long sleeper.

A thorough history is essential. For example, early morning awakening (terminal insomnia) is a common feature of depression; anxiety will often cause difficulty falling asleep (initial insomnia); and excessive daytime sleepiness may be encountered in narcolepsy. Additional features of narcolepsy include positive family history, sleep paralysis, hypnagogic hallucinations, and sudden loss of muscle tone with startle or emotion (cataplexy). Sleep history from the patient (and often a bed partner) will guide the examiner in diagnosis. One must inquire about medications, alcohol, weight gain, and snoring.

When sleep disturbance is significant, appropriate consultation should be obtained. Sleep laboratory studies including the all-night polysomnogram (PSG), the multiple sleep latency test (MSLT), and the maintenance of wakefulness test (MWT) are used in studying sleep disturbances.

Medications, such as stimulants and antidepressants, generally preclude certification when narcolepsy or psychiatric conditions are responsible for the sleep disturbance. If depression and/or anxiety resolves with treatment and medication is discontinued, certification may be considered. Successful treatment of sleep apnea with continuous positive airway pressure (CPAP) or bilevel positive airway pressure (BIPAP) may allow aeromedical certification.

Cervical and Lumbar Radiculopathies

Cervical and lumbar radiculopathies may temporarily compromise aviation safety when acutely symptomatic with pain or accompanied by significant neurologic deficit such as foot drop. Causes include degenerative disc disease in the cervical or lumbar spine, osteophytes impinging upon nerve roots, or ruptured intervertebral discs causing nerve root compression and neurologic deficit in an extremity. Pain may be severe, with weakness and sensory loss appropriate to the involved nerve root. In addition, ligamentous hypertrophy, osteophytic narrowing, and degenerative disc disease may compromise the cervical or lumbar spinal canal, resulting in stenosis. Cervical spinal cord compression may cause spasticity in the lower extremities, ataxia, and loss of posterior column sensation (vibratory and position sense). Lumbar stenosis causes bilateral hip and proximal leg pain with walking that is relieved by rest.

Cervical radiculopathies are accompanied by complaints of neck pain and limitation of motion, radicular pain in the distribution of the nerve root involved, and possibly weakness and sensory loss if nerve root compression is sufficiently severe. Medial scapular pain is a hallmark of cervical radiculopathy. Sixty percent of cervical nerve root compressions involve the seventh cervical nerve root, with pain radiating into the hand and index finger a common complaint. There may be triceps, pronator, or finger flexor weakness and a loss of the triceps reflex.

Lumbar radiculopathies are characterized by pain radiating into the big toe (L5 nerve root) or sole and lateral aspect of the foot (S1 nerve root), and less commonly anterior thigh (L4). Pain is often worsened with cough, sneeze, bend, and strain, and may be worse at night. Standing, lying, or sitting may increase the pain. A foot drop (inability to walk on the heel) and numbness of the big toe would signify an L5 radiculopathy, whereas inability to walk on the toes (gastrocnemius weakness) and numbness of the lateral foot would indicate an S1 radiculopathy. With S1 nerve root lesions, the ankle reflex may be absent.

Most radiculopathies can be managed conservatively with heat, massage, ultrasound, traction, and physical therapy. Muscle relaxants and analgesics may also be employed. When conservative therapy is unsuccessful, epidural steroid injection at the appropriate level may provide relief. Surgery is reserved for situations in which there is severe, intractable pain unresponsive to physical therapy, significant neurologic deficit (motor weakness), or frequently recurrent episodes that interfere with lifestyle.

Although radiculopathies may be temporarily disabling while acute there is no difficulty with aeromedical certification once they have resolved. Furthermore, it is unusual to encounter significant permanent neurologic deficit that might compromise aviation safety. Spinal column integrity might deserve special consideration in specific settings, such as exposure to ejection seat aircraft.

Peripheral Neuropathies

There are numerous causes of peripheral neuropathy including diabetes, alcohol, nutritional deficiency, vitamin deficiency, renal failure, and hereditary disorders. Neurologic manifestations of peripheral neuropathy include pain, sensory loss, motor deficit, and depressed or absent reflexes, characteristically involving the lower extremities. Many cases are mild, causing little or no functional impairment, thereby posing no threat to aviation safety. Periodic monitoring would be necessary for early identification of significant impairment. Prominent pain requiring narcotic or mind-altering medication, severe sensory loss, or significant motor deficit might preclude aeromedical certification. The AME/FS must consider the underlying condition, if known, as well in determining aeromedical certification.

Myopathies and Disorders of the Neuromuscular Junction

Because early onset muscular dystrophies commonly cause severe disability early in life, they are not an aeromedical certification issue. However, late onset dystrophy, such as limb-girdle dystrophy, occurring in adulthood, may cause proximal muscular weakness sufficient to compromise aviation safety. These disorders are slowly progressive, and there is no available treatment. Early on, the weakness may be so mild that medical certification is possible. It is essential, however, that these individuals be periodically monitored, since they will usually reach a stage that demands disqualification.

Myasthenia gravis is an autoimmune disorder involving the neuromuscular junction, in which autoantibodies inhibit acetylcholine receptor binding. This results in weakness, which may involve bulbar, axial, or extremity skeletal muscles. Diplopia, a common presenting symptom, is of obvious aeromedical concern. Thymic hyperplasia or thymic tumor (thymoma) may accompany the disease. CT imaging of the mediastinum is often necessary to demonstrate the lesion. Although there may be long periods of remission, recurrence is common, and myasthenic crisis with profound weakness may be triggered by infection or other environmental stimuli. Treatment of myasthenia includes cholinesterase inhibitors, corticosteroids, and immunosuppressive agents. An excess of cholinesterase inhibitors may result in cholinergic crisis, also attended by profound weakness. Because active myasthenia gravis requiring use of anticholinesterases is unpredictable, disqualification is the rule. If a sufficient period of remission is achieved either spontaneously or with treatment, certification could be considered.

References

1. Rapin I. Static disorders of brain development. In: Rowland LP, ed. *Merritt's Textbook of Neurology*. 9th ed. Baltimore: Williams & Wilkins; 1995:507.

2. Rapin I. Static disorders of brain development. In: Rowland LP, ed. *Merritt's Textbook of Neurology*. 9th ed. Baltimore: Williams & Wilkins; 1995:509.

3. Greer M. Structural malformations. In: Rowland LP, ed. *Merritt's Textbook of Neurology*. 9th ed. Baltimore: Williams & Wilkins; 1995:520-524.

4. Miller JR, Jubelt B. Infections of the nervous system. In: Rowland LP, ed. *Merritt's Textbook of Neurology*. 9th ed. Baltimore: Williams & Wilkins; 1995:109.

5. Jansen RS. Epidemiology and neuroepidemiology of human immunodeficiency virus infection. In: Berger JR, Levy RM, eds. *Aids and the Nervous System*, 2nd ed. Philadelphia: Lippincott-Raven; 1997:13-29.

6. Castro GC, Ward JW, Slutsker L, Buehler J, Jaffe H, Berkelman R. 1993 Revised Classification System for HIV Infection and Expanded Surveillance Case Definition for AIDS Among Adolescents and Adults. Centers for Disease Control and Prevention, Morbidity and Mortality Weekly Report, Vol. 41, No. RR-17, Dec. 18, 1992. Atlanta, Georgia: U.S. Department of Health and Human Services, Public Health Service.

7. Dornadula G, Zhang H, VanUitert B, Stern J, Livornese L, Ingerman M, Witek J, Kedanis RJ, Natkin J, DeSimone J, Pomerantz R. Residual HIV-1 RNA in blood plasma of patients taking highly active antiretroviral therapy. *JAMA*. 1999;282:1627-1632.

8. Becker DP, Grossman RG, McLaurin RL, Caveness WF. Head injuries—Panel 3. Neurological and neurosurgical conditions associated with aviation safety. *Arch Neurol*. 1979;36(special issue):750-757.

9. Evans RW. The postconcussion syndrome and the sequelae of mild head injury. In: Evans RW, ed. *Neurologic Clinics: The Neurology of Trauma*. Philadelphia: Saunders; 1992: 10(4); 816.

10. Evans RW. The postconcussion syndrome and the sequelae of mild head injury. In: Evans RW, ed. *Neurologic Clinics: The Neurology of Trauma*. Philadelphia: Saunders; 1992;10(4):879-893.

11. Fetell MR. Tumors. In: Rowland LP, ed. *Merritt's Textbook of Neurology*. 9th ed. Baltimore: Williams & Wilkins; 1995:313.

12. Fahn S. Parkinsonism. In: Rowland LP, ed. *Merritt's Textbook of Neurology*. 9th ed. Baltimore: Williams & Wilkins; 1995:71.

13. Mohr JP, Gautier JC, Pessin MS. Internal carotid artery disease. In: Barnett HJM, Mohr JP, Stein BM, Yatsu FM, eds. *Stroke: Pathophysiology, Diagnosis and Management*. 2nd ed. New York: Churchill Livingstone; 1992:311.

14. Robertson JT, Barnett HJM. Surgery for symptomatic disease due to arteriosclerosis of the carotid artery. In: Barnett HJM, Mohr JP, Stein BM, Yatsu FM, eds. *Stroke: Pathophysiology, Diagnosis and Management*. 2nd ed. New York: Churchill Livingstone; 1992:1005-1008.

15. Mohr JP, Gautier JC, Pessin MS. Internal carotid artery disease. In: Barnett HJM, Mohr JP, Stein BM, Yatsu FM, eds. *Stroke: Pathophysiology, Diagnosis and Management*. 2nd ed. New York: Churchill Livingstone; 1992:309.

16. Mohr JP, Gautier JC, Pessin MS. Internal carotid artery disease. In: Barnett HJM, Mohr JP, Stein BM, Yatsu FM, eds. *Stroke: Pathophysiology, Diagnosis and Management*. 2nd ed. New York: Churchill Livingstone; 1992:1023.

17. Albers GW, Tijssen JGP. Antiplatelet therapy: New foundations for optimal treatment decisions. *Neurology*. 1999;53(supp 4):S25-S31.

18. Sacco RL, Wolf PA, Gorelick PB. Risk factors and their management for stroke prevention: Outlook for 1999 and beyond. *Neurology*. 1999;53(supp 4):S15-S24.

19. Youl BD, Coutellier A, Dubois B, Leger JM, Bousser MG. Three cases of spontaneous extracranial vertebral artery dissection. *Stroke*. 1990;21:618-625.

20. Schievink WI, Mokri B, O'Fallon W. Recurrent spontaneous cervical artery dissection. *N Engl J Med*. 1994;330(6):393-397.

21. Toffol GJ, Biller J, Adams H. Nontraumatic intracerebral hemorrhage in young adults. *Arch Neurol*. 1987;44:483-485.

22. Drachman DA, Apfelbaum RI, Posner JB. Dizziness and disorders of equilibrium, panel 8. Neurological and neurosurgical conditions associated with aviation safety. *Arch Neurol*. 1979;36(special issue):806-810.

23. Hodges JR. Transient amnesia, clinical and neuropsychological aspects. In: Lord Walton of Detchant, Warlow CP, eds. *Major Problems in Neurology*. Vol. 24. Philadelphia: Saunders; 1991:65.

24. Ross RT. Syncope. In: Walton Sir J, ed. *Major Problems in Neurology*. Vol. 18. Philadelphia: Saunders; 1988:19.

25. Ross RT. Syncope. In: Walton Sir J, ed. *Major Problems in Neurology*. Vol. 18. Philadelphia: Saunders; 1988:13-17.

26. Grubb BP, Olshansky B, eds. *Syncope: Mechanisms and Management*. Armonk, New York: Futura Publishing Co; 1998:2.

27. Mansourati J, Blanc JJ. Tilt test procedure: Angle, duration, positivity criteria. In: Blanc JJ, Benditt D, Sutton R, eds. *Neurally Mediated Syncope: Pathophysiology, Investigations, and Treatment*. Vol. 10. The Bakken Research Center Series. Armonk, NY: Futura Publishing Co; 1996:79-83.

28. Kapoor WN, Smith MA, Miller NL. Upright tilt testing in evaluating syncope: A comprehensive literature review. *Am J Med*. 1994;97:78-88.

29. Brooks R, Ruskin JN, Powell AC, Newell J, Garan H, McGovern BA. Prospective evaluation of day-to-day reproducibility of upright tilt-table testing in unexplained syncope. *Am J Cardiol*. 1993;71:1289-1292.

30. Raviele A, Themistoclakis S, Gasparini G. Drug treatment of vasovagal syncope. In: Blanc JJ, Benditt D, Sutton R, eds. *Neurally Mediated Syncope: Pathophysiology, Investigations, and Treatment*. Vol. 10. The Bakken Research Center Series. Armonk NY: Futura Publishing Co; 1996:113-117.

31. Petersen MEV, Chamberlain-Weber R, Fitzpatrick AP, et al. Permanent pacing for cardioinhibitory malignant vasovagal syncope. *Br Heart J*. 1994;71:274-281.

32. Daubert JC, Mabo P, Gras D, Baisset JM. Role of permanent cardiac pacing in vasovagal syncope. In: Blanc JJ, Benditt D, Sutton R, eds. *Neurally Mediated Syncope: Pathophysiology, Investigations, and Treatment*. Vol. 10. The Bakken Research Center Series. Armonk, NY: Futura Publishing Co; 1996:119-126.

33. Engel, J Jr. *Seizures and Epilepsy*. Philadelphia: FA Davis Co; 1989:3.

34. Hauser WA. Epidemiology of seizure disorders and the epilepsies. In: Santili N, ed. *Managing Seizure Disorders: A Handbook for Health Care Professionals*. Philadelphia: Lippincott-Raven; 1996:11.

35. Hauser WA, Rich SS, Lee JRJ, Annegers JF, Anderson VE. Risk of recurrent seizures after two unprovoked seizures. *N Engl J Med*. 1998;338:429-434.

36. Hauser WA, Rich SS, Annegers JF, Anderson VE. Seizure recurrence after a first unprovoked seizure: An extended follow up. *Neurology*. 1990;40:1163-1170.

37. Fisch, BJ. Neurological aspects of sleep. In: Aminoff MJ, ed. *Neurology and General Medicine*. 2nd ed. New York: Churchill Livingstone; 1995:499.

Chapter 5
Ophthalmology

Since the earliest days of aviation, AMEs and flight surgeons have recognized that normal vision is essential for safety in flight operations. In defining ***normal vision***, we include not just visual acuity, but rather all the manifold functions of the eye important to aviators: near vision for seeing instruments; distant vision for seeing other aircraft; depth perception for formation flying, air-to-air refueling, and landing; color vision for map reading and beacon light and target identification; night vision for nighttime flying; and fusion for prevention of diplopia.

Flight safety demands that ophthalmologic function be normal (and in military aviation, target acquisition is just as vital), and to ensure this, considerable attention is paid to the eye during the physical examination. A battery of tests is available to measure near and distant visual acuity, refractive error, visual fields, color vision, night vision, depth perception, degree of phoria and tropia, diplopia, and accommodation. Over the years, ophthalmologists with a special interest in aviation medicine have developed these tests to evaluate ophthalmologic function, and these doctors also established the minimum standards acceptable for flight certification as delineated in the physical standards manual of every aviation medical department.

Aviators who cannot meet the standards for ophthalmologic function—whether due to impairment from disease or due to the aging process—may be disqualified from flying until the underlying disease process, if curable, is treated and full visual function is restored. However, if full restoration of visual function cannot be achieved, medical waivers can be granted on an individual basis. Factors to consider include the extent and degree of abnormality, the status of the uninvolved eye, the prognosis, and the demands of flight operations. Also it should be remembered that an abnormality of the eye is frequently a manifestation of underlying systemic disease. Because a detailed discussion of ophthalmologic diseases is beyond the purview of this book, only a few general remarks about ophthalmologic physical standards follow, along with a discussion of several eye disorders of special aeromedical interest.

Visual Acuity

Reading instruments and sighting other aircraft obviously require normal near and distant vision. Even with 20/20 visual acuity, at a speed of 500 knots the aircraft would fly approximately ¾ of a nautical mile by the time a pilot sees an outside object, identifies it, and takes appropriate action.[1] An aviator with vision poorer than 20/20 would present more of a threat to flight safety because the reaction time would be even slower and the distance traversed correspondingly much greater.

Although 20/20 vision is required for entry into some flight training programs, many aviators will eventually require corrective lenses for myopia, hyperopia, and presbyopia, especially as they age. In most cases, use of corrective lenses would not contraindicate flight duties as long as visual acuity meets minimum acceptable standards. However, if corrective spectacles are necessary, it should be emphasized that they must be worn at all times while on flight duty, since accidents have occurred in which the pilot forgot or ignored the requirement to wear them while on duty.[2] For example, a hyperopic pilot who was not wearing his spectacles on duty placed a critical toggle switch in the wrong position resulting in the loss of an aircraft. Other examples of crew negligence in wearing spectacles are on record, with some resulting in poor landings and aircraft damage.

A special case in point is the older pilot with presbyopia. Cases have been reported in which presbyopic pilots, who were either wearing the incorrect pair of spectacles or not wearing any, inadvertently turned the wrong switches, resulting in accidents. Consequently, the AME/FS must ensure, through consultation with the optometrist, that the pilot has the proper set of spectacles (usually bifocals) that will allow the aviator to clearly see the instrument panel as well as outside the aircraft.

If an aviator's visual acuity cannot be corrected to minimum acceptable limits with corrective lenses, medical waivers should be granted only selectively and in accordance with medical department policy. (The use of contact lenses and keratotomy for correction of visual acuity will be discussed separately.)

Visual Field Defects

As a general rule, aviators should have neither visual field defects nor scotomata. A full, normal field of vision is necessary to allow adequate central and peripheral vision, particularly at night. If visual field defects or scotomata are detected, the etiology should be sought since they may reveal serious underlying diseases such as glaucoma, chiasmal lesions, vascular disease, multiple sclerosis, and migraine headaches. Besides the ophthalmologic dysfunction, these underlying conditions might affect other systems causing symptoms which would contraindicate flight status. Medical waivers could be granted if the scotomata or visual field defects are not associated with serious underlying pathology, are transient or static, and are not extensive enough to significantly interfere with visual function.

Color Vision

The necessity for normal color vision for safe aviation has long been debated. Some believe it is necessary for the identification of lights of different colors (navigation lights, airport beacons, approach and taxiway lights), map reading and, in military operations, target identification. During the Vietnam War, forward air controllers [FACS] frequently described targets by their color and marked them with colored smoke bombs for incoming strike aircraft. Even if one concedes that normal color vision is not always essential for safe flight, it does give the pilot an extra edge which could be vital under certain conditions.

Abnormal color vision can be congenital or acquired secondary to brain injury, central serous retinopathy, optic neuritis, central nervous system disease, or drug or toxic substance poisoning. Most cases are congenital with the vast majority found among males. This visual defect can be mild, moderate, or severe in degree and is classified as anomalous trichromatism, dichromatism, and monochromatism, respectively, with patients in the latter category only able to distinguish white and shades of gray. Dichromats can only discern 2 of the basic hues, whereas anomalous trichromats, although able to discern all 3 basic hues, have problems perceiving one of them. There are various tests available to detect defective color vision, including pseudoisochromatic plates and the Farnsworth lantern.

A number of studies have been done to determine if defective color vision is truly a hazard to flying safety.[3] Although it was found that the accident rate for pilots with abnormal color vision is twice that of pilots with normal color vision, it could not be unequivocally demonstrated that the deficit in color vision actually caused the difference in accident rates.

Because the potential danger from abnormal color vision is so controversial, determination of flight certification is best made on the basis of operational requirements as well as through diagnosis of the extent of the deficit. For example, a pilot with anomalous trichromatism could function safely working in general aviation while a military fighter pilot with monochromatism would be at a clear disadvantage. More scientific evidence is needed before consensus can be reached about the danger posed by abnormal color vision.

Night Blindness

Little need be said here about night blindness or nyctalopia due to the obvious danger it poses to flight safety. Because most cases of night blindness are inherited, aviator candidates so afflicted are usually identified and eliminated at the time of their initial physical examination. However, nyctalopia can be acquired later in life, for example because of vitamin A deficiency, retinitis pigmentosa, or hepatic cirrhosis. Medical waivers for nyctalopia should not be granted except in the rare case in which an underlying disease process is identified and treated with subsequent restoration of normal night vision, or if a pilot is restricted to daytime flight duty only.

Tropias and Phorias

The complex subject of tropias and phorias is beyond the purview of this book. The AME/FS, however, must fully understand the nuances of these dysfunctions, which are described in standard ophthalmology texts. Tropias may be due to a congenital CNS lesion or may be acquired by injury or various disease processes such as multiple sclerosis and diabetes. Regardless of etiology, the presence of a tropia is abnormal and, if severe, is a clear threat to flight safety because it can cause diplopia, amblyopia, and loss of accommodation.

Besides possible manifest ocular deviation of a tropia, almost all individuals have a degree of latent ocular deviation or phoria, which may or may not be abnormal depending upon its dioptric degree. It can be observed in patients only when normal fusional impulses are interrupted such as with a Maddox rod test. It has also been demonstrated that phorias can be induced in some individuals by fatigue, alcohol intake, or hypoxia—all possible stressors in aviation. A threat to flight safety exists if the phoria is excessive because, like a tropia, it can cause diplopia. For these reasons aviation medical departments should examine all aviators for tropia and phoria and establish acceptable standards for certification.

Depth Perception

Depth perception in the aviation environment depends on monocular and binocular cues. The monocular cues include retinal image size, aerial perspective, linear perspective, overlapping contours, and motion parallax. The most important binocular cue is stereopsis which allows distance judgment up to 200 m. Because the relative importance of monocular and binocular cues is somewhat conjectural, members of the aviation medical community do not always agree that binocular vision is absolutely essential for conventional cockpit duties. For example, some believe that a pilot with one functioning eye is at no disadvantage in flight and can function adequately utilizing monocular cues for depth perception. Although it could be argued that this might be true for general aviation, it is less convincing for specialized flight situations, such as military operations, aerial spraying, or any other type of mission requiring high-speed, low-level maneuvers. Another concern is the absence of a second eye as a backup should something happen to the single functioning eye. Like so many other ophthalmic conditions affecting flight operations, flight certification must be determined in part by the flight operations of each organization.

Glaucoma

The ciliary body produces aqueous humor, which normally flows from the posterior chamber to the anterior chamber, and then through the canal of Schlemm. Interruption of this flow results in an abnormal accumulation of aqueous humor and increased intraocular pressure, which can damage the optic nerve causing decreased visual acuity and eventually blindness.

Glaucoma is classified as narrow-angle, secondary, and open-angle. In the narrow-angle variety, the outflow of aqueous humor is impeded because of an anatomic defect which partially obstructs the canal of Schlemm. The factors precipitating attacks of narrow- or closed-angle glaucoma are not well understood, although there is an association with pupillary dilatation, stress, and excitement. These attacks may also be triggered by the mydriatic effects of medications such as atropine, which causes dilatation of the iris, further obstruction of aqueous outflow, and a sudden and precipitous rise in intraocular pressure. As a result, patients complain of acute onset of incapacitating ocular pain, decreased visual acuity, and seeing halos around lights. Fortunately, narrow-angle glaucoma is not a common disease, but when it does occur it is usually treated surgically with peripheral iridectomy. Aviators could be considered for medical waivers if surgery is successful, normal intraocular pressure is restored, and there is no other ophthalmologic dysfunction.

Unlike narrow-angle glaucoma, secondary glaucoma is always due to an underlying process such as trauma, uveitis, cataracts, or a tumor. Once the underlying cause is treated, restoration of normal intraocular pressure can be expected, and at that time a request for medical waiver may be granted.

By far the most common form of glaucoma the AME/FS will encounter is the open-angle variety, which is rarely seen before age 40, but is the second leading cause of blindness in the United States.[4] Although its etiology is unknown, there appears to be interference with the outflow of aqueous humor in the trabecular meshwork near the canal of Schlemm. Open-angle glaucoma is frequently asymptomatic for as long as 10 years, and thus is almost always diagnosed not by patient complaint, but by increased intraocular pressure determined by a screening tonometric examination. Although open-angle glaucoma causes no obvious early symptoms, it will eventually lead to visual field defects, decreased visual acuity, and blindness from increased pressure on the optic nerve and retina. Hence, early detection and treatment is essential. For this reason tonometric determinations by Schiotz tonometry, puff tonometry, or applanation should be performed periodically on aviators over age 40.

Glaucoma is characterized by damage to the optic nerve causing a progressive visual field loss. It is more likely to occur when the intraocular pressure (IOP) exceeds 21 mm Hg, although the disease process sometimes occurs with lower IOPs. In any event treatment should begin if ocular pathology is noted by ophthalmoscopy or visual field loss. Some ophthalmologists would also prescribe therapy if the IOP were elevated with no other abnormalities.

Treatment is usually medical although in some cases surgery is indicated. It is important that treatment begin as early as possible to prevent further progression of the disease process and possible blindness.

There are several varieties of medication prescribed for open-angle glaucoma, and they act by either decreasing aqueous humor production or enhancing aqueous outflow. Most are topicals that are absorbed to some degree and may cause adverse systemic side effects that could affect pilot performance. These agents include beta-blockers, miotics, parasympathomimetics, sympathomimetics, and prostaglandin analogs. Another therapeutic modality is use of oral carbonic anhydrase inhibitors.[4]

Beta-blockers such as timolol or betaxolol are the mainstay of treatment. They generally cause few undesirable side effects but should be used with caution in patients with asthma or diabetes. Timolol is particularly suitable for aviators because it effectively lowers IOP while causing few side effects. Studies have shown that this medication causes no change in pupil size, only a slight decrease in pulse, and no significant changes in blood pressure.[5,6]

Although pilocarpine, a parasympathomimetic that facilitates aqueous outflow by pupillary constriction, is an excellent medication for open-angle glaucoma, its use by aviators should be restricted because of its potential side effects. It may cause miosis and spasm of the ciliary body, which in turn produces impaired night vision, loss of accommodative power, blurred vision, and pseudomyopia, any of which create a hazard to flight safety. An exception might be made for Ocusert®, which slowly releases pilocarpine when it is inserted into the eye. For some reason the intraocular pressure is brought under control by this medicating device, but the usual parasympathomimetic side effects are almost completely eliminated.[7]

Sympathomimetics such as epinephrine are also effective. Although they do not significantly affect visual acuity, night vision, or accommodation, there is the potential for increased blood pressure, headaches, and arrhythmias,[4] so they should be used with caution. A new class of medication for open-angle glaucoma are the prostaglandin analogs, which show therapeutic promise with few side effects. More studies are needed before their efficacy and side effect profile is completely understood.

Acetazolamide, a carbonic anhydrase inhibitor, is not often prescribed, and the AME/FS should be cautioned that patients may complain of a number of side effects including nausea, vomiting, diarrhea, abdominal pain, paresthesias, and possible kidney stones. Another theoretical disadvantage to its use in aviators is its disturbance of the body's acid-base balance causing a metabolic acidosis and shift in the oxyhemoglobin dissociation curve.

In the event that medical management is not effective, 2 surgical procedures are available: argon laser trabeculoplasty and filtration surgery. Unfortunately, with the former procedure 50% of eyes have recurring increased IOP within 5 years. With the latter, long term control may be achieved but only with postsurgical glaucoma medication.[8]

In summary, it is advisable to periodically check the IOP of aviators after age 40 because of the insidious nature of open-angle glaucoma and the risk of blindness. Once glaucoma is diagnosed and treatment prescribed, follow-up is essential to ensure that the disease process has been arrested and that there are no unwanted side effects from the medication. Although most of the medications available (with the exception of pilocarpine) have minimal side effects, it is recommended that aviators first be ground tested for 30 days. Timolol is probably the most desirable medication for aviators while pilocarpine would be the least desirable.

Uveitis

Uveitis is the all-inclusive term for inflammation of any part of the uveal tract: the iris, ciliary body, choroid, and retina. Histologically the inflammatory process can be classified as nongranulomatous or granulomatous. The nongranulomatous type is of unknown etiology although some investigators believe that it is due to a sensitivity reaction. The disease usually involves the anterior uveal tract, ie, the iris and ciliary body, causing an acute inflammatory reaction with severe pain, photophobia, blurred vision, and redness. The treatment of choice is steroid therapy which usually brings about remission. In general, the prognosis for nongranulomatous uveitis is good, although recurrences are common.

The granulomatous form, on the other hand, is usually due to an underlying process such as tuberculosis, toxoplasmosis, syphilis, or histoplasmosis, but in many cases no causative organism is found. The lesions may occur in the anterior or posterior uvea, although there is a definite predilection for the latter. The symptoms are usually insidious with patients complaining of pain, photophobia, and blurred vision. Treatment consists of therapy for any underlying diseases, as well as symptomatic medications such as mydriatics, analgesics, and steroids. The prognosis for the granulomatous form of the disease is not as good as that of the nongranulomatous form, because in the former symptoms may last for months to years with periods of remissions and exacerbations. Furthermore, if the macula is involved there may be a permanent decrease in visual acuity.

The AME/FS is concerned with uveitis regardless of its etiology because of its possible complications and sequelae. For example, the formation of anterior or posterior synechiae may impede the flow of aqueous humor resulting in secondary glaucoma; cataracts may develop because of interference with lens metabolism; and most importantly, it may impair visual acuity by retinal detachment or macular degeneration. Uveitis might also be a manifestation of a serious underlying disease process which may require disqualification from flight duty. Therefore, if a medical waiver is to be requested for uveitis, it is recommended that the AME/FS conform to the following guidelines.

- A search for an underlying disease must be made and if detected, it must be treated and cured.
- The uveitis must be in full remission.
- Visual acuity must be restored to acceptable standards without other visual dysfunction that could compromise flight safety.

Central Serous Chorioretinopathy

Central serous chorioretinopathy (CSC), a disease of unknown etiology, causes ocular symptoms due to increased vascular permeability of the choroid with a resultant fluid leak and detachment of the retina in the macular area. It is most frequently found in healthy adults, mainly males, in their thirties and forties. CSC usually has an acute onset involving one or both eyes. Patients with CSC usually complain of diminished or blurred vision, scotomata, and abnormal color vision. Depth perception also becomes abnormal and visual acuity can deteriorate to as low as 20/100. The disease can be diagnosed by ophthalmoscopy (there is a loss of the foveal light reflex with a circle of edema around the macula) or fluorescein angiography. The course is one of remissions and exacerbations with 80% of eyes undergoing spontaneous complete remission and restoration of normal visual acuity and depth perception within 6 months.[9] However, there is the occasional case which will remain active for a long time and cause some degree of residual ophthalmologic dysfunction such as scotomata or color vision deficiency.

There is no known medical treatment for CSC, although photocoagulation sometimes shortens the course of the detachment; most patients regain their visual acuity with or without treatment. The recurrence rate is 20%-30% and is not influenced by laser photocoagulation therapy.[9]

Forty-seven USAF aviators with CSC were followed at the USAF School of Aerospace Medicine. Major complaints included blurred vision, distorted images, micropsia, central scotomata, and changes in color vision.[10] Most cases resolved spontaneously but about 50% had recurrences. Ninety-seven percent of the aviators returned to the cockpit.

Aviators with active CRC should be restricted from flight duty. Once remission occurs—usually within several months—and the patient has regained normal visual acuity and depth perception, a request for a medical waiver can be granted. However, because there is a significant recurrence rate, close following is recommended.

Cataracts

Cataract formation or opacification of the lens can develop at any age and is most commonly associated with congenital factors, trauma, inflammation, and advancing age. If it appears in a younger aviator, the AME/FS should try to determine its etiology since treatment of the underlying disease may reverse its development. In general, cataracts are not particularly serious unless they are progressive and interfere with normal vision. The natural course of cataracts (ie, those with no underlying pathologic condition such as infection) is not entirely predictable. Some may remain small and static and not impair vision; others may later progress to the point of serious visual impairment. Therefore the presence of a cataract does not necessarily require restriction from flight duty as long as adequate visual acuity is maintained. In such cases periodic ophthalmologic examination is necessary to ensure that there has been no progression.

It may become necessary for some aviators to have cataract surgery (extraction or phacoemulsification) once the disease process has become severe enough to impede normal vision. With surgical removal of the lens, the patient becomes apha-kic and requires insertion of intraocular lenses (IOLs). If IOLs are unsuitable for any reason, spectacles or contact lenses are necessary to correct vision. Unfortunately, the spectacles necessary for aphakics are extremely thick and heavy (sometimes referred to as "coke bottle lenses") and cause some distortion, rendering the aviator unsuitable for some types of flight duty. (Contact lenses are discussed below.)

Fortunately, the insertion of IOLs is possible for most aphakics, and the lenses are safe and effective. IOLs are made of polymethylmethacrylate (PMMA) and can be inserted into the anterior chamber (in front of the iris) or posterior chamber (behind the iris). The latter procedure is more popular because anterior chamber placement results in far more complications.[11] In any event, possible complications include malposition of the lenses resulting in glare and seeing halos and flashing lights. Also, cystoid macular edema causing photophobia, fluctuating visual acuity, and pain can occur months to years later. Other adverse sequelae include capsular opacification and retinal detachment. Consequently it is advisable to ensure close follow-up of aviators who elect to have this procedure.

Interestingly and not surprisingly there is increasing use of IOLs in civil avia-tors.[12] Reports indicate that the population of these aviators has a higher accident risk than does the total population of aviators. However, the use of IOLs was not found to be causal.[13] Even though IOLs can be ground to fit the patient's individual needs, aviators should have them ground with a diopter power to correct distant vision (in this case spectacles would be needed for reading). The results of IOL surgery have generally been good, with 85% of patients in one study achieving 20/40 or better visual acuity.[13] Of the 45,000 cases studied, only a small percentage had complications such as macular edema, secondary glaucoma, hyphema, and lens dis-location. In another study of 1000 cases, complications reported included malposi-tion of the lens (0.3%), inflammation or infection (3.3%), macular edema (3.3%), and retinal detachment (0.3%).[14]

These data indicate that the utility and efficacy of IOLs as well as their low com-plication rate make them suitable for aviators. Regarding high-performance aircraft and the effects of acceleration on the IOLs, studies at the USAF School of Aerospace Medicine indicated that high G loads (up to $+12G_z$) will not displace the lenses in monkeys.

If a flight organization approves use of IOLs for its aviators, it should ensure that the lenses are endorsed by the appropriate regulatory agencies (such as the FDA in the U.S.), that an adequate healing period of up to several months has elapsed after surgery, and that the resultant refractive error and visual acuity have stabilized and are within acceptable standards.

Retinal Detachment

Although retinal detachment can be caused by a multitude of underlying processes such as tumors of the eye, trauma, and inflammation of many different types, many cases are spontaneous and idiopathic. There is also evidence that aphakia and high myopia are predisposing conditions. Regardless of the cause, the retina separates from the choroid thereby losing its blood supply at the site of the detachment. If the detachment is in the area of the fovea, serious central field defects may result including blindness. If the fovea is spared, the patient will have peripheral field defects with varying degrees of visual impairment. The diagnosis of retinal detachment can be made by history—the patient usually complains of flashes or spots in front of the eyes or the sensation of a curtain coming down obscuring the field of vision—and by ophthalmoscopic examination. The treatment of retinal detachment includes photocoagulation, cryosurgery, and scleral buckling as well as specific therapy for any amenable underlying cause. If treatment is not instituted soon after detachment occurs, permanent impairment of visual acuity or blindness could result.

The success rate for surgical management of retinal detachment is 85%-90% depending on the procedure. If the macula is involved, the prognosis is less optimistic. Another factor to consider is the high incidence of retinal detachment in the opposite eye, usually within 10 years.[15]

Therefore the AME/FS has several concerns for the aviator with retinal detachment who has been treated surgically. Has visual acuity been restored to acceptable standards? Will there be a recurrence? Will retinal detachment occur in the other eye? If the answer to the first question is yes, a recommendation for a medical waiver should certainly be considered. As for the latter two considerations, which are unpredictable and not particularly uncommon, a waiver could be requested as long as the patient is followed closely. Even with a recurrence inflight, normal function in the opposite eye should preclude complete incapacitation.

Keratoconus

Keratoconus is a disease of unknown etiology although hereditary factors possibly play a role. The pathologic process, a thinning and conelike protrusion of the cornea, causes an irregular myopic astigmatism usually first apparent in late puberty or early adulthood. Keratoconus should be suspected when a young adult presents with these findings and referred to an ophthalmologist who can confirm the suspicion with slit lamp, keratoscopy, and keratometry examinations. Keratoconus is usually a bilateral disease and, although many cases remain static, is often progressive.

The treatment options for keratoconus include spectacles, contact lenses, and corneal transplant (keratoplasty). Because of the degree of astigmatism that usually develops with this disease, spectacles will not provide satisfactory correction for most patients; contact lenses may be needed to restore normal visual acuity. Keratoplasty, the third option, offers an excellent chance of cure. The success rate for corneal transplant is 90%-96% although it may take up to 6 months for complete visual recovery,[15,17] and up to 50% of patients may still need some correction with contact lenses.[16] Complications are uncommon, but include corneal rejection, post-operative astigmatism, and recurrence. Pilots who can be corrected to acceptable visual standards with contact lenses or by keratoplasty can be granted a medical waiver. It is advisable to follow-up closely for 6 months.

There is another interesting aspect of keratoconus the AME/FS must address. Most prospective aviators with keratoconus are probably disqualified on initial physical examination for entry into flight training unless the disease goes undetected or unless the individual has been wearing contact lenses for some time prior to the examination. It is well known that individuals with astigmatism due to keratoconus who wear contact lenses for some months are able to score 20/20 visual acuity even with the contact lenses removed. This incongruity is explained by corneal molding, a process by which the curvature of the cornea is "molded" or shaped by the inner surface of the contact lens, permitting normal uncorrected visual acuity. If the AME/FS suspects keratoconus and corneal molding, a referral to an ophthalmologist is advisable because contact lenses sometimes leave telltale lesions on the cornea detectable with a slit lamp. Furthermore, medical records containing previous visual acuity and refraction studies would betray the individual who has been wearing contact lenses surreptitiously through the inconsistent findings on sequential examinations.

Contact Lenses

Contact lenses are sometimes prescribed because of certain diseases (all rare in a screened aviation population) such as aphakia, keratoconus, irregular astigmatism, and corneal scarring, because they cause a refractive error that cannot be corrected to 20/20 with regular corrective lenses. However, in the majority of cases prescriptions for contact lenses are written at the patient's request, for cosmetic rather than medical reasons.

Contact lenses do offer distinct advantages to the aviator. Unlike spectacles, there is no problem integrating them with cockpit equipment such as helmets, oxygen masks, and pressure suit and chemical defense ensembles. Also, they permit a full field of vision and will not fog—all benefits to aviators flying high-performance aircraft. Over the past few decades there have been great technical advances in the design and manufacture of contact lenses. We have advanced from the early scleral contacts to the present-day soft contact lenses (SCLs), hard contact lenses (HCLs), rigid gas-permeable, and disposable contacts made of better-tolerated materials that permit extended wear for weeks at a time.

For many years contact lens use was prohibited by most flight organizations due to fears of slippage or loss inflight, bubble formation, foreign body irritation, and keratoconjunctivitis due to infection or irritation, to name only a few. The military services were particularly restrictive in this respect. However, these fears have been allayed by the results of numerous studies which have prompted a reversal of policy by many military and civil flight organizations.

Illustrative of this is a study of 124 aviators wearing either SCLs or HCLs.[18] Only a few reported a foreign body that was easily removed inflight; some described eye discomfort or irritation probably secondary to dryness; others experienced decentering mainly due to lens manipulation or rubbing of the eyes (only one was attributed to acceleration); and several had corneal abrasions. Overall the contact lenses were well tolerated with only minor problems, none of which impaired or endangered flight safety. Only 4 aviators had to be temporarily disqualified from flying. Another study was published with similar findings.[19]

From a strictly military point of view, the flight surgeon should be concerned with bubble formation under the lens, dislodgment secondary to accelerative forces, and pain, discomfort, or decreased visual acuity in flight due to decreased partial pressure of oxygen and/or low cockpit humidity. Pursuant to these concerns there has been considerable research done to better understand these problems. In one study, 51 subjects with soft or rigid gas-permeable contacts were taken in an altitude chamber to as high as 7625 m (25,000 ft) including rapid decompression from 2438 m (8000 ft) to 6706 m (22,000 ft).[20] In 2 of 5 subjects wearing rigid gas-permeable contacts, bubble formation was noted centrally whereas for those wearing soft lenses, gas bubbles were observed in 24% of the 92 eyes examined, although the bubbles were in the limbus rather than centrally located. Consequently, there was no effect on vision. In other studies, no bubbles were seen in subjects wearing soft contact lenses taken to as high as 11,278 m (37,000 ft) in an altitude chamber.[21] Hence, it would appear that bubble formation under contacts is not an operational problem, at least for aviators with soft lenses.

Acceleration studies were conducted to see if high G forces could cause decentering or dislodgment of hard and soft contact lenses. For those with soft lenses, there was no lens movement with forces as high as $8+G_z$, although there was significant decentering with reduced vision for subjects wearing hard contacts.[22] Again, soft contact lenses appeared to have passed the test.

Because some flight crew members who wear contact lenses inflight have complained of eye discomfort, probably due to drying (some aircraft have extremely low humidity), decreased ambient partial pressure of oxygen, or cigarette smoke, studies have been done on long distance missions. In one study, 10 subjects wearing soft contact lenses and 6 controls were examined inflight on a C-5 transport aircraft during a trans-Pacific round trip between San Antonio, Texas and Korea. Although some subjects demonstrated conjunctival injection, discomfort was minimal and there were no significant changes in visual acuity. The investigators concluded from this long and stressful trip that there was no degradation of performance and no reason to preclude use of contacts in transport aircrew.[23]

These and other studies have demonstrated that the wearing of contact lenses does not pose a threat to flight safety as was originally thought. However, the lenses must be fitted properly and procured from approved sources, and aviators must be informed about their proper wear, handling, and cleaning. It is also advisable that spectacles be carried on all flights as backup in case the contact lenses are dislodged or lost.

Disease of the External Eye

The AME/FS will frequently diagnose and treat various disorders involving the external portion of the eye. Blepharitis, keratitis, dacryocystitis, conjunctivitis, and hordeolum are examples commonly encountered in office practice. Furthermore, patients will occasionally be treated for various degrees of trauma ranging from minor corneal abrasions to severe acid or alkali burns.

Although some diseases of the external eye may not impair visual dysfunction (acid or alkali burns being an exception), others may cause pain, excessive tearing, or annoying sensations which may act to impair visual acuity. Therefore, a minor condition which in other patients might be ignored can be significant in a cockpit environment. In general, the treatment for these conditions consists of irrigation, ophthalmologic topicals (antibiotics or steroids), systemic antibiotics, and patching. In most cases there is full remission after a few days to a few weeks of treatment. Aviators should be temporarily disqualified from flight duty if the disease causes significant decrement of visual acuity or if the prescribed medications have side effects that may impair visual function significantly.

Refractive Surgery

Radial keratotomy (RK), photorefractive keratectomy (PRK), and laser in-situ ker-atomileusis (LASIK) are surgical procedures mainly performed to correct myopia. If successful, the patient may no longer need spectacles or contact lenses for correction. The allure of a surgical procedure which promises to normalize myopic vision is particularly tantalizing to aviators and student pilot applicants. Unfortunately these procedures may have complications that would pose an added hazard to flight safety.

RK is performed by making a number of radial incisions on the periphery of the cornea causing it to flatten somewhat. Although the refractive error and visual acuity may be improved, a number of patients will develop anisometropia (a difference in the refractive power of the two eyes), sensitivity to glare, and diurnal visual acuity and refractive error changes. Consequently, some flight organizations disqualify anyone who had this procedure from entry into both flight training and retention as fully trained aviators. Other organizations, particularly in civil aviation, are less restrictive. However, RK is being performed less and less today due to the advent of PRK and LASIK therapy.

In PRK, an excimer laser is used to reshape the anterior cornea to correct the refractive error. Correction stabilizes in 3-6 months for low myopia and 6-18 months for high myopia.[24] Although the outcome varies from center to center, 75%-100% of patients will attain 20/40 or better uncorrected visual acuity,[25] with 58%-75% attaining 20/20 visual acuity.[26] Consequently, some patients need to continue wearing either contact lenses or spectacles postsurgery.

The following complications of PRK of concern to the AME/FS have been reported[24-27]:

- Corneal haze. This usually clears within 12 months in most patients, but in some it may take up to 2 years to clear.
- Corneal scarring or opacities. Wound healing response can cause this, but it does not necessarily affect visual acuity.
- Seeing halos around light sources. This is a common complaint and can be severe in some cases.
- Diurnal fluctuation of refractive error and visual acuity. In one study of 135 patients, this complication persisted in 14% of cases for 6 months and in 4% for 1 year.[25]
- Undercorrection or overcorrection. This is dependent in part on the skill of the surgeon and in some cases requires a second procedure.

- Decreased contrast sensitivity.
- Glare. Glare can be particularly bothersome and occurs in about 50% of cases for as long as 2 years postsurgery.[26]
- Loss of best corrected visual acuity. This can occur in as many as 8% of patients.[24]

There have also been anecdotal reports of fluctuation of vision, suggesting that a hypoxic environment may be detrimental to vision in aviators who have had refractive surgery. More research is needed to resolve this.

Although this is a long list of possible complications of PRK, we have accumulated enough experience to know most patients have excellent results without significant adverse effects. Hence, many aviators having PRK could be qualified for flight as long as close follow-up is ensured.

Another procedure related to PRK is laser in-situ keratomileusis, better known as LASIK. It differs from PRK in that a corneal flap is created and retracted just before excimer laser ablation. The flap is then returned to its original position. Although this is a fairly new procedure, it appears to be as effective as PRK with similar but fewer complications.[28,29] Because of limited experience with this procedure, flight qualification is still problematic.

RK, PRK, and LASIK are procedures that effectively correct myopia. New techniques will no doubt be developed in the near future that will be even more effective. Nevertheless, the postsurgical complications, particularly problems seeing glare and halos, fluctuating refractive error and diurnal visual acuity, impaired night vision, and decreased contrast have clear aeromedical implications. There are also the poorly known effects of accelerative forces (mainly in aerobatic and military flying), hypoxia, and very low humidity on the postsurgical cornea. Determination of aeromedical disposition of aviators undergoing these procedures is difficult because of the variability of results and the ill-defined incidence of complications. If aeromedical disposition is decided on a case-by-case basis, it is advisable to wait at least 6-12 months after surgery since most complications seem to disappear in that time period. Close follow-up including an ophthalmological examination with keratometry and corneal topography is essential.

References

1. Tredici TJ. Ophthalmology in aerospace medicine. In: DeHart RL, ed. *Fundamentals of Aerospace Medicine*. 2nd ed. Philadelphia: Williams & Wilkins; 1996.
2. Rayman RB. Aircraft accidents/incidents among aircrewmen flying with medical waiver. *Aerospace Med*. 1972;43(11):1265-1269.

3. Zentner AB. A proposal for diagnostic color vision standards for civil airmen. *Aviat Space Environ Med*. 1988;59(8):770-775.

4. Lewis PR, Phillips TG, Sassani JW. Topical therapies for glaucoma: What family physicians need to know. *AFP*. 1999;59(7):1871-1879.

5. Allen RC, Hertzmark E, Walker AM, et al. A double-masked comparison of betaxolol versus timolol in the treatment of open angle glaucoma. *Am J Ophthal*. 1986;101:535-541.

6. LeBlanc RP, Kripp G. Timolol: Canadian multicenter study. *Ophthalmol*. 1981;88(3):244-248.

7. Tredici TJ. Screening and management of glaucoma in flying personnel. *Mil Med*. 1980;145(1):34-38.

8. Rosenberg LF. Glaucoma: Early detection and therapy for prevention of vision loss. *AFP*. 1995;52(8):2289-2298.

9. Hardy RA. Central serous chorioretinopathy. In: Vaughn D, Asbury T, Riordan-Eva P, eds. *General Ophthalmology*. 14th ed. Norwalk, Conn: Appleton & Lange; 1995.

10. Green RP, Carlson DW, Diekert JP, Tredici TJ. Central serous chorioretinopathy in US Air Force aviators: A review. *Aviat Space Environ Med*. 1988;59:1170-1175.

11. Kanski JJ. *Clinical Ophthalmology*. 3rd ed. London: Butterworth-Heinemann; 1994.

12. Nakagawara VB, Loochan FK, Wood KJ. Aphakia and artificial lens implants in the civil airman population. *Aviat Space Environ Med*. 1993;64:932-938.

13. Nakagawara VB, Montgomery RW, Wood KJ. An assessment of aviation risk of aphakic civil airmen by class of certificate held and by age: 1982–85. DOT/FAA/AM-95/11. Federal Aviation Administration, Civil Aeromedical Institute, Oklahoma City. March 1995.

14. DeLuise VP. Complications of intraocular lenses. *Int Ophthalmol Clin*. 1987;27(3):195-204.

15. Newell FN. *Ophthalmology: Principles and Concepts*. 6th ed. St. Louis: CV Mosby Co; 1986.

16. Rabinowitz YS. Keratoconus. *Surv Ophthalmol*. 1998;42:299-319.

17. Weston BC, White GL. Corneal transplantation. *AFP*. 1996;54(6):1945-1948.

18. Dennis RJ, Tredici TJ, Ivan DJ, Jackson WG. The USAF aircrew medical contact lens study group. *Aviat Space Environ Med*. 1996;67:303-307.

19. Dennis RJ, Apsey DA, Ivan DJ. Aircrew soft contact lens wear: A survey of USAF eyecare professionals. *Aviat Space Environ Med*. 1993;64:1044-1047.

20. Flynn WJ, Miller RE, Tredici TJ, et al. Contact lens wear at altitude: Subcontact lens bubble formation. *Aviat Space Environ Med*. 1987;58(11):1115-1118.

21. Tredici TJ, Flynn WJ. Contact lens wear for visual disorders in USAF aviators. USAFSAM TR-86-23. USAF School of Aerospace Medicine, Brooks AFB, Texas. September 1986.

22. Flynn WJ, Block MG, Tredici TJ, et al. Effect of positive acceleration ($+G_z$) on soft contact lens wear. *Aviat Space Environ Med*. 1987;58(6):581-587.

23. Dennis RJ, Flynn WJ, Oakley CJ, et al. A field study on soft contact lens wear in USAF military transport aircraft. USAFSAM TR-88-4. USAF School of Aerospace Medicine, Brooks AFB, Texas. April 1988.

24. Nakagawara VB, Wood KJ. The aeromedical certification of photorefractive keratectomy in civil aviation: A reference guide. DOT/FAA/AM-98/25. Civil Aeromedical Institute, Oklahoma City. September 1998.

25. Seiler T, McDonnell PJ. Excimer laser photorefractive keratectomy. *Surv Ophthal*. 1995;40(2):89-118.

26. Ivan DJ, Tredici TJ, Perez-Beurra J, et al. Photorefractive keratectomy (PRK) in the military aviator: An aeromedical perspective. *Aviat Space Environ Med*. 1996;67:770-776.

27. Ellerton CR, Krueger RR. Postoperative complications of excimer laser photorefractive keratectomy for myopia. *Ophthal Clin North Am*. 1998;11(2):165-181.

28. Sanchez-Thorin JC, Barraquer-Granados JI. Myopic laser-assisted keratomileusis: An overview of published results. *Int Ophthal Clin*. 1996;36(4):53-63.

29. Carr JD, Stulting RD, Thompson KP, Waring GO. Laser in-situ keratomileusis. *Ophthal Clin North Am*. 1997;10(4):533-542.

Chapter 6
Otolaryngology

Proper function of the ears, nose, and throat is indispensable to the aviator. Changes in air pressure and the disorienting effects of flight demand a healthy system of tubes, ostia, cavities, and labyrinths. Can the Valsalva maneuver be performed? When subjected to varying pressures, can the middle ears and sinuses equalize? Is labyrinthine function normal? Because dysfunction of any of the fundamental anatomic parts of the otolaryngologic system can cause incapacitation, indeed often sudden incapacitation, as a result of pain or disorientation, the granting or denial of approval of medical waivers for otolaryngologic conditions is based on such considerations. Of particular interest to the AME/FS are vertigo, otosclerosis, Meniere's disease, and air sickness. Discussion of these and other relevant subjects follows.

Vertigo

Dorland's Medical Dictionary defines vertigo as a hallucination of movement: a sensation as if the external world were revolving around the patient (objective vertigo) or as if the patient were revolving in space (subjective vertigo). Care must be taken when eliciting the history not to confuse this symptom with dizziness or giddiness. There are many causes of vertigo, some rather benign and self-limiting, while others are of a more serious nature. The differential diagnosis includes labyrinthine disease, vertebrobasilar artery insufficiency, vascular accidents, multiple sclerosis, epilepsy, and posterior fossa tumors, among others. Regardless of etiology, the suddenness of vertigo as well as its potentially overwhelming effects are particularly threatening not only during the most critical phases of flight (ie, takeoff, landing, low level flight), but also during climb out, cruise, or descent.

Aviators who experience vertigo must undergo a thorough evaluation in order to determine its etiology because diagnosis rather than symptoms will dictate whether or not flight duty can continue safely. A discussion follows of the more common causes of vertigo.

Meniere's Disease

High on the list of the differential diagnosis of vertigo is Meniere's disease or endolymphatic hydrops. Although its etiology is not known, the symptoms are caused by distention of the endolymphatic system due to an overproduction of endolymph. The symptom triad of vertigo, tinnitus, and low frequency sensorineural hearing loss, along with nausea, vomiting, aural fullness, and spontaneous nystagmus are the hallmarks of this disease, but the AME/FS will rarely encounter such a classical presentation. Most patients instead will complain of one symptom, vertigo or hearing loss for example, which should raise the suspicion of Meniere's disease. It may take months or even years for other symptoms that would confirm the diagnosis to develop. When vertigo does occur, the attacks are sudden and usually last 2 to 6 hours, and occur unpredictably days, weeks, or months apart.[1] Because patients usually only have complaints of vertigo or hearing loss, the definitive diagnosis of Meniere's disease is therefore often tentative. Signs that may aid in confirming the diagnosis are the demonstration of recruitment and a hypoactive caloric response in the involved ear. In one study of 574 patients with Meniere's disease, over 300 had vertiginous attacks lasting 30 minutes to 12 hours.[2] Over half the cases had between 1-4 attacks/week and 1-10 attacks/day, and 94% had some degree of hearing loss.

The medical treatment for acute episodes includes benzodiazepines, anticholinergics, and antihistamines. For maintenance or prophylaxis, dietary therapy (restricted sodium intake) and diuretics are reported to be very effective in 58% of cases.[3]

For patients with severe vertigo or vertigo unresponsive to medical therapy, there are several surgical procedures that can give some relief. Endolymphatic sac procedures with shunt, labyrinthectomy, and vestibular neurectomy are surgical options. With the shunt procedure, good control of vertigo was reported in 65% of cases at 3 years and 50% at 10 years.[1] Although vertigo can be eliminated or at least ameliorated in many cases, there may be only marginal improvement in hearing, so as with medical treatment, surgery leaves much to be desired.

Positional Vertigo

Positional vertigo is usually a benign, self-limiting illness with full remission within a few months, although it can also be a manifestation of serious underlying central nervous system disease or trauma. It is of paramount importance to make this differentiation.

Individuals afflicted with benign positional vertigo will experience an attack with quick movements of the head or when the head is placed in a certain critical position. The onset is sudden and attacks usually last for 10-15 seconds with spontaneous remission. There is no tinnitus, decreased auditory acuity, or neurologic dysfunction. The diagnosis is made by history and a positive Hallpike test. The test is considered positive if there is severe vertigo and nystagmus when the head is placed in the critical position. Characteristically, there is fatigability if the test is done repetitively. However, if the critical position is assumed 1 hour later, the vertigo will once again occur.

Although most cases of benign positional vertigo remit spontaneously, vestibular suppressants and antiemetics can be prescribed for amelioration of symptoms. For refractory cases there are 3 surgical options: neurectomy (with a 10%-20% incidence of postsurgery sensorineural hearing loss); retrosigmoid vestibular nerve section (an intracranial procedure); and posterior canal occlusion, the procedure of choice (with a 5% incidence of postsurgery sensorineural hearing loss).[4] Although all 3 procedures effectively cure the vertiginous attacks, the possible adverse sequelae must not be ignored.

Labyrinthitis

Labyrinthitis, a disease of the inner ear that causes severe incapacitating vertigo, can be classified as toxic, serous, or infectious. The toxic form is caused by a number of well-known antibiotics—streptomycin and kanamycin first come to mind—which affect the vestibular apparatus and cochlea, causing not only vertigo, but also tinnitus and hearing loss. Upon withdrawal of the offending agent, there may be complete remission of these symptoms, but in some cases the damage may be permanent. Serous labyrinthitis is sometimes a sequela of trauma to the vestibule, for example poststapedectomy, which usually resolves in a short time without residua. And finally, infectious labyrinthitis is either bacterial or viral in origin and probably accounts for the vast majority of cases. Bacterial infection of the labyrinth is a serious condition that may result from otitis media, mastoiditis, or head trauma. Patients will become violently ill with nausea, vomiting, and vertigo, and vigorous treatment with antibiotics and surgical drainage is usually necessary. Fortunately, bacterial or purulent labyrinthitis is relatively uncommon.

Of all forms of labyrinthitis, the one most commonly seen by the AME/FS is the viral form. In some cases there is involvement only of the vestibular nerve or nucleus, in which case the diagnosis is vestibular neuronitis, which for practical purposes is indistinguishable from labyrinthitis. In either case, almost half the patients will complain of an antecedent upper respiratory infection followed by nausea, vomiting, and vestibular symptoms. Symptoms are so severe that even when reclining in bed the patient will often hold onto the mattress in order to keep from "falling." The crisis lasts several days with gradual remission over a period of weeks. Viral labyrinthitis is treated symptomatically with antiemetics and labyrinthine depressants. Within 4-6 weeks of onset there is usually spontaneous remission without recurrence.

Acoustic Neuroma

Acoustic neuroma, a slow-growing tumor of the eighth cranial nerve, accounts for 8%-10% of all brain tumors. The earliest symptoms are unilateral sensorineural hearing loss, tinnitus, and dysequilibrium. Common complaints include hearing loss (95%), tinnitus (70%), dysequilibrium (70%), and headache (40%).[5] Because of the proximity of the fifth, sixth, and seventh cranial nerves to the acoustic nerve, the progressively enlarging neuroma may eventually impinge on them, causing sensory disturbances of the face, weakness or paralysis of the facial muscles, and diplopia. The diagnosis can best be made by MRI. Audiometry, brainstem-evoked responses, and caloric testing are useful adjunctive modalities.

The treatment of acoustic neuroma is surgical resection with the objective of tumor removal while preserving hearing and facial nerve function. The postsurgery results vary from center to center and depend to some extent on the size of the tumor. Although some patients will enjoy complete cure, others may have recurrence or complications. In one series of 162 cases, 2 patients (0.81%) had recurrence, 19% had facial nerve paralysis, hearing was lost in 91%, and 23% had balance impairment at 2 years.[6] So even after treatment the aeromedical disposition must be given careful consideration.

Alternobaric Vertigo

Alternobaric or pressure vertigo was first recognized in 1957. It is an occupational hazard in aviators because the vertiginous attacks are caused by a sudden increase in pressure within the middle ear. This typically occurs during 2 phases of flight: during ascent as the ambient pressure decreases and during descent when aviators frequently perform a Valsalva maneuver. It is thought that this increased pressure in the middle ear is transmitted to the labyrinth through the oval window by the footplate of the stapes, resulting in transient vertigo in certain susceptible individuals. This propensity is compounded if the individual has an upper respiratory infection or has obstruction of the eustachian tube.

Although the vertigo is frequently fairly brief (ie, several seconds), there is a clear threat to flight safety. Interestingly, in several surveys 10%-17% of pilots admitted that they had experienced alternobaric vertigo during their careers.[7]

Treatment of alternobaric vertigo is based on prevention. Avoiding flight when suffering from an upper respiratory infection is an admonition well known to the AME/FS and aviator. It is also recommended that during descent, pressure in the middle ear be equilibrated in small increments by repeating the Valsalva maneuver every few seconds rather than allowing a large pressure buildup before performing the maneuver.

Aeromedical Disposition of Vertigo

Attacks of vertigo can be disorienting and are extremely dangerous should they occur in flight. Even a mild episode occurring in a critical phase of flight could be disastrous. Therefore aviators experiencing vertigo must be fully evaluated to ascertain the cause of the vertiginous attack and to determine the probability of recurrence. A careful history and thoughtful ordering and interpretation of diagnostic procedures are paramount if the AME/FS is to accurately assess the differential diagnosis of vertigo.

In some cases the cause of vertigo may remain indeterminate despite an exhaustive evaluation. Without a diagnosis, the aeromedical disposition is difficult because the risk of recurrence cannot be ascertained. Until more sophisticated diagnostic techniques are available, the aeromedical disposition of aviators with vertigo of undetermined cause must be left to the empirical dictates of each aviation medicine department.

On the other hand if a diagnosis can be made, enough is known of the natural history of the various entities causing vertigo to permit enlightened aeromedical disposition. For example, aviators with Meniere's disease should be disqualified from flying because the vertiginous attacks recur at indefinite and totally unpredictable intervals. And in addition to vertigo other symptoms of the disease, including sudden decrease of auditory acuity and spontaneous nystagmus, pose an unacceptable risk to flight safety. Even with medical or surgical treatment a significant number of patients experience recurrent symptoms.

As for benign positional vertigo, most aviators can eventually return to flight duty because the condition is self-limiting and not recurrent. As long as there are symptoms temporary restriction is clearly necessary. Patients should be followed by the AME/FS until there is complete remission, which may take weeks or months. If surgery is performed, the patient must be fully recovered and have acceptable auditory acuity.

The outlook for labyrinthitis or vestibular neuronitis is also favorable since most cases are due to viral infection, are self-limiting, and have little chance of spontaneous recurrence. So a return to the cockpit would be in order once treatment is completed and there is assurance of complete remission, usually after 4-6 weeks. An exception might be made for patients with permanent damage to the vestibular system from toxic drugs or a severe bacterial infection that caused extensive suppuration.

Although acoustic neuroma is a slow-growing tumor with an insidious onset of symptoms, the inevitability of vertigo is reason enough to disqualify aviators from flying. A medical waiver should only be considered once the tumor is surgically removed and the patient's auditory and vestibular functions have been restored.

The aeromedical disposition of aviators with alternobaric vertigo can be difficult and should be determined on a case-by-case basis rather than by rigid policy. As a rule, aviators with frequently recurring alternobaric vertigo should probably be disqualified from flying. Vertiginous attacks with altitude changes would be undesirable, particularly in high-performance aircraft. However, occasional episodes that are clearly associated with upper respiratory infection could be waived as long as the condition is fully understood and there is assurance that the aviator will comply with an order not to fly with an upper respiratory infection.

Otosclerosis

Otosclerosis is a disease that causes a progressive loss of hearing usually seen in young adults. A bony dystrophy develops, most often involving the footplate of the stapes, resulting in a conductive hearing loss. Although patients can usually function normally early in the course of the disease, the pathologic process will eventually affect the speech range frequencies. At some point, depending on the extent of hearing loss and the individual's needs, a hearing aid or a corrective surgical procedure may become necessary. Both options have aeromedical implications of which the AME/FS must be aware.

In spite of technological advances in the design of hearing aids, they still have deficiencies rendering them of marginal use in the cockpit. The normal sense of hearing allows us to filter out unwanted noise during conversation, which is why speech is understandable to us even in a noisy room, but a hearing aid cannot do this. Instead, all sound in the environment of the listener is amplified and distorted, causing great difficulty in understanding the speaker. Similarly, when using headphones in the cockpit an aviator may hear static and messages on the same frequency meant for other aircraft. The aviator must be able to "tune out" or suppress the unwanted transmissions and extract only those relevant to his aircraft. Hence, the use of a hearing aid in flight could be a great liability.

If hearing aids are deemed unsatisfactory, the alternative is corrective surgery. Due to unsatisfactory results, the older procedures, fenestration of the semicircular canal and stapes mobilization, have been largely replaced by stapedectomy. Although there are numerous techniques used for this procedure, all of them basically involve removing part or all of the stapes, sealing the oval window with a membrane (vein, perichondrium, or fascia) and restoring ossicular continuity by connecting the incus to the oval window with a prosthesis (teflon, stainless steel, or platinum). Gelfoam seals are no longer used because they are associated with fistula formation.[8]

The purpose of this procedure is to improve the patient's auditory acuity and in many cases normal hearing is indeed restored. However, there are possible complications of stapedectomy that must be considered. These include further hearing loss due to cochlear damage, injury to the facial nerve, infection of the middle ear or labyrinth, and disturbances of equilibrium. Clearly, any of these postoperative sequelae could compromise an aviator's ability to function, but since they usually occur shortly after the operation, well before an aeromedical waiver request is made, there is no threat to flying safety.

The most serious long-term complication of stapedectomy, at least for aviators, is perilymph fistula because it can cause sudden, severe vertiginous attacks. With fistulization, there is an abnormal communication through the oval window allowing perilymph to leak from the vestibule into the middle ear. This complication can occur not only during the immediate postoperative period, but also months, and in some cases years, after the operation. It should be suspected whenever a post-stapedectomy patient complains of fluctuating hearing loss, tinnitus, vertigo, or dysequilibrium. The incidence of perilymph fistula varies from 0.6%-3.5%, depending on the skill of the surgeon and the type of prosthesis-graft. As ENT surgeons have become more skilled in performing stapedectomies this complication has become more rare. For example, in one large cohort of 828 cases, there was perilymph leakage and vertigo in only 0.3%.[9] ENT surgeons emphasize that the occurrence of perilymph fistula as well as other complications of stapedectomy is dependent above all on the experience and skill of the surgeon.

There is also the danger of fistulization and vertigo due to dislodgment of the prosthesis caused by sudden pressure changes in the middle ear. It could conceivably be caused by rapid ascent or descent, rapid decompression, or even a Valsalva maneuver, all of which pose a threat, particularly in high-performance aircraft.

In summary, perilymph fistula can occur following any type of stapedectomy procedure although the incidence is low when the operation is performed by an experienced surgeon. Fistulization can occur not only as a sequela of surgery, but also with sudden changes of pressure in the middle ear. The most significant aeromedical implication of perilymph fistula is the possibility of severe, incapacitating vertigo. Thus aviators with stapedectomy should be selected for waiver using the following criteria to minimize the risk of vertigo and sudden incapacitation.

- The patient must be at least 1 year postsurgery.
- The operation should be performed by an experienced surgeon.
- Hearing must have been restored to acceptable standards.
- The patient must be completely free of vestibular symptoms (such as vertigo, dizziness, and nausea) and must demonstrate normal eustachian tube function.
- The patient should be periodically evaluated by the AME/FS to ensure a perilymph fistula has not developed.

The External and Middle Ear

Common diseases of the external and middle ear include otitis externa, acute otitis media, chronic otitis media, and barotitis media. Patients can usually be cured by prescribing appropriate medication, although they must temporarily be disqualified from flying for a short time until recovery is complete.

Otitis externa is an infection of the skin of the external auditory canal most commonly caused by gram-negative rods and *Staphylococcus* species. It is particularly common in hot, humid weather or in areas where people frequently swim. Patients complain of mild to severe pain in the afflicted ear, otorrhea, and decreased auditory acuity. Occasionally there are also systemic manifestations of fever, malaise, and enlarged regional nodes. Most cases can be rapidly cured by cleaning the external auditory canal and applying topical agents containing antibiotics and steroids. In many cases, aviators with otitis externa can continue to fly. However, in others temporary removal from the cockpit may be salutary, particularly if symptoms are severe enough to cause a systemic reaction. The AME/FS should keep in mind that the use of headsets or helmets can exacerbate or prolong the infection by their occlusive effect on the external auditory canal.

Acute otitis media is an infection of the middle ear caused by streptococci, staphylococci, pneumococci, and *Haemophilus influenzae*. It can be readily diagnosed in patients who complain of pain and fullness in the ear, hearing loss, and fever, as well as by pathologic changes in the tympanic membrane. Treatment usually consists of systemic antibiotics, decongestants, and antihistamines. Aviators with acute otitis media should not fly for several reasons. First, these patients always have a certain degree of discomfort that may cause performance decrement. Second, fluid in the middle ear and obstruction due to inflammation of the lateral portion of the eustachian tube does not permit normal equilibration of the barometric pressure with changes of altitude. On descent the pressure dysequilibrium may cause even more fluid accumulation. And third, decongestants, particularly those combined with antihistamines, may cause undesirable side effects such as drowsiness. For these reasons, before an aviator with acute otitis media is allowed to fly, their condition should be in full remission with all medication discontinued.

Chronic otitis media can be a greater problem than acute otitis media because complications such as a perforated tympanic membrane and cholesteatoma formation may develop. However if the perforation is central and the infection is in remission, there is no need to deny flight status. In fact, a hole in the eardrum would facilitate air exchange during changes in barometric pressure thereby reducing or eliminating the risk of developing barotitis media. But eventual repair of the perforation is desirable to improve hearing and to eliminate the possibility of reintroducing infection through the accumulation of dirt and sweat, particularly when the aviator is using headsets. Furthermore, a peripherally located perforation may induce a cholesteatoma that can slowly enlarge, eroding bone and leading to vertigo, destruction of the middle ear, and intracranial infection. It would therefore be imperative to remove these individuals from the cockpit until the condition is cured. In most patients a surgical procedure is necessary, either simple mastoidectomy, modified radical mastoidectomy, or radical mastoidectomy. A return to flight status could be considered (assuming cure has been effected with restoration of auditory acuity to acceptable standards) following surgery. However an exception may have to be made for aviators who have had a radical mastoidectomy because this procedure entails dissection of the ossicles within the middle ear. This extent of violation of the middle ear is frequently followed by residual vertigo that poses a risk to flight safety.

Barotitis media is an entity peculiar to the occupations of aviation and underwater diving in that it is caused by changes in air or water pressure. It is defined as an acute or chronic inflammation caused by a pressure differential between the tympanic cavity and the surrounding atmosphere. The middle ear communicates with the nasopharynx via the eustachian tube, a bony and membranocartilaginous structure. The membranocartilaginous portion has a one-way flutter valve which opens into the nasopharynx readily allowing equilibration when the pressure within the middle ear exceeds the ambient barometric pressure. As an aircraft gains altitude, a pressure differential between the middle ear and outside atmosphere develops, causing air to escape via the eustachian tube. However, the one-way valve does not readily allow air flow in the reverse direction, that is, from the nasopharynx to the middle ear. This reverse flow is needed for equilibration to occur when the outside atmospheric pressure exceeds that of the middle ear. This phenomenon of negative pressure within the middle ear occurs when an aircraft descends. The one-way valve can be opened to allow reversed air flow only by maneuvers such as yawning, chewing, or the Valsalva maneuver.

Problems with barotitis media arise if equilibration cannot be achieved during descent. This may occur if the aviator does not voluntarily force the eustachian tube flutter valve open or if there is a disease process which impedes its normal function. For example, an upper respiratory infection or allergic rhinitis may cause inflammation and edema that prevents opening the valve even with forceful maneuvers (hence the perennial admonition of the AME/FS to aviators not to fly with a cold).

If barotitis media occurs, the negative pressure in the middle ear will cause retraction of the tympanic membrane, engorgement of blood vessels, and the accumulation of serous or hemorrhagic fluid. In severe cases, it may also cause the tympanic membrane to rupture. As a result, the aviator may experience a painful ear, a feeling of fullness, decreased auditory acuity, and tinnitus.

The objective of treatment of barotitis media is the equilibration of pressure by opening the eustachian tube. This can best be done by prescribing topical (nasal spray) and systemic decongestants. Politzerization is frequently a helpful adjunctive procedure. Most patients require a few days to a few weeks of therapy depending on the severity of the original insult.

Aviators with barotitis media should be restricted from flying for the duration of their treatment and until normal eustachian tube function can be demonstrated. To continue flying would only exacerbate the condition and prolong recovery. Furthermore, many systemic decongestants contain antihistamines that may induce drowsiness. And finally, although barotitis media is usually a mild condition, there is the possibility of sudden inflight incapacitation due to sudden, severe ear pain. (The USAF has such cases on record.)

Diseases of the Nasal Passages and Sinuses

Conditions well known to the AME/FS that cause blockage of the eustachian tubes and interruption of air flow during changes in altitude include the common cold, allergic rhinitis, and deviated nasal septum. Because an aviator flying with any of these conditions could develop barotitis media, temporary restriction from flying is advisable until the treatment is completed and the disease is in remission. Because topical decongestants are frequently prescribed for these patients, a word of caution is in order. Aviators frequently use excessive amounts of nasal spray and nose drops to keep the nasal passages and sinuses clear without realizing the potential harm from overuse of these drugs. Overuse can be extremely irritating to mucous membranes, causing rhinitis medicamentosa with its attendant swelling and secretions. Thus nasal spray abuse can cause that which its proper use seeks to prevent.

Allergic Rhinitis

Allergic rhinitis or hay fever is a bothersome disease causing itchy nose, sneezing, excess nasal secretion, and blockage of the air passages. Symptoms are frequently seasonal and are triggered by various antigens such as grasses, pollens, and dusts.

This illness has long been the bane of aviators not only because its annoying symptoms are usually recurring, but also because the older, rarely-used antihistamines cause sedation and drowsiness, necessitating at least temporary removal from the cockpit. This problem has largely been overcome by the availability of second-generation antihistamines that do not cross the blood-brain barrier and thus do not cause drowsiness. Because they effectively relieve symptoms and cause no adverse side effects they are suitable for use by aviators. The FAA's *Guide for Aviation Medical Examiners* states that such nonsedating antihistamines may be used while flying after adequate individual experience has determined that the medication is well tolerated without significant side effects.[10]

Other treatment regimens include cromolyn and topical nasal steroids. Cromolyn is a liquid spray that is not recommended for treatment, but rather as a preventive agent to greatly decrease rhinorrhea, nasal stuffiness, and sneezing. It is primarily a topical agent with little absorption, and that which is absorbed causes no systemic effects. Cromolyn liquid spray is well tolerated with some patients complaining of only transient nasal stinging, irritation, and burning, rendering it safe and effective for allergic rhinitis.

Topical steroids, are also extremely effective in the prevention of the bothersome symptoms of allergic rhinitis. Although these are steroids, very little if any is absorbed through the nasal mucosa. In any event, there is no significant effect on the hypothalamus-pituitary-adrenal axis.

Based on the information now available on cromolyn, beclomethasone, and flunisolide, it would seem that aviators could continue with flight duties as long as these medications effectively control their symptoms.

Finally, hyposensitization may be indicated for patients in which the allergen is identified by skin testing. This may require weekly injections for months to years. Although the aviator could continue cockpit duties, it is prudent, at least early in the treatment program, to restrict the aviator on days of injection in order to obviate a possible inflight reaction.

For the aviator treated with the older antihistamines, restriction from flying is recommended whenever medication is prescribed because of the side effect of drowsiness. However, with the newer nonsedating antihistamines, topical steroids, cromolyn, and hyposensitization, most aviators should be able to continue flight duty without compromising safety.

Deviated Nasal Septum and Nasal Polyposis

Airway obstruction is sometimes encountered because of structural abnormalities such as deviated nasal septum and nasal polyposis. Either one can cause mechanical blockage of the sinus ostia located in the meatus, the space just inferior to each turbinate. If air cannot move freely in and out of the sinuses with changes in altitude, barosinusitis will result. Deviated nasal septum is thought to be due to birth injury or later trauma. Regardless of etiology, the nasal passage on the side of the deviation will be partially obstructed. If the patient has a concomitant URI or allergic rhinitis, the nasal passage is further narrowed because of edema and secretions thus compounding the problem.

For aviators with minor septal deviations that do not impede air flow, treatment is usually unnecessary and there is no contraindication to flying. However, for lesions severe enough to interfere with ventilation of the nasal passages or sinuses, restriction from flying would be advisable due to the danger of developing barosinusitis during flight. Once surgical correction is accomplished (septoplasty or submucosal resection) and the free movement of air through the nasal passages and sinuses is assured, a return to the cockpit is in order.

Likewise a polyp that arises in the nasal or sinus mucosa can also interfere with breathing and blockage of the sinus ostia by acting as a ball-flap valve. They may be single or multiple and of varying size. Aviators with polyps should have a polypectomy to prevent mechanical obstruction of the sinuses and ensuing barosinusitis.

Barosinusitis

The sinuses are encased in bone and communicate with the nasopharynx via their respective ostia. However, unlike the eustachian tube, there is no one-way valve that may be opened forcefully by doing a Valsalva maneuver. The flow of air into and out of the sinuses via the ostia is passive and moves from areas of high pressure to areas of low pressure. Therefore as an aircraft ascends, the positive pressure in the sinuses causes outflow until there is equilibrium with the ambient pressure. During descent there is increasing negative intrasinus pressure, so ambient air seeks entrance into the sinuses to equilibrate. For air to flow unimpeded the sinuses and nasopharynx must be free of any disease or obstruction, such as that caused by upper respiratory infection, allergic rhinitis, deviated nasal septum, polyps, and sinusitis.

If disease is present barosinusitis can occur, particularly during descent. Air seeking to enter the sinuses from the nasopharynx via the narrow ostia may be blocked by edema, inflammation, or a polyp, resulting in increasing negative pressure as the aircraft descends. Although symptoms vary depending on the circumstances, there is a possibility of sudden, severe pain that may be incapacitating. So barosinusitis poses a threat to flight safety particularly if it occurs during descent just prior to landing or, in a military environment, during a dive-bombing maneuver.

Treatment of barosinusitis consists of measures to relieve pain, promote drainage from the sinuses, and prevent infection, so analgesics, topical and systemic decongestants, and antibiotics are usually prescribed. Once the patient is asymptomatic, a search for underlying disease should be undertaken and if found, corrected.

The proper aeromedical disposition of aviators with barosinusitis demands temporary disqualification until treatment is complete and the patient is asymptomatic. Furthermore, if any underlying condition thought to have contributed to the onset of barosinusitis is found, such as nasal polyposis or deviated nasal septum, disqualification from cockpit duty should continue until it is also treated and cured.

References

1. Know GW, McPherson A. Meniere's disease: Differential diagnosis and treatment. *AFP*. 1997;55(4):1185-1190.

2. Haid CT, Watermeier D, Wolf SR, Berg M. Clinical survey of Meniere's disease: 574 cases. *Acta Otolaryngol*. 1995;520(suppl):251-255.

3. Slattery WH, Fayad JN. Medical treatment of Meniere's disease. *Otolaryngol Clin North Am*. 1997;30(6):1027-1037.

4. Schwaber MK. Vestibular disorders. In: Hughes GB, Pensak ML, eds. *Clinical Otology*. 2nd ed. New York: Thieme; 1997.

5. Lustig LR, Jackler RK. Benign tumors of the temporal bone. In: Hughes GB, Pensak ML, eds. *Clinical Otology*. 2nd ed. Thieme: New York; 1997.

6. Harner SG, Ebersold MJ. Management of acoustic neuroma 1978–1983. *J Neurosurg*. 1985;63:175-179.

7. Benson AJ. Pressure (alternobaric) vertigo. In: Ernsting J, King P, eds. *Aviation Medicine*. 2nd ed. London: Butterworths; 1988.

8. Slattery WH, House JW. Prostheses for stapes surgery. *Otolaryngol Clin North Am*. 1995;28(2):253-264.

9. Glasscock ME, Storper IS, Haynes DS, Bohrer PS. Twenty-five years of experience with stapedectomy. *Laryngoscope*. 1995;105:899-904.

10. Federal Aviation Administration. *Guide for Aviation Medical Examiners*. Washington, DC: Author; October 1999.

Chapter 7
Cardiology

eart disease is of particular interest to the aviation medicine practitioner (AME/FS) because there are many cardiac disorders whose natural history includes events that might be suddenly incapacitating. Heart disease, especially atherosclerotic coronary heart disease, is very prevalent in industrialized countries. Examples of such possible incapacitating events include sudden cardiac death, syncope, presyncope, myocardial infarction, angina, tachyarrhythmias, bradyarrhythmias, and thromboembolic events. These and other cardiac events are viewed as safety issues because of their sudden, unpredictable, and possibly incapacitating nature. Clinicians typically do not consider many of these events to be suddenly incapacitating, but in critical situations such as the acute phases of flight (takeoff and landing), these cardiac events could suddenly and significantly compromise the performance of flight duties. In addition to these safety considerations, there is also the potential for an aviator to permanently lose flight status due to chronic progression of heart disease.

Cardiology is a rapidly changing field with incredible advances occurring literally on a daily basis. A detailed clinical and aeromedical discussion of every cardiac disorder is beyond the scope of this book and would require an entire textbook to cover aviation cardiology alone. Nor is it possible to offer specific flying status recommendations for the entire spectrum of private, commercial, and military aviation. Rather this chapter will discuss in a broad fashion common cardiac disorders likely to be of interest to the AME/FS. Clinical features, natural history, and aeromedical considerations will be discussed. An aeromedical disposition process is suggested below as a means to reasonably address issues of qualification for flying duties for cardiac diagnoses. This suggested process and the following discussions of cardiac disorders is intended to provide a framework that can be tailored by the AME/FS or licensing agency into an aeromedical disposition policy for their particular aviation operation. This process, or a modification of it, may be used to address other cardiac disorders not discussed herein and can be applied to the broad range of aeromedical cardiology concerns for military and commercial aviation medicine. The principles can also be applied to general aviation or private flying.

A general description of the aeromedical disposition process follows. For a specific cardiac disorder, one should address several points. ***First***, determine a threshold of acceptable risk for events that may be suddenly incapacitating. That is, select a threshold annual rate of suddenly incapacitating events that is aeromedically acceptable for continuation of flying duties or entry into flight training and above which continued duties or training would not be acceptable. This threshold should be fixed and applicable to all cardiac disorders considered for possible flight duty. An aeromedical risk threshold of 1% per year for potentially suddenly incapacitating events is recommended for considering aeromedical disposition of cardiac diagnoses. This is adapted from the "1% rule" of European civilian aviation standards, the development and evolution of which was well described in the first and second European aviation cardiology workshops.[1-4] The "1% rule" as proposed for European civilian aviation standards was intended to represent a 1% per year ***mortality rate*** for the cardiac diagnosis under consideration. Their recommendations were meant to apply to civilian, especially commercial, aviation with the recognized safety factor of pilot redundancy in the commercial airliner cockpit. It may be aeromedically more prudent to consider all potentially suddenly incapacitating events, especially for military aviation, aerobatic flying, and civilian single pilot aircraft.

Second, define the aeromedical endpoints of concern for the particular cardiac diagnosis under consideration. These are endpoints that might be suddenly incapacitating or significantly degrade performance if they occurred during flight, and may be quite different from endpoints typically of clinical concern. For example, in the cardiac literature regarding nonsustained ventricular tachycardia, sudden cardiac death is considered to be the sole endpoint. But lesser hemodynamic events such as syncope, presyncope, and lightheadedness would also be of considerable aeromedical concern.

Third, determine the annual event rate for the selected endpoints. Ideally, this would come from a review of the clinical cardiology literature and a database of aviators. When relying on the cardiology literature, as much as possible one must isolate a subset of the population that closely resembles aviators or another low-risk subset that is potentially aeromedically comparable. This can be a very difficult task. Ideally, annual event rates should be derived from long-term follow-up studies of at least 5 years' duration. Highly acclaimed new procedures may seem promising in allowing continuation of aviation duties, but usually the literature initially provides only 6-12 months of follow-up on cohorts of relatively small size. Aeromedical disposition policies should not be based solely on such limited data regardless of how promising they might appear.

Fourth, decide whether there are special considerations such as ejection seat versus nonejection seat aircraft, single versus multiple pilot aircraft, high-performance (jet fighter) versus low-performance (private civil, commercial airliner, tanker, transport, bomber, rotary wing) aircraft, and very high altitude reconnaissance aircraft. Another special consideration might be continued flight duties for a trained aviator versus initial entry into flight training.

Fifth, define a reevaluation and recertification policy if continued flying duties are allowed. This policy should specify both type and frequency of required testing.

Sixth, consider the impact of other aeromedical endpoints that are not suddenly incapacitating. These other aeromedical endpoints of attrition, such as chronic progression from mild to severe aortic regurgitation, may affect policies regarding entry into flight training or continued flying duties if the rate of progression is high. They should at least be considered in defining reevaluation and recertification policies.

Seventh, consider how treatment, especially medical therapy, affects fight duty eligibility. This chapter will not discuss in detail the occupational impact and considerations of all cardiac medications prescribed for various cardiac disorders. The usual medical therapeutic options will be mentioned for the various diagnoses, along with an indication of whether the natural history literature annotates medication use in its databases. A brief discussion of cardiovascular medications appears at the end of the chapter. Surgical or other interventional therapy (eg, coronary angioplasty, mitral valve repair) should be viewed as a new diagnosis and considered independently via this process. The above steps are summarized below:

1. Determine threshold of acceptable risk for suddenly incapacitating events.
2. Define suddenly incapacitating aeromedical endpoints of concern.
3. Determine annual event rate for the selected endpoints.
4. Define and examine any special considerations (eg, single versus multiple pilot aircraft).
5. Define a recertification and reevaluation policy.
6. Consider other aeromedical endpoints.
7. Consider impact of medical therapy.

There are two cautions to keep in mind before investigating the clinical literature for outcomes or natural history data to set guidelines for determining aeromedical disposition. *First*, much of clinical knowledge is derived from hospital-based, symptomatic patient populations, especially from tertiary referral centers. As such, these data may suffer from significant referral bias and reflect higher event rates and worse prognosis than is applicable to more general outpatient populations, including the aviator population. The medical and aeromedical communities need studies with unselected, community-based populations to obtain more applicable information. Fortunately, there has been a recent trend toward such studies in the literature for several major cardiac disorders. **Second**, there may be an opposite bias, a survivor bias, in some studies of community-based populations if these populations are comprised of older subjects. In this case, this aged cohort might only represent the natural history of lower-risk survivors of the disease. Using such data could underestimate the prognosis of the disease in younger subjects.

As a final note, proper sources should be consulted in developing aeromedical standards and disposition policies. Certainly, this and other aeromedical textbooks are good resources, as is the aviation, space, and occupational medicine literature. Policies of military and civilian aviation licensing authorities from various countries may also be consulted. Many of these are published in some form or are accessible on the Internet. Although the standard cardiac literature often lacks data on specific aeromedical endpoints, it still contains a wealth of information. Many aviation databases and papers are published in the cardiology literature rather than the aeromedical literature. Outstanding examples are the two European aviation cardiology workshops referenced above.[1-4] Recent community-based population studies and other natural history studies may also provide valuable information for aeromedical disposition policy determinations.

Cardiology, preventive, and sports medicine societies have published recommendations for preparticipation cardiac screening and guidelines for continued participation in competitive sports for athletes with cardiac disorders. Although not always directly applicable, these resources have occupational considerations similar to those of aviation medicine and offer excellent advice. Over the past decade or more, cardiology societies in several countries have published guidelines on cardiac diagnostic and interventional procedures and the management of various cardiac diagnoses. These opinions from respected cardiology organizations may be useful as references, for ordering tests for occupational indications in today's climate of increasing oversight by third-party payers, and for developing evaluation and reevaluation policies. The information is not always immediately obvious, and it may require some effort to find and decipher appropriate data for use in aeromedical disposition, but a wealth of assistance is available to the determined aviation medicine practitioner.

Electrocardiographic Abnormalities

Introduction

Appropriate aeromedical disposition of electrocardiographic (ECG) findings can be a vexing problem for the AME/FS. This section reviews common ECG findings from an aeromedical perspective. In standard ECG textbooks and literature, the significance of ECG findings is usually based on data from clinical populations, often from tertiary referral centers, and these data may not be applicable to aviator populations. Policies for the aeromedical disposition of ECG findings should be based as much as possible on observations within aviator populations. The value of comparison with previous ECGs cannot be overemphasized; a change from prior ECGs may be more significant than a nonspecific finding on an isolated ECG. A detailed discussion of the diagnostic criteria for the various ECG findings is beyond the scope of this work; the reader is referred to standard ECG textbooks for such information. Common ECG abnormalities are discussed below, and the various tachyarrhythmias, such as atrial fibrillation and supraventricular and ventricular tachycardia, are discussed in a later section on tachyarrhythmias.

The United States Air Force (USAF) implemented an ECG program for its aviators in April of 1957. ECG findings of the first 67,375 aviators[5] and later the first 122,043 aviators[6] were reported. These two landmark studies, still referenced in ECG textbooks and publications today, described in detail the full spectrum of ECG findings in an apparently healthy and asymptomatic USAF aviator population. USAF policies regarding the aeromedical disposition of ECG findings in military aviators have been previously published.[7,8] The reader is also referred to three other excellent resources. The first provides guidelines for the performance of ECGs and contains an excellent review of the history of the electrocardiograph, as well as recommendations regarding the use of the ECG as a screening test in asymptomatic individuals.[9] The second resource is an excellent literature review of ECG findings in healthy subjects, including data from studies of military aviators as well as general civilian populations.[10] The third useful report reviews ECG variants and arrhythmias occurring in athletes.[11] It is quite reasonable to use data from cardiac literature on athletes to help guide aeromedical policies in at least some aviator populations such as military aviators, particularly single-seat jet fighter pilots.

Normal Variants

Many ECG findings are not technically normal, but also do not indicate underlying heart disease in a generally healthy and asymptomatic aviator. These findings may be considered normal variants that usually do not require further investigation by the AME/FS. Below is a list of common normal variants.

- Sinus bradycardia and sinus arrhythmia
- Sinus pause <2-3 seconds
- Wandering atrial pacemaker
- Ectopic atrial and junctional rhythms (rate <100 beats per minute)
- Idioventricular rhythm
- Nonspecific intraventricular conduction delay (QRS interval <120 msec all leads)
- Incomplete right bundle branch block
- First degree atrioventricular block
- Mobitz type I second degree atrioventricular block (Wenckebach block)
- ST segment elevation due to early repolarization
- rSR' pattern in V_1/V_2 with QRS interval <120 msec
- R>S in V_1 without other evidence of right ventricular hypertrophy or inferior infarction
- Right axis deviation without other evidence of right ventricular hypertrophy
- Indeterminate axis
- Supraventricular or ventricular escape beats
- Rare isolated supraventricular and ventricular premature ectopy

Chamber Dilation and Hypertrophy

Considerations include ECG signs of left and right atrial abnormality and left and right ventricular hypertrophy. There are no ECG signs of ventricular dilation per se. The definitive study for all of these ECG abnormalities is echocardiography.

Atrial Abnormality

Atrial abnormality was reported in only 5 of 122,043 military aviators (0.04/1000).[6] Atrial abnormality on ECG may be due to pressure or volume overload resulting in atrial hypertrophy, atrial dilation, or both. The ECG changes may also be present in the absence of any apparent disease. The ECG criteria for atrial abnormality are relatively nonspecific in the absence of symptoms or signs of underlying cardiac disease that might cause atrial enlargement or hypertrophy. Echocardiography can assess the presence of atrial enlargement and most underlying causative diseases. In the presence of underlying disease, aeromedical disposition should be determined by the severity of the causative process. Otherwise, the aeromedical issue would be the disposition of echocardiographic atrial dilation in the absence of demonstrated pathology. This would likely be mild enlargement of one or both atria and should probably be treated as a normal variant without further assessment or treatment.

Ventricular Hypertrophy

Right ventricular hypertrophy occurred in only 1 of 122,043 military aviators (0.008/1000), and left ventricular hypertrophy occurred in 5 of 122,043 aviators (0.04/1000).[6] ECG criteria for right ventricular hypertrophy, biventricular hypertrophy, and left ventricular hypertrophy with secondary ST-T changes (strain) are rarely seen in the aviator population, and are likely due to underlying cardiac or pulmonary disease. Echocardiography should be performed and appropriate medical treatment and subsequent aeromedical disposition pursued based on the findings.

The AME/FS is more likely to see left ventricular hypertrophy based on voltage criteria alone, without secondary supportive ECG findings such as ST-T wave changes. Several voltage criteria exist for left ventricular hypertrophy; all are nondiagnostic or nonspecific in a relatively young, healthy, and nonobese population such as aviators. Again, echocardiography is diagnostic. If left ventricular hypertrophy is present, echocardiography will exclude or diagnose coexisting aortic stenosis or classic hypertrophic cardiomyopathy as a cause, and blood pressure checks can exclude hypertension. The more common dilemma in an aviator is mild concentric left ventricular hypertrophy in the absence of aortic stenosis or hypertension: Is it physiologic (ie, athletic heart) or "mild" hypertrophic cardiomyopathy? It cannot be overemphasized that the differentiation between the two is critical—one is a normal physiologic variant and the other a disqualifying disease entity. A detailed exercise history and careful consideration of the left ventricular wall measurements are very important in making this differentiation.

The normal range of left ventricular wall thickness is generally considered to be 7-11 mm on echocardiography. Reported measurements from screening echocardiograms in 480 Canadian military pilot candidates ranged from 6-10 mm in females (n = 32) and 7-12 mm in males (n = 448).[12] Of a total of 1476 screening echocardiograms, only 5 (0.3%) had left ventricular hypertrophy by standard criteria. Another study compared sedentary, athletic, and hypertrophic cardiomyopathy subjects.[13] Mean septal/posterior left ventricular wall thicknesses were 8/8, 13/13, and 15/12 mm, respectively, for the 3 subject groups. Increased left ventricular wall thickness occurs in both aerobic and anaerobic athletes and is greatest in athletes in mixed sports such as rowing and cycling. The increase is usually small, within the range of normal values, rarely exceeds 14 mm, and represents a 10%-20% increase over baseline thickness. These exercise-induced hypertrophic changes may significantly decrease within 1-4 weeks of abstinence from exercise. This regression would not occur with hypertrophic cardiomyopathy.

Although there is overlap between athletic hypertrophy and hypertrophic cardiomyopathy, it seems reasonable to consider mild concentric hypertrophy of 12-13 mm a normal physiologic response to exercise in a physically active aviator without underlying hypertension or aortic stenosis. On the other hand, wall thickness greater than 11 mm could be considered abnormal and evaluated further. Measurements of 14 mm or greater should definitely be pursued to differentiate physiologic hypertrophy from mild hypertrophic cardiomyopathy. Repeat echocardiography at least 4 weeks after complete discontinuation of exercise should demonstrate at least some regression of athletic physiologic hypertrophy. In some individuals a longer period of abstinence may be necessary. Exercise must be completely stopped; a reduction in exercise level is not sufficient to cause regression. Again, hypertrophic cardiomyopathy would not be expected to regress during abstinence from exercise.

Conduction Disturbances

Topics of aeromedical concern include the atrioventricular (AV) blocks, nonspecific intraventricular conduction delays, bundle branch blocks, hemiblocks, and axis deviation.

First Degree AV Block and Mobitz I Second Degree AV Block (Wenckebach Block)

These two findings have been reported to occur on ECG in 0.6% and 0.004% of aviators, respectively,[10] and are generally normal variants caused by increased resting vagal tone, especially in physically active individuals. No evaluation is routinely recommended for these findings, although further testing may be performed in an individual case at the discretion of the interpreting physician. Extreme degrees of these findings, such as a greatly prolonged PR interval (eg, >0.30 sec) or frequent Wenckebach episodes while awake may warrant evaluation, especially if it is a new finding or if it occurs in an older aviator (eg, over age 40). Demonstrating resolution with exercise is usually sufficient evaluation.

Mobitz II Second Degree AV Block and Third Degree (Complete) AV Block

Prevalence of these abnormalities in aviators has been reported as 0.003% and 0.004%, respectively, on resting ECG.[10] Acquired third degree block and Mobitz II second degree block put the patient at risk for continued and more advanced AV block and bradycardia-related symptoms. When considering aeromedical disposition, this risk must be considered in relation to the adequacy of heart rate and other cardiac responses to the stresses of the aviation environment. Cardiovascular compensatory mechanisms would be compromised, especially with aerobatic and some military flying.

Most authorities would consider either of these diagnoses an indication for permanent pacing. Some controversy exists regarding permanent pacing for asymptomatic Mobitz II and acquired third degree block, but the bulk of the evidence and expert opinion favors permanent pacing. This requirement for permanent pacing and the risk of sudden hemodynamic symptoms or impairment warrant permanent disqualification from flying. Aeromedical considerations of cardiac pacemakers are discussed in a later section.

Right Bundle Branch Block (RBBB)

RBBB has been reported to occur in 0.2%-0.4% of military aviators,[6,10] and prevalence in civilian populations has been reported to be 0.2%-2.0%.[10] RBBB seems to impart minimal risk of advanced conduction system disease or coronary heart disease. A study of 394 aviators with RBBB demonstrated this relative benignity.[14] Complete evaluation was performed on 372 of the 394 cases. Ninety-four percent were normal, only 3% had coronary heart disease, and 3% had other abnormalities. Over 10 years of follow-up, only 1 of the 372 aviators tested developed third degree AV block, 2 of them experienced syncope, 4% died, 6% developed coronary heart disease, and 6% developed hypertension.

There appears to be no increased risk of progressive conduction system disease, and the future occurrence of other cardiac problems is no different from that of a healthy aviator without RBBB. Consequently, no more than a noninvasive evaluation would seem warranted in an asymptomatic aviator with new RBBB. Echocardiography and graded exercise testing should be sufficient as first line testing. Twenty-four-hour ambulatory ECG monitoring might also be considered to exclude transient, more extensive conduction defects. Aviators with RBBB and no evidence of underlying cardiac disease by noninvasive testing can fly safely without restriction. Periodic reevaluation may be performed but is probably not necessary.

Left Bundle Branch Block (LBBB)

LBBB has been reported in 0.01%-0.1% of healthy military aviators and in 0.2%-0.7% of various civilian populations.[6,10] LBBB was rare in military aviators under age 35, but its prevalence increases with advancing age, as does the prevalence of coronary heart disease and hypertension. In a report of 125 military aviators with LBBB, complete evaluation of 121 of the 125 revealed no underlying disease in 101 (89%), coronary heart disease in 11 (9%), and mild to moderate hypertension in 8 (7%).[14] There was also one case of idiopathic dilated cardiomyopathy. Over 9 years of follow-up, 1 of 114 aviators developed complete heart block associated with an acute myocardial infarction, 8% died, 5% developed coronary heart disease, and 6% developed hypertension. There were also 2 new cases of symptomatic idiopathic dilated cardiomyopathy. In later USAF experience, approximately 15% of aviators with LBBB have had underlying coronary heart disease.

LBBB is more often associated with underlying cardiovascular disease than RBBB and therefore aeromedically of greater concern. At minimum, a thorough noninvasive evaluation, including nuclear or echocardiographic stress imaging, should be performed. Considering the above noted possibility of underlying coronary heart disease and the inaccuracy of many noninvasive tests in the presence of LBBB, coronary angiography might also be warranted for definitive diagnosis, especially in older or high-risk aviators. In the absence of underlying cardiac disease return to unrestricted flying is acceptable. However, although the risk of progressive conduction system disease is not increased, periodic noninvasive reevaluation as described should be performed to exclude developing cardiac disease, especially coronary heart disease and dilated cardiomyopathy. Reevaluation every 1-3 years is suggested.

Nonspecific Intraventricular Conduction Delay (IVCD)

IVCD with QRS duration less than 120 msec is considered a normal variant in an asymptomatic, apparently healthy individual. IVCD with QRS interval ≥120 msec occurred in 0.4% of aviators.[6] The QRS morphology usually resembles LBBB more than RBBB. The likelihood of underlying heart disease is uncertain for an IVCD with QRS ≥120 msec duration. Therefore, the aeromedical significance of this finding is unclear, but it is of more concern if it is a new finding in an older aviator rather than an extant condition of long standing, or an isolated finding in a young aviator. When underlying heart disease is present, there is often associated cardiomegaly, so it is prudent to further evaluate aviators with this finding. Echocardiography for younger aviators (ie, age <35 years) or echocardiography plus graded exercise testing with nuclear or echocardiographic stress imaging is probably sufficient to exclude underlying heart disease. Twenty-four-hour ambulatory ECG monitoring might also be considered. In the absence of underlying cardiac disease, return to unrestricted flying is acceptable. There are few if any reports regarding the long-term prognosis of IVCD with QRS duration of 120 msec or longer. Periodic reevaluation, as recommended above for LBBB, therefore seems to be aeromedically prudent.

Left Anterior and Posterior Hemiblocks (LAHB, LPHB) and Bifascicular Block

Prevalence of LAHB and LPHB was reported as 0.9% and 0.1%, respectively, in one study of military aviators[6]; in another study of military aviators the prevalence of each type of hemiblock was only 0.01%.[14] In civilian populations, LAHB has been reported in 1%-14%.[10] Prognosis appears to be good in individuals with LAHB or LPHB if no underlying heart disease is found after a thorough noninvasive evaluation.

For the purpose of this discussion, bifascicular block is defined as RBBB plus either LAHB or LPHB. Prevalence figures for bifascicular block in aviators or healthy populations are not readily available. However, in the above referenced study of 394 military aviators with RBBB, the incidence of cardiac disease was no different for RBBB with normal axis versus RBBB with LAHB or LPHB (bifascicular block).[14]

Thus, LAHB, LPHB, and bifascicular block do not seem to carry an increased risk of cardiac death or other adverse events in otherwise normal individuals. Noninvasive evaluation as recommended above for RBBB is therefore likely to be sufficient. However, most clinical references ascribe a higher likelihood of underlying cardiac disease for both types of hemiblock than for RBBB with normal axis. A more thorough noninvasive evaluation, such as that recommended above for non-specific IVCD, might therefore be preferred, especially for military aviators or higher-risk civilian aviators. Periodic reevaluation would also then be indicated. If isolated LAHB or LPHB occurs in a young aviator (eg, age 30-35 years or less) with a low cardiac risk profile, graded exercise testing is unlikely to be helpful.

Axis Deviation

As reported, left axis deviation (LAD) occurred in 0.9% of aviators and right axis deviation (RAD) in 0.07%.[6] Due to different criteria for simple axis deviation versus hemiblocks, the literature on these two findings is probably quite mixed. The primary aeromedical concern would again be presence of underlying cardiac disease, and, for RAD, pulmonary disease. Emphasis should be placed on comparison with prior ECGs. Gradual leftward axis shift over time is often a normal occurrence of advancing age, but an abrupt axis shift compared to prior ECGs may be more compelling for further assessment.

A report on 69 consecutive military aviation training candidates who had echocardiography performed to evaluate RAD >95 degrees found only one candidate with a disqualifying cardiac finding, a large atrial septal defect also detectable by abnormal auscultatory findings.[15] In a cohort of 1700 Japan Airlines pilots 35 years of age or older, 30 were found to have marked LAD (axis more negative than −30 degrees), a prevalence of 1.8%.[16] Average age at the time of initial employment with Japan Airlines was about 22 years and mean follow-up was 22.6 years. Marked LAD was present at the time of initial employment in 12 of 30 (40%); the other 18 initially had a normal axis (6/30, 20%), or mild LAD (12/30, 40%, axis 0 to −30 degrees). During follow-up there were no cardiac events or new cardiac diagnoses in the 30 aviators except for two cases of borderline hypertension. One of these two also had mild left ventricular hypertrophy on echocardiography. In addition to periodic examinations and ECGs, all 30 had graded exercise testing without evidence of ischemia and 26/30 had echocardiography. On routine serial ECGs 70% (21/30) demonstrated a progressive leftward axis shift with advancing age.

History should exclude pulmonary disease of any aeromedical or clinical significance, but chest x-ray and spirometry are certainly easily obtained if needed. Echocardiography and, in the case of LAD, graded exercise testing, should be adequate to exclude underlying cardiac disease. If LAD is present in a young aviator (age 30-35 or less) with a low cardiac risk profile, graded exercise testing is unlikely to be helpful. If evaluation discloses no underlying disease, unrestricted flying without need for future reassessment is advised.

Supraventricular and Ventricular Ectopy

Isolated ectopy and paired ectopy (couplets) on an ECG includes premature supraventricular and premature ventricular contractions (PVC). In this discussion, the term ectopy will refer to both supraventricular and ventricular *ectopy* unless otherwise specified. Supraventricular ectopy includes premature atrial contractions (PAC) and premature junctional contractions. The term *PAC* will be used to refer to all supraventricular ectopy. If isolated or paired ectopy itself causes hemodynamic symptoms, then aeromedical disposition is determined by the symptoms as well as by the presence and severity of underlying heart disease. In the absence of hemodynamic symptoms, there are two basic aeromedical concerns regarding isolated and paired ectopy: Is the ECG ectopy predictive of sustained tachyarrhythmias, and is it predictive of underlying disease? If the answer to these two questions is no, then there really is no basis for aeromedical concern. On 12-lead ECG, PACs occurred in about 0.6% of aviators and 0.4%-3.0% of civilian populations. PVCs occurred in about 0.8% of aviators and 2.0%-7.0% of various civilian populations.[6,10]

In a study of 430 military aviators evaluated for nonsustained or sustained supraventricular tachycardia (SVT), neither frequent PACs, PAC pairing, nor nonsustained SVT was predictive of hemodynamically symptomatic SVT or of recurrent sustained SVT.[17] In a similar study of 193 military aviators with nonsustained ventricular tachycardia, neither frequent PVCs nor PVC pairing predicted sustained ventricular tachycardia, or associated hemodynamic events of sudden death, syncope, or presyncope.[18] Data from these two reports indicates that frequent isolated ectopy and paired ectopy do not present an increased risk for sustained supraventricular or ventricular tachycardias.

The predictive value of supraventricular or ventricular ectopy on ECG for underlying cardiac disease is less clear. The considerable frequency and variability of ectopy in normal subjects makes it difficult to determine its predictive value for disease. PACs may occur in association with some disease states, such as mitral valve prolapse, but prognosis is not related to the PACs. On the other hand, frequent and complex PVCs in the presence of coronary and some other heart diseases clearly confer a poorer prognosis. In an aeromedical context, one might evaluate ECG ectopy with 24-hour ambulatory monitoring, and pursue further evaluation (eg, with echocardiography and graded exercise test) based on the frequency and complexity of ectopy found on the ambulatory monitoring, and on other evidence of disease from history and examination. Alternatively, one might restrict such investigation to aviators at increased cardiac risk based on age, gender, and classic risk factors.

Pending more information from the aviator population, it is suggested that ectopy on ECG be evaluated by 24-hour ambulatory monitoring. Rare or occasional ectopy (≤1% of total beats on ambulatory monitoring) would not warrant further evaluation or any restriction of flight duty. Further assessment could be limited to aviators with frequent ectopy (>1% of total beats) or any pairing occurring on ambulatory monitoring. Adequate assessment would include echocardiography and graded exercise testing. More extensive noninvasive evaluation might be considered for very frequent ectopy (>10% of total beats) or frequent pairing (>10 pairs total) on ambulatory monitoring. If there are no associated hemodynamic symptoms and the noninvasive evaluation discloses no underlying cardiac disease, then continuation of unrestricted flying is acceptable. Periodic reevaluation may be considered for very frequent ectopy and for frequent pairing.

Possible Myocardial Ischemia

ECG changes suggestive of myocardial infarction should be investigated, with the extent of investigation dependent on the degree of certainty of the ECG changes. Comparison with prior ECGs is very helpful. Graded exercise testing is often performed for evaluation, but it is not a good choice as the sole test; it is quite possible to have had a prior myocardial infarction and still have a normal treadmill. One would only be testing for residual ischemic lesions, not the presence of an infarction. Echocardiography to detect abnormal regional wall motion or a radionuclide myocardial perfusion scan to detect a resting perfusion defect would be more appropriate to diagnose or exclude myocardial infarction. A more comprehensive evaluation would include stress echocardiography or exercise radionuclide perfusion scan to exclude both myocardial infarction and residual ischemia. Even ECG changes considered diagnostic of myocardial infarction should be further evaluated prior to definitive aeromedical disposition.

A more common ECG dilemma would be small, nondiagnostic Q waves in the inferior leads and poor R wave progression in the anterior precordial leads. These findings might be due to myocardial infarction, but are more likely normal variants or caused by lead misplacement. They may nevertheless require clarification. Comparison with old ECGs and prudent judgment should determine whether and to what extent an evaluation should be performed. For poor R wave progression, a reasonable initial step would be repeat ECG with careful attention to proper placement of the precordial leads. The above noted noninvasive testing may be necessary in selected instances.

ST-T wave changes indicating possible myocardial ischemia may also warrant further investigation. Two previous studies of aviator ECGs reported ST-T wave changes in 0.9% of military aviators and T wave changes in 1.2% of military aviators, respectively.[5,6] ST-T wave changes are a very nonspecific finding in asymptomatic subjects, yet ST changes do have some predictive value for underlying coronary heart disease. This is particularly true if the ST changes are new compared to prior ECGs. Unfortunately, the incidence of both coronary heart disease and ST-T abnormalities increases with age. Published medical guidelines recommend a baseline screening ECG in asymptomatic subjects of any age whose cardiovascular performance is linked to public safety (eg, aviators), and regular follow-up ECGs in asymptomatic subjects older than 40 years.[9] Periodic screening ECGs due to occupational indications are therefore reasonable.

The disposition of ST-T changes should be guided by the aviator's age and risk profile for coronary heart disease. Menstruating females and males younger than age 35-40 with a low risk profile are unlikely to have coronary heart disease and further evaluation may be unnecessary. Further noninvasive testing should be considered for young males with a high coronary risk profile, males older than 35-40 years, and postmenopausal female aviators with *new* ST-T wave changes. ST-T wave changes may be transient and caused by a variety of factors, including the nonfasting state. First, determine that the changes are new compared to prior ECGs. If so, the ECG should be repeated, ensuring that it is done in the fasting state. If the changes persist, then further noninvasive testing to exclude coronary heart disease should be considered. The reader is referred to the next section for a discussion of the screening tests available and their predictive values.

Screening for Coronary Artery Disease

Introduction

This section will not discuss the pros and cons of screening for coronary heart disease (CHD). Assuming that there are indications, or at least a perceived need, to screen some groups of aviators for asymptomatic or subclinical CHD, this section will briefly discuss the concept and review some commonly used tests that might be used for CHD screening of aviators. Screening for a disease, CHD in this case, implies that the subjects under consideration are asymptomatic and do not appear to have CHD. Screening is generally inappropriate unless identification of the disease in its early, asymptomatic state may lead to therapy that may improve the clinical prognosis. Early detection of asymptomatic CHD fits this criterion, and it has significant potential to improve health because primary and secondary prevention of CHD are effective in many risk groups. Also, the initial clinical presentation of CHD is often abrupt and catastrophic, eg, sudden cardiac death and myocardial infarction. In aviation medicine, identifying the aviator with asymptomatic significant CHD and terminating or restricting his flight duties might be considered a "therapeutic intervention" with potential to improve occupational outcome.

Before considering a CHD screening program for an aviator population, one must answer several questions. ***First,*** what tests are available for CHD screening? Screening tests should be readily available and locally accessible to the AME/FS and the aviator being screened. They should also be relatively inexpensive. ***Second,*** how accurate are these tests? What is the positive predictive value of an abnormal/positive test? ***Third,*** what course of action will be taken for those with abnormal tests? Risk factor management, more extensive noninvasive evaluation, and diagnostic coronary angiography are all options. ***Fourth,*** should the entire aviator population be screened? Or should the population be stratified into higher-risk subsets for screening? What is the impact of risk stratification for CHD screening?

Significant CHD is generally defined as at least one atherosclerotic lesion causing a 50% or greater reduction of coronary artery diameter, as diagnosed by coronary angiography. Classically, CHD screening has been used to detect asymptomatic significant CHD. Traditional screening tests such as the treadmill or cycle ergometer detect stress-induced myocardial ischemia, which is caused by significant lesions. However, there may be aeromedical (and clinical) value to detect early, nonsignificant CHD lesions as well. It is now well known that myocardial infarctions and unstable angina frequently occur at the site of nonsignificant lesions (<50% reduction of coronary artery diameter). Also, the expected natural history for nonsignificant CHD would be progression to significant CHD. And one might expect more favorable results of risk factor modification if it is begun early, when the CHD is non-significant, prior to the onset of symptoms or other clinical presentation.

Screening Tests

Electrocardiography

Electrocardiography (ECG) is very nonspecific as a screen for CHD but has nevertheless traditionally been a fundamental part of routine surveillance programs in aviators. Published guidelines for the performance of ECGs recommend screening ECGs in persons over age 40.[9] As noted earlier, in the ECG abnormalities section, nonspecific ST-T wave changes have been shown to increase with advancing age, as does the incidence of CHD. Forty publications were reviewed to address the utility of ECG as a screening tool.[19] Although Q waves and nonspecific ST-T waves had a relative risk of CHD mortality up to 4.6, the reviewers concluded that ECG was of screening value only in the presence of significant CHD risk factors. In a report of 16,000 ECGs performed on 14,000 aviators and air traffic controllers, minor ST-T wave changes in 103 subjects were investigated with graded exercise testing, and 19 were found to be abnormal.[20] Eleven of the 19 had no further evaluation, and 5 of the remaining 8 were subsequently shown to have CHD. In spite of the association of advancing age, CHD, and ECG changes, the resting ECG is not a valuable screening tool. It is probably more appropriate to consider the ECG an extension of the cardiac history and physical examination, similar to laboratory testing for lipid profiles. Along with classic CHD risk factors, the ECG may help to identify a subset of higher-risk aviators for whom CHD screening might be performed.

Graded Exercise Testing

Graded exercise testing with treadmill or cycle ergometry and ECG monitoring is the classic test for CHD screening and likely the most commonly used modality after history, physical examination, lipid profile, and ECG. A committee of experts published guidelines for the performance of exercise testing, giving a Class II recommendation for screening exercise testing in males over age 40 and women over age 50 who are engaged in special occupations in which impairment might impact public safety.[21] A Class II recommendation means that the committee review found conflicting evidence and/or had a divergence of opinion about the usefulness or efficacy of the procedure. In other words, some, but not all, of the committee members felt that these were appropriate indications for exercise testing. Earlier guidelines published in 1986 also reviewed the literature on screening exercise testing, reporting that the positive predictive value of an abnormal treadmill test for significant CHD in men averaged about 21%, with values ranging from 5%-46%, but in most studies were less than 25%.[22] Their findings were similar to those of the later guidelines—a Class II recommendation for men over age 40 with 2 or more additional risk factors or engaged in a special occupation that might impact public safety. These recommendations from two panels of experts and the heightened aeromedical concern about CHD support the use of screening exercise testing in selected circumstances.

However, the poor yield of exercise testing due to the relatively low prevalence of CHD in the healthy aviator population must be recognized. In an 8-year follow-up report of 548 military aviators who had graded exercise testing, only 4.2% (23/548) had an abnormal test,[23] and clinically evident CHD developed in 6.9% (38/548). Sensitivity and positive predictive value of an abnormal treadmill test to detect these events was only 16% and 26%, respectively. Another group of researchers similarly followed 1390 military aviators for 6 years after exercise testing.[24] An abnormal test had only a 20% probability for development of clinical CHD. And a third report followed 888 men and women for 5 years after a screening treadmill test.[25] In women and in men age 40 or younger, classic abnormal ST segment depression on treadmill test was of no value for predicting subsequent CHD; in men over age 40, the positive predictive value was 17%.

Other experience with military aviators has demonstrated similar positive predictive values for angiographic CHD. In unselected male aviators, an abnormal screening treadmill test had only a 10% positive predictive value for significant CHD at angiography.[26] And an abnormal screening treadmill test performed on male aviators with new ST-T wave changes on routine ECG was only 25% predictive of angiographic significant CHD.

The positive predictive value of an abnormal treadmill test for angiographic or clinically significant CHD in an asymptomatic male aviator would seem then to be only about 20%-25%. Results for cycle ergometry would presumably be similar. These relatively poor results for screening treadmill tests are a marked contrast to results with angina populations, an expected consequence of testing an asymptomatic population with a relatively low prevalence of CHD. Nevertheless, graded exercise testing remains the fundamental screening tool for CHD and it is also readily available and relatively inexpensive.

Imaging for Coronary Artery Calcification

Detection of coronary artery calcification adds an additional dimension to CHD screening. Whereas other testing modalities attempt to detect evidence of transient myocardial ischemia induced by exertion (a physiologic or functional test), detection of coronary calcification is more an anatomic or structural test, detecting calcification in existing atherosclerotic plaques regardless of the severity of luminal stenosis. Coronary calcium detection has potential value for predicting the presence of both significant and nonsignificant CHD in asymptomatic subjects. Although detection of coronary calcium by electron beam computed tomography (EBCT) has been a topic of great interest in the recent literature, this concept is far from new. Detection of coronary calcification by standard, image-intensified fluoroscopic examination (coronary artery fluoroscopy or CAF) has been used as a diagnostic tool since the 1960s and is relatively accurate at predicting the presence of some degree of CHD. But CAF is much less helpful in predicting severity of disease.

In an era when interest favored detecting and treating significant disease, CAF was largely abandoned by clinicians in favor of exercise testing and other physiologic tests designed to detect myocardial ischemia. In a report of CAF experience, 1466 military aviators were screened by CAF and 613 subsequently had coronary angiography for abnormal CAF, treadmill exercise test, and/or exercise thallium scintigraphy.[27] The positive predictive value of CAF was 38% for significant CHD and 69% for any measurable CHD (nonsignificant and significant). Even in the subset with positive CAF but normal treadmill test and normal thallium scintigraphy, 27% had significant CHD. For any measurable CHD, the positive predictive values of treadmill and thallium scintigraphy were only 33% and 35%, respectively; the data presented did not allow calculation of positive predictive values of these two tests for significant CHD.

The interest in primary prevention of CHD and the ability of EBCT to detect and quantitate coronary calcium burden has dramatically changed views and practices about CHD screening. Calcium burden, assessed by EBCT as a calcium score, may predict future cardiac events and both the presence and severity of angiographic disease. At the time of this writing we are seeing an explosion of interest, research, and literature regarding the correlation of EBCT with both coronary angiographic findings and CHD events. It is not surprising that most of the literature involves symptomatic or older, high-risk patients, given the high prevalence of disease in such populations. The role of EBCT in screening younger, healthy, asymptomatic populations (eg, aviators) for CHD has yet to be determined, but it is extremely promising. The United States Army has recently begun a long-term follow-up study to help define the role of EBCT in predicting cardiac events in young asymptomatic military personnel.[28] While this is not an aviator population, the demographics are very applicable to aviators—apparently healthy military personnel aged 40-45.

Again, a screening test should be relatively inexpensive and readily accessible to the physician and patient. At a cost of less than $500, EBCT probably meets the former criterion, but it is not readily accessible to all aviators and the servicing AME/FS. This will probably change in the near future as this field rapidly develops. Both the clinical and aeromedical communities are eagerly awaiting further definition of the role of EBCT for screening asymptomatic individuals.

Stress Radionuclide Imaging

Thallium exercise scintigraphy and other methods of radionuclide stress imaging are not usually considered first level screening tests, but rather second level tests done after an initial abnormal screening test such as a treadmill test. However, it is advisable to briefly address these tests in reference to aviators. One study evaluated planar thallium exercise scintigraphy in 845 asymptomatic male military aviators undergoing coronary angiography for abnormal noninvasive tests suggesting CHD.[29] The positive predictive value of abnormal thallium scintigraphy for significant CHD was only 25%, a value identical to that of graded exercise testing as discussed above.

Single photon emission computed tomography (SPECT) is a more recently used imaging technique most authorities consider to be more accurate than planar imaging, but there are few, if any, reports regarding its predictive value in large groups of asymptomatic aviators.

Stress Echocardiography

Stress echocardiography, like radionuclide imaging, is also best considered a second level screening test. Stress echocardiography has better sensitivity and specificity than graded exercise testing and is comparable to radionuclide imaging in most reports. In a recent review of stress echocardiography, the sensitivity of treadmill or cycle ergometry stress echocardiography for significant CHD ranged from 74%-97%, and specificity ranged from 64%-96%.[30] But stress echocardiography is less accurate for detecting single vessel CHD, moderate CHD lesions, and CHD without prior infarction. Unfortunately, these categories of CHD are more likely in the asymptomatic aviator than severe stenoses, multivessel disease, and prior infarctions. Sensitivity for single vessel disease ranged between 33% and 92%, and for subjects without prior infarction between 53% and 91%.

Compared to stress echocardiography, exercise radionuclide imaging with SPECT is more sensitive for detection of single vessel and moderate disease, but has lower specificity. These studies involve symptomatic, clinical patient populations. There are no published data for stress echocardiography in aviator populations. If used for screening asymptomatic aviators, both stress echocardiography and stress radionuclide imaging will suffer from the same problem as graded exercise testing—relatively poor positive predictive value due to relatively low prevalence of CHD.

Noninvasive Coronary Angiography

This final element in CHD screening is mentioned only to pique the reader's interest—coronary angiography by EBCT, magnetic resonance angiography (MRA), or other as yet undeveloped techniques to noninvasively image the coronary arteries.

In the relatively near future it should be possible to obtain images of the coronary artery system by EBCT or MRA and exclude or diagnose significant CHD with high reliability compared to standard invasive coronary angiography. What role will this assume in an asymptomatic aviator population? As this technology matures and becomes more available, aviation licensing authorities will have to decide what level of accuracy compared to the gold standard of coronary angiography is acceptable for their particular aviation environments. Another issue would be whether it is acceptable to detect or exclude only significant disease, or if the presence of non-significant disease must also be determined, for example, in aerobatic or high-performance jet pilots with high CHD risk profiles.

Risk Stratification

The prevalence of CHD in an asymptomatic military aviator population is low, probably less than 10%, more likely on the order of 5%, because of the high physical standards set for military service and aviation and the relatively younger age and overall good health of military aviators. Commercial civilian pilots and certainly civilian private pilots may have a prevalence of CHD closer to that of the general population. Nevertheless, performing screening tests in any unselected aviator population will yield many "false positive" tests and a low predictive value for significant CHD. This poor performance is due to the low prevalence of the disease sought, and not to inadequacy of the test itself or of the providers performing and interpreting the tests.

Sensitivity and specificity of screening treadmill tests are about 60% and 90%, respectively. In a hypothetical population with a significant CHD prevalence of 50%, treadmill testing would then have a positive predictive value of 86% for significant CHD. However, in a population with a prevalence of only 5%, an abnormal screening treadmill would be only 24% predictive of significant CHD. This has obvious implications for unnecessary subsequent testing, including invasive coronary angiography.

Risk stratifying the aviator population prior to performing screening tests is necessary to improve positive predictive value. As noted above, performing screening treadmill tests in unselected asymptomatic male military aviators has a very poor predictive value (10%) for angiographic significant CHD. Even this group was minimally risk stratified by gender (male only) and age (37 years or older). Stratifying the population further to include only those with new resting ST-T wave changes on ECG improved positive predictive value to 25%. Further analysis of subgroups by number of classic CHD risk factors yielded positive predictive values of an abnormal treadmill test ranging from 9%-64%.[26] The review of thallium scintigraphy discussed earlier provides a similar example of this lesson.[29] The positive predictive value of an abnormal thallium scintigram in asymptomatic male aviators was only 25% overall for significant CHD, but the positive predictive value ranged from 8%-43% across different subgroups stratified by age and the ratio of total cholesterol to HDL cholesterol.

From these brief observations, it is clear that if one contemplates CHD screening for asymptomatic aviator populations or for an individual aviator, these issues of disease prevalence and predictive values of the tests used must be carefully considered. For a given military or civilian aviation environment, one must strive to appropriately balance the ability to both detect disease and to exclude nondisease. History, physical examination, ECG, and assessment of classic CHD risk factors are the appropriate tools for risk stratifying aviators prior to performance of screening tests.

In an excellent overview of the considerations involved in designing an effective CHD screening program, the reviewers stated that identifying atherosclerotic plaque, such as by detection of coronary calcification, should be more successful than tests that detect the effects of ischemia, although these tests are useful in identifying severe disease.[31] They concluded by suggesting the use of a combination of coronary artery calcification detection and graded exercise testing as a sensible screening method. The United States Army has used such a program with its aviators for several years. Risk stratification is performed at the time of routine flight physical examination, with total cholesterol, ratio of total cholesterol to HDL cholesterol, and a calculated Framingham risk index. If the male aviator fails the specified threshold of any 1 or more of these 3 parameters, and is over age 40, then local health care providers perform a graded exercise test and CAF for detection of coronary artery calcification. In this program, the positive predictive value of CAF has been 83% for measurable CHD and 46% for significant CHD. Corresponding values for treadmill test were 53% and 32%, respectively.[32] These excellent results of screening tests are the product of well conceived and implemented risk stratification prior to testing.

Coronary Heart Disease

A Review

Introduction

Atherosclerotic coronary heart disease (CHD) is a leading cause of morbidity and mortality in industrialized nations. This fact alone should make CHD a primary health concern of the AME/FS. And its modes of presentation (sudden cardiac death, myocardial infarction, unstable and stable angina, and ischemic arrhythmias) are certainly of paramount concern because of possible sudden incapacitation or performance decrement. Therefore, CHD is undoubtedly one of the most common and important topics of aeromedical decision making.

CHD is also a leading cause of denial or loss of licensure in both civilian and military aviators. In a report on permanent groundings and restricted flying qualifications in Canadian Forces military aviators over a 10-year period, CHD was the most common disqualifying diagnosis.[33] CHD accounted for 25% of all permanent groundings, and other cardiovascular disorders accounted for an additional 17%.

Background prevalence rates for clinically manifest CHD in some general populations, by age and gender groupings, are available in the literature but may not be applicable to the overall healthier aviator population. Although the aviator lifestyle is often said to be conducive to poor health habits, in countries where CHD is a prominent health problem, aviators tend to be healthier than the general population. This is due to many factors, including better education, higher socioeconomic status, better information on the health benefits of proper diet and exercise, and greater motivation to pursue a healthy lifestyle. In countries where CHD is less of a health problem, the health parameters of aviators often more closely reflect those of their general populations.

Autopsy reports of 710 commercial pilots involved in fatal aviation accidents were reviewed.[34] Some degree of coronary atherosclerosis was present in 69%, but it was considered severe in only 2.5%. Prevalence of severe disease increased with age, from 0.6% in pilots younger than age 40, up to 7.4% in pilots aged 50 years or older. Another study reviewed autopsy findings of 288 aviators killed in aircraft accidents, including military, commercial, and private aviators, and compared them to a control group of 132 apparently healthy males aged 18-62 years who suffered accidental deaths.[35] Prevalence of significant CHD was not substantially different among the four groups—17% in military aviators, 24.5% in commercial aviators, 22% in private aviators, and 18% in the control group. Mean ages for the four groups were 29.1, 39.7, 37.2, and 29.9 years, respectively.

Mortality statistics from 1952 through 1988 for 2327 Japan Airlines aviators were compared to those of the general Japanese population.[36] Leading causes of death were accidental trauma, malignancy, and cardiovascular disease. Total mortality was significantly lower in the aviators. Accidental deaths were significantly higher, malignancy deaths were similar, and cardiovascular deaths were lower in the aviators compared to the general population. Another study reported cardiac events (myocardial infarction, angina, and sudden cardiac death) occurring from 1988 through 1992 in apparently healthy military aviators on unrestricted flying status.[37] Five-year average annual event rates by age group were 0.0054% (30-34 years), 0.018% (35-39 years), 0.038% (40-44 years), 0.14% (45-49 years), and 0.13% (50-54 years). The overall average was 0.02% per year. The mean age of aviators suffering a cardiac event was 44 years (range, 31-53). Most disturbing was the finding that 82% of the events were myocardial infarction (61%) or sudden cardiac death (21%); only 18% presented as angina. This suggests a serious problem with underreporting or denial of angina by this aviator population.

These studies provide ample evidence that CHD certainly warrants consideration in any discussion of aeromedical dispositions. Following a brief review of natural history, long-term outcome data will be discussed for normal coronary angiography populations, clinically nonsignificant CHD and significant CHD.

Natural History

Clinical literature focuses primarily on cardiac death, sudden death, and fatal and nonfatal myocardial infarction as clinical endpoints. Depending on the particular aviation environment, aeromedical endpoints may include these, along with unstable or stable angina, heart failure, progression of disease (worsening of existing lesions and development of new significant lesions), need for revascularization, and use of antianginal medications. Therapy of CHD includes medications and revascularization, with choice of therapy depending primarily on the extent of CHD as assessed by angiography, the status of left ventricular function, and severity of symptoms. Revascularization, whether by surgery or catheter-based technique (eg, angioplasty, stent), is a unique topic unto itself and will be discussed separately.

Normal Coronary Angiography. Several groups have reported long-term studies of populations with normal coronary angiography, demonstrating annual cardiac event rates of 0%-0.65% per year over approximately 10 years of follow-up.[38-40] Events in these reports are generally sudden cardiac death, fatal and nonfatal myocardial infarction, and development of angina with documented significant CHD. In the United States, various population studies report annual cardiac event rates of about 0.5% per year for apparently healthy males aged 35-54 years. And as noted above, annual event rates for apparently healthy male military aviators have been reported as less than 0.15% per year for the same age range.[37] Along with the selected threshold (eg, 1% per year), these event rates may be compared to event rates in clinical and aviator cohorts with nonsignificant and significant CHD.

Nonsignificant CHD. On coronary angiography, lesions are graded by the percentage of reduction in diameter of the vessel lumen by comparing the minimum lumen diameter of the lesion to the lumen diameter of the adjacent normal artery segment. The percentage of reduction of the lesion increases with increasing severity. For example, a 20% lesion is mild CHD, representing only a 20% reduction in diameter of the vessel lumen, whereas a 90% lesion is severe CHD, representing a 90% reduction in diameter of the vessel lumen. Anatomically significant disease is generally considered to be one or more lesions of 50% or greater diameter reduction.

Discussions in this text referring to **_significant_** CHD use this definition. **_Nonsignificant_** CHD then refers to a lesion of less than 50% reduction in diameter. Annual event rates for established CHD progressively increase with increased severity of disease, even within the range of clinically nonsignificant disease. Therefore, one must consider event rates of different categories of severity of CHD—nonsignificant (often termed mild or minimal) CHD with worst lesion less than 50%, and significant CHD with worst lesion 50% or greater. Even within these two categories of CHD, annual event rates increase with increasing severity of disease as determined both by maximum single stenosis and total number of lesions or coronary arteries affected.

Long-term studies of nonsignificant CHD patients report annual cardiac event rates of about 1.5%-3.0% per year over approximately 10 years of follow-up in different subcategories of nonsignificant CHD.[39] Unfortunately, some of these studies include maximum lesions of 50% in their cohort, a lesion severity generally considered and defined in this text as significant disease. It is interesting that noninvasive test results (eg, abnormal treadmill, abnormal thallium scintigram) at the time of index catheterization do not predict future CHD events or survival for patients with nonsignificant CHD. Rather, classic CHD risk factors and the extent of nonsignificant CHD at index coronary angiography predict future events.

This range of annual cardiac event rates for nonsignificant CHD may not be applicable to the aviator, especially the asymptomatic aviator with nonsignificant CHD diagnosed as a result of the careful aeromedical scrutiny of periodic flight examinations or a formal CHD screening program. These clinical cohorts predominantly involve patients with a chest pain syndrome that ultimately prompted coronary angiography for definitive diagnosis. Aviator population characteristics that might result in a lower annual event rate for similar anatomic disease include relatively younger age, fewer comorbid diagnoses, better CHD risk profiles, and absence of angina. Annual cardiac event rates in some military aviators with nonsignificant CHD have been reported as less than 1% per year.[41] In the subset with a maximum lesion of 40% stenosis, annual cardiac event rates were 0.6% and 0.4% per year at 5 and 10 years of follow-up, respectively, with no cardiac deaths.

Figures limited to survival also demonstrate a graded prognosis depending on severity of disease. One study demonstrated 96% survival at 7 years for normal coronary angiography versus 92% survival for CHD with worst lesion less than 50%.[42] Another study reported 99.2% survival at 10 years for normal angiography or worst lesion less than 30%, but 83.5% survival for CHD with worst lesion 30%-50%.[39] And a third study reported a 10-year survival of 98% for CHD with maximum lesion less than 25% versus 90% survival for a 25%-50% maximum lesion.[43] A very thorough and excellent review of the natural history of CHD from an aeromedical perspective focused primarily on survival and included many of these same references.[44] The authors concluded that aviators with CHD with maximum lesion less than 50%, no evidence of ischemia, and normal left ventricular function, could be considered for special issuance to fly as or with copilot. Data regarding the ischemic potential and danger of nonsignificant disease in the high $+G_z$ cockpit is lacking, but several factors warrant disqualification from high $+G_z$ flight. Among these are the uncertainty of risk itself, the fact that these aircraft (except for trainers) are usually single seat, the increased cardiac demands of high $+G_z$, and the awareness that acute events often occur with nonsignificant stenoses and that asymptomatic progression to significant disease may occur.

Significant CHD. The prognosis of significant CHD is more widely studied and reported than that of nonsignificant CHD because it is of greater interest to the clinician. Again, these clinical cohorts are predominantly symptomatic (angina) and many of the study subjects have had a prior myocardial infarction. Event rates depend on how many of the 3 major coronary arteries are involved, the presence or absence of left main coronary artery disease, and the status of left ventricular function. In the cardiac literature, annual ***mortality*** rates for all categories of medically treated significant CHD are approximately 3.0%-3.5% per year over 10 years of follow-up.[45-47]

For the purpose of aeromedical disposition, however, one should examine the better prognostic subgroups—normal left ventricular function (especially without prior myocardial infarction) and single or double vessel disease. Annual ***event*** rates for the best comparison significant CHD subgroups from these referenced reports are approximately 3.0%-7.5% per year at 3, 5, and 10 years of follow-up.[45-47] These events include cardiac death, myocardial infarction, and angina requiring revascularization. Certainly the excluded events of stable angina, new onset angina, and medically controlled angina would also be of aeromedical concern. A related aeromedical concern would be the impact of significant CHD on exercise tolerance and other measures of physical endurance and performance ability, particularly for military aviators. Annual cardiac event rates of asymptomatic military aviators with a maximum lesion of only 50%, and with normal left ventricular function, but no prior myocardial infarction, have been reported as 2.9% and 2.3% per year at 5 and 10 years of follow-up, respectively.[41]

Progression of Angiographic CHD. A major aeromedical concern regarding CHD is progression of disease—the progression of existing nonsignificant lesions to significant lesions and the development of new significant lesions. One of the most compelling demonstrations of this problem comes from a revascularization trial.[48] The investigators compared late outcomes of treatment with medical therapy alone versus angioplasty or bypass surgery in patients with significant single vessel disease of the proximal left anterior descending coronary artery, stable angina, and normal left ventricular function. Per study design, most of the study subjects also had follow-up coronary angiography 2 years after their index angiography and treatment randomization. A new significant lesion in a previously normal coronary artery segment appeared in 36% of medical therapy subjects, 36% of angioplasty subjects, and 29% of bypass surgery subjects within only 2 years.

Similar progression rates are documented for nonsignificant CHD in chest pain populations.[39,40,49,50] The progression rates in most studies are difficult to interpret, however, because most of the subjects did not have follow-up angiography. Routine repeat angiography was not part of the study protocol; the procedure was performed only for clinical indications. The progression rates reported in the revascularization trial described above are more reliable because repeat angiography was part of the original study design.[48] What is lacking for aeromedical purposes is progression rates in a large cohort of aviators with nonsignificant CHD.

Post Myocardial Infarction. The existence of myocardial infarction would seem to imply underlying significant CHD. However, it has been proven that infarction is often caused by an insignificant lesion, although significant lesions are frequently present in other coronary arteries. If significant CHD is present at other sites, then the prognosis indicated by the anatomy, with and without infarction, should determine aeromedical disposition. Isolated nonsignificant CHD with myocardial infarction puts the aviator at higher risk than asymptomatic nonsignificant CHD without any prior cardiac events. Another aeromedical concern postinfarction is the status of left ventricular function and possible ventricular arrhythmias.

A cohort of 799 patients with myocardial infarction treated with thrombolysis was followed for an average 1.6 years.[51] In subjects with a residual infarction lesion of less than 50% stenosis, 2.4% died and 5% experienced recurrent myocardial infarction. In those with a significant residual lesion of 50% or greater stenosis, 3.5% died and 5% had a second infarction. Some subjects with a residual stenosis less than 50% had significant disease elsewhere, but 35% of them had no significant disease elsewhere, and 47% had significant disease in only one artery. In another report of 74 patients with myocardial infarction and normal coronary angiography, 15% died during a mean follow-up of 10.5 years.[52] Most deaths (9/11) were cardiovascular and 6 were sudden. A second myocardial infarction occurred in 2 survivors and in 3 non-survivors. And in a report on 145 U.S. Navy pilots suffering a cardiovascular disease event or diagnosis, 58/145 had an acute myocardial infarction or chronic ischemic heart disease.[53] Subsequent death, hospitalization, or physical disability occurred in 40% with infarction and 57% with chronic ischemia, usually within 1 year of the incident event. Another consideration in aeromedical disposition is that most clinical guidelines recommend at least beta-blocker therapy and often ACE inhibitor therapy as standard care after myocardial infarction. Use of these medications would also be a consideration in any policy regarding flight certification.

Summary and Aeromedical Recommendations

Use of antianginal medications (long-acting nitrates, calcium channel antagonists, beta-blockers, and short-acting sublingual nitroglycerin) must be carefully considered in the aviator. Certainly these medications may cause side effects, including subtle effects on performance, in the individual aviator. Also, their use for the treatment of angina implies an underlying active ischemia substrate, and the presence of this underlying ischemia may preclude a return to flight duty. Current licensing policies for civilian aviation operations generally reflect this opinion. Special issuance policies generally require there be no evidence of ischemia by symptoms or exercise testing, with the exercise testing performed off cardioactive medications. Medication use is discussed further in a later section of this chapter. In the recommendations suggested below for the aeromedical disposition of CHD, with or without revascularization, medical therapy for the treatment of ischemic symptoms is not recommended for any category of flying.

However, some allowance might be made to use these medications for indications other than treatment of ischemic symptoms. For example, beta-blockers and calcium channel antagonists might be appropriately used for treatment of coexisting hypertension. And most treatment guidelines recommend use of beta-blockers and possibly ACE inhibitors routinely after myocardial infarction for prognostic indications. Aspirin is aeromedically acceptable and should generally be used in all CHD patients unless otherwise contraindicated.

If flight certification is considered for any degree of CHD, with or without revascularization, then secondary preventive efforts become of critical importance. Indeed, documentation of continuing successful modification of risk factors might be considered a criterion for certification by some licensing authorities. Military and civilian commercial aviators often have lower CHD risk characteristics than the general population. Referenced works from the two European workshops in aviation cardiology make the very valid point that data from available clinical trials are not applicable to aviators. The aeromedical community needs comparable aviator databases to better address these issues.

Annual cardiac event rates are comparable and less than 1% per year for normal coronary angiography subjects, apparently healthy populations, healthy military aviators, and military aviators with nonsignificant CHD. Aviators and other clinical populations with significant CHD have annual event rates of at least 2.5% per year, increasing with greater extent or severity of disease. For consideration of return to flight duties, it is not adequate to only document that an aviator is presently asymptomatic without objective evidence of ischemia, because many other factors affect annual event rates for appropriate aeromedical endpoints. Of paramount concern is establishing an acceptable threshold for annual events, as well as identifying possible low-risk subgroups from the general literature and, ideally, from aviator populations. Following are suggested aeromedical disposition guidelines for this very difficult topic.

Nonsignificant CHD. Return to high-performance military and aerobatic flying is not recommended. Return to low-performance, multipilot military and commercial flying and return to general, private flying are recommended. There should be no history of angina or prior myocardial infarction, no objective evidence of ischemia in the distribution of the affected coronary artery, and left ventricular function should be normal. Annual review with noninvasive testing is recommended. If annual review shows significant degradation of noninvasive test results, repeat angiography should be considered. Progression to significant CHD may occur without symptoms and noninvasive testing may not detect it. Therefore, routine repeat coronary angiography should be considered at 3-5 year intervals in at least some aviator categories, such as military aviators. Aspirin therapy and aggressive risk factor modification are also recommended. Licensing authorities may choose to consider the individual aviator's risk factor profile and the success of risk factor modification when making decisions regarding return to flight duty or for timing of reevaluation.

Significant CHD. With or without a history of ischemic symptoms, a return to flying is generally not recommended for significant CHD that has not been revascularized. Revascularized CHD is discussed below. An exception might be return to general private flying, or limited multipilot commercial flying (eg, flight duty excluding passenger flights) for ***asymptomatic*** moderate disease with a single significant lesion in the range of 50%-70% stenosis. If certification is being considered, there should be no history of angina and no objective evidence of ischemia in the distribution of the affected artery by noninvasive testing off cardioactive medications, preferably graded exercise testing with radionuclide perfusion scintigraphy. Left ventricular function should be normal with no significant regional wall motion abnormalities. Repeat graded exercise testing at 6-12 month intervals is recommended with full noninvasive review annually. Periodic repeat coronary angiography at 2-3 year intervals should also be considered.

Post Myocardial Infarction. Return to military or aerobatic flying is not recommended. Return to multipilot commercial flying and general, private flying may be permissible for select cases. If considered, a nonflying observation period of at least 6 months is recommended. Post observation there should be no ischemia by symptoms or by noninvasive testing. For commercial flying, graded exercise testing with radionuclide perfusion scintigraphy is recommended. A small area of periinfarction reversible ischemia may be acceptable. Exercise testing should be performed off cardioactive medications with a target heart rate of 100% predicted for age. Overall left ventricular function should be normal with no left ventricular aneurysm or major regional wall motion abnormality. Twenty-four-hour ambulatory monitoring to assess for ventricular arrhythmias should also be considered. Coronary angiography is recommended, at least for commercial flying, especially if carrying passengers. Coronary angiography should demonstrate no significant stenoses other than at the infarction site. A patent infarct-related artery carries a better prognosis than a completely occluded artery; licensing authorities may choose to consider this in a disposition decision. Repeat graded exercise testing at 6-12 month intervals and annual full review are recommended. Periodic repeat coronary angiography at 2-3 year intervals may be prudent, at least for commercial flying. Allowance of return to flying after myocardial infarction should also permit some medications for secondary prevention purposes. For example, in addition to lipid modification, most treatment guidelines recommend beta-blocker therapy, and possibly ACE inhibitor therapy (unless contraindicated in an individual patient) after myocardial infarction, for their demonstrated ability to improve prognosis. As discussed earlier, medical therapy should not be utilized to treat postinfarction ischemic symptoms.

Surgical- and Catheter-Based Intervention

Introduction

Addressing the topic of return to flying after coronary artery revascularization is difficult and often emotionally charged. Many civilian licensing authorities have approved certification for general aviation and for restricted commercial aviation duties in multicrew aircraft after successful revascularization. Stipulations for certification may include a nonflying observation period of at least 6 months after the procedure, no symptoms, normal or near normal left ventricular function, good exercise tolerance, and no evidence of residual ischemia by noninvasive testing. Coronary angiography may be required for definitive assessment of the results of revascularization prior to certification, and periodic follow-up coronary angiography may be required for reassessment. Periodic review, usually annually, and including repeat noninvasive testing, is also required. The low rate of commercial aircraft accidents involving cardiac events in aviators certified to fly after revascularization attests to the effectiveness of the certification policies in that aviation environment.

Aeromedical disposition depends to a large extent on the philosophy of the licensing authority, the particular aviation environment under consideration, the level of acceptable percent-per-year threshold risk, and exactly which cardiac endpoints are considered within that threshold risk. Civilian recertification policies generally consider cardiac mortality less than 1% per year and cardiac mortality plus myocardial infarction less than 2% per year as threshold criteria. Inherent within these policies for civilian commercial recertification is the acknowledged safety advantage of redundancy in the cockpit.

This topic has been reviewed from an aeromedical perspective for military aviation with proposed guidelines for restricted flying duties for low-risk aviators after coronary artery bypass grafting (CABG) or single vessel angioplasty.[54] This review of major trials concluded that an asymptomatic military aviator with no prior infarction or heart failure who successfully modified his risk factor profile had a sufficiently low risk to warrant return to restricted flying duties as or with copilot. Specific stipulations for initial and subsequent assessment were similar to those noted above for commercial aviators. However, the more stringent standards for both military service and military aviation, and the demands of the combat mission, may warrant a more cautious approach and a broader definition of aeromedical endpoints considered within the threshold of acceptable risk. If significant CHD without revascularization is considered permanently disqualifying for certain aviator types such as military aviators, then the risk of development of new significant CHD lesions in revascularized subjects might also be considered an aeromedical endpoint. Repeat revascularization rates should then be considered because this implies the presence of significant CHD.

Significant CHD treated by revascularization may be a different consideration than untreated or medically treated CHD, and should in a sense be considered a different diagnosis for aeromedical decision making. The primary question is whether the risk for revascularized significant CAD is comparable to that for nonsignificant CHD. For example, is a 75% lesion which has been dilated by angioplasty down to a 20% residual lesion equivalent aeromedically, or even clinically, to an untreated 20% lesion? Or, is a 75% lesion with a single arterial bypass graft comparable to a 25% lesion in the same location with respect to subsequent 5- to 10-year annual cardiac event rates? Revascularized significant CHD should not be more favorably considered than untreated or medically treated significant CHD unless its event rates are greatly improved and comparable to those of nonsignificant CHD. The fact that the aviator feels well, the perception on the part of the aviator that he or she has been "fixed," and the reassurance from the attending cardiologist that the individual is now "low risk" and doing well without evidence of ischemia ***at the present time*** may be insufficient grounds for return to flight duty, especially military and commercial flying. Unfortunately, these are the pressures that are too frequently placed on the attending AME/FS and the licensing authority.

Catheter-Based Intervention

The angioplasty literature was reviewed for late outcomes, in an attempt to identify a patient subset similar to the military aviator population, and determine whether the risk was low enough to allow return to military flying.[55] Cardiac events considered were cardiac death, myocardial infarction, and need for revascularization due to restenosis or progression of disease. The target annual event rate was less than or equal to 1% per year. Angina was not considered but occurred in 13%-43% of patients within 3-6 years. The review concentrated on late outcomes occurring 1 year or more after angioplasty. Beginning 1 year after successful angioplasty, annual event rates were 2.4%-4.1% per year and stable out to 5 years of follow-up. The highest event rate was from a study that only accepted patients without prior myocardial infarction. Patients younger than 40 years of age had the highest rate of repeat revascularization for restenosis or for new significant disease. Development of new significant disease at other sites and in other vessels (progression) occurred at about 7% per year, such that by 5-8 years postangioplasty, 39%-45% of *asymptomatic* patients had developed significant disease elsewhere. Risk of the selected endpoints was not reduced by age younger than 40 years, absence of symptoms before or after angioplasty, absence of myocardial infarction, single vessel disease, or postangioplasty target lesion less than 30% stenosis. A subset of aviators with risk sufficiently low to warrant return to military flight duties was not identified.

The second European workshop in aviation cardiology provided an excellent review of late outcomes of angioplasty and coronary stents.[56] Certification for civilian commercial and private licensure was addressed using thresholds of less than 1% per year late death rate and less than 2% per year death or myocardial infarction rate. From this perspective, it was concluded that treatment of single vessel, native vessel disease (ie, not of a bypass graft) with angioplasty or stent met the threshold criteria. It was also concluded that treated simple 2-vessel disease might be favorably considered, but that more severe 2-vessel disease and 3-vessel disease treated by these methods was incompatible with relicensure. Simple 2-vessel disease excluded severe proximal left anterior descending coronary artery disease. Additionally, excellent advice was given for appropriate methods to review the literature for aeromedical disposition purposes. The recommended protocol for relicensure and periodic review was similar to that already established for CABG. It is of significant interest that in this review of angioplasty/stent versus CABG trials, annual rates of late death and of death/infarction for multivessel CABG averaged 1.5% and 3.3% per year, respectively, with no trials meeting the above criteria of less than 1% and less than 2% per year, respectively.

Balloon angioplasty is the basic catheter-based intervention technique. Therefore, more data with longer follow-up are available for this procedure compared to newer techniques. With proper case selection, angioplasty is very successful initially when performed by an experienced cardiologist. One of its major drawbacks is early restenosis, which occurs within a few months; hence the 6 month minimum nonflying observation period generally recommended prior to recertification for civilian flying. Various intervention trials report early restenosis rates of 30%-35% or more. Overcoming this early restenosis problem is the major reason for developing better methods of catheter-based intervention, such as atherectomy, laser, rotational devices, and stents. Some have not resulted in a significant improvement over angioplasty, while others (eg, stents) have reduced the restenosis rate significantly, to a range of about 20%. This is a tremendous clinical advance, but is of relative insignificance for aeromedical disposition, because licensing authorities should only consider recertification for successful interventions. Newer methods that decrease the restenosis rate thus reduce the rate of needed repeat revascularization of the original site. They have not significantly reduced the incidence of late events of cardiac death, myocardial infarction, angina, or revascularization, because these late events are probably due primarily to the unrelenting progression of CHD, as discussed previously in this section. Coronary stents currently hold the most promise, both clinically and aeromedically.

Coronary Artery Bypass Grafting

CABG has long been considered incompatible with military aviation, at least by most armed forces, but has for several years been accepted for recertification for civilian flying under carefully specified conditions. The problem and approach are like that of catheter-based intervention, depending largely on the chosen threshold of annual event rate and the selection of endpoints. Aeromedical endpoints for CABG are identical to those of catheter-based intervention, with the substitution of late graft closure for late restenosis. Late cardiac death, myocardial infarction, repeat revascularization, progression of disease, angina, and antianginal medications are all possible events to consider.

Much of the recent data regarding CABG comes from trials comparing catheter-based interventions to CABG. These have relatively short-term follow-up data. A metaanalysis of 8 major trials reported a mean follow-up for the combined analysis of 2.7 years (range, 1-4.7 years).[57] Two of the studies involved only patients with single vessel disease, and in a third trial 45% had single vessel disease. Late events after 1 year of follow-up for CABG were 1.9% cardiac death or myocardial infarction and 3.5% repeat revascularization. Angina occurred in 10.8% and 12.7% at 1 and 3 years, respectively. Late events in single vessel disease were 1.7% cardiac death or myocardial infarction, 3.9% repeat revascularization, and 6.5% and 12.5% angina at 1 and 3 years, respectively.

A previously referenced study comparing medical, angioplasty, and surgical therapy of single vessel left anterior descending disease documented development of new significant lesions in 30% of the CABG cohort within only 2 years after surgery.[48] This was one of the single vessel disease studies included in the above metaanalysis. In the surgical cohort during 3.5 years follow-up, 3% experienced death, infarction, or repeat revascularization. In 2.5 years of mean follow-up, the other single vessel disease study reported death in 1.5%, infarction in 3.0%, repeat revascularization in 4.5%, and angina in 11%.

Internal thoracic artery grafts have a significant advantage over saphenous vein grafts due to their extraordinary long-term patency rates of greater than 90% at 10-20 years. In some studies, the presence of a thoracic artery graft increases survival 10%-30% over saphenous vein grafts, and the presence or absence of a thoracic artery graft is a more potent predictor of survival than even left ventricular function. The above mentioned single vessel disease trials from the metaanalysis used internal thoracic artery grafts. Another study reported survival rates of 749 thoracic artery bypass graft patients with or without associated saphenous vein grafts.[58] Cumulative death rates at 4, 8, 12, and 16 years were 5%, 13%, 23%, and 36%, respectively. In an earlier study, the same group reported clinical event rates on 490 CABG patients with internal thoracic artery grafts.[59] At 5 and 10 years the following events had occurred: cumulative deaths 9% and 25%, late myocardial infarctions 6% and 18%, angina 25% and 40%, and reoperation 1% and 3%.

Excellent reviews of CABG from the civilian aeromedical perspective have been published.[60,61] CABG trials before and after the widespread use of internal thoracic artery grafts are well described. Generally, the results from these two reviews and the above discussed reports are clinically very favorable, especially for internal thoracic grafts. However, the total event rates may be inappropriate for some aviation considerations. The problems are extracting annual rates for appropriate events and selecting a subset of patients comparable to aviators. The above noted metaanalysis of 8 major trials does present favorable late event rates, if one considers the acceptable threshold to be cardiac death less than 1% per year and cardiac death/myocardial infarction less than 2% per year.[57] When angina, antianginal medication use, repeat revascularizations, and the 7%-15% per year risk of progression of significant disease at other sites is considered, the potential aeromedical risk rises significantly.

A fascinating subset of the CASS (Coronary Artery Surgery Study) Registry was analyzed to address the question of post-CABG airline pilots returning to flying.[62] From 10,312 patients in the registry, the researchers selected 2326 who had clinical and postoperative characteristics similar to those of commercial airline pilots. Among other characteristics considered, they excluded myocardial infarction, hospitalization for chest pain, congestive heart failure, rhythm disturbance, or stroke occurring within 12 months after CABG. Mean follow-up was 52 months. The 1207 patients without preoperative myocardial infarction had a 5-year probability of 1.6% per year of sudden death, myocardial infarction, or acute coronary insufficiency. For the 122 patients who additionally had never smoked and had no history of hypertension, the 5-year probability risk was only 0.4% per year.

Summary and Aeromedical Recommendations

Aeromedical endpoints for revascularization include those discussed earlier for nonsignificant and significant CHD. In addition there is the problem of short- and long-term graft closure for CABG, and acute and subacute restenosis for angioplasty and other catheter-based revascularization. But the real concern is the development of new significant lesions within 2-3 years. As noted above,[48] approximately 30%-35% of single vessel left anterior descending disease treated medically, by angioplasty, or by internal thoracic artery graft, had new significant disease within 2 years of the index angiography. And in an angioplasty review,[55] new significant lesions developed at a rate of about 7% per year over approximately 5 years of follow-up. As already discussed, normal coronary angiography populations, apparently healthy civilian populations aged 35-54 years, apparently healthy military aviators, and military aviators with nonsignificant CHD, have annual CHD event rates less than 1% per year, whereas significant CHD without revascularization has event rates of 2.5% per year or greater.

Postrevascularization annual CHD event rates seem to be in the range of 2.5%-5.0% per year, even for the better prognostic subgroups with normal left ventricular function, no prior myocardial infarction, and only single or double vessel disease. This considers angina, progression, and revascularization as late events, in addition to cardiac death and infarction. Event rates of revascularized significant CHD do not match those of nonsignificant CHD. Whether those event rates are acceptable again depends on the particular aviation environment in question, the threshold of annual risk considered acceptable, and exactly which events are considered in that threshold. These may vary, especially for considerations of civilian versus military aviation.

Following are suggested recommendations for the aeromedical disposition of CHD after successful revascularization. The general recommendations discussed above for CHD without revascularization also apply here.

Catheter-Based Intervention. Return to military or aerobatic flying is not recommended. Return to multipilot commercial flying and to general, private flying may be permissible for successful single or double vessel intervention. If considered, a nonflying observation period of at least 6 months is recommended. Postintervention there should be no ischemia by symptoms or by noninvasive testing. For commercial flying, graded exercise testing with radionuclide perfusion scintigraphy is recommended. Exercise testing should be performed off cardioactive medications with a target heart rate of 100% predicted for age. Overall left ventricular function should be normal with no significant regional wall motion abnormalities. Twenty-four-hour ambulatory monitoring to assess for ventricular arrhythmias is also a consideration. Coronary angiography is recommended, at least for commercial flying, especially if carrying passengers for hire. Coronary angiography should demonstrate continued success of the intervention (≤30% residual stenosis suggested) and no significant stenoses elsewhere. Repeat graded exercise testing at 6-12 month intervals and annual full review are recommended. Periodic repeat coronary angiography at 2-3 year intervals is recommended for commercial flying.

Coronary Artery Bypass Grafting. Return to military or aerobatic flying is not recommended. As with catheter-based intervention, return to multipilot commercial flying and to general, private aviation may be permissible, especially if one or more internal thoracic artery grafts were used. Other stipulations are the same as for catheter-based intervention as outlined above. Coronary angiography should demonstrate patency of all grafts.

Primary Prevention of Coronary Heart Disease

Although the rates of various measures of CHD morbidity and mortality have declined in the United States and some other countries, CHD continues to be a leading cause, if not the leading cause, of adult death and disability in many industrialized nations. Furthermore, CHD is a frequent cause of medical disqualification of airline pilots and military aviators. Thus CHD is clearly a major public health concern as well as a significant aeromedical concern. The obvious solution for the general public as well as the aviator population is to prevent the occurrence of CHD. Primary prevention of CHD should become a basic responsibility of the AME/FS to his or her aviators.

The number of risk factors potentially affecting CHD is lengthy and continually growing. New and emerging risk factors such as homocysteine, fibrinogen, C-reactive protein, and infectious agents, to name only a few, are topics of considerable current research. Classic modifiable risk factors include smoking, elevated total and LDL cholesterol, low HDL cholesterol, and hypertension. Diabetes mellitus, obesity, sedentary lifestyle, and postmenopausal status are others. The impact of modification varies, depending on the particular risk factor involved, and socioeconomic and ethnic factors. Nonmodifiable risk factors are age, gender, and family history of premature CHD.

Cigarette smoking, through several mechanisms of action, has clearly been shown to be an important risk factor for CHD and other atherosclerotic vascular diseases in both men and women. Smoking cessation quickly produces significant and lasting decreases in CHD morbidity and mortality. The magnitude of the impact of smoking may vary in different ethnic population groups but the adverse health effects seem clear. Counseling and encouragement to stop smoking, as well as formal smoking cessation programs should be an integral part of any primary prevention effort. Hypertension is discussed separately in another section. The remainder of this brief discussion will be directed toward abnormal lipid profiles.

Much has been written about the primary and secondary prevention of CHD, especially regarding lipid-lowering therapy. Primary prevention of CHD has been clearly shown to be effective in many risk subgroups, including women and individuals with only mildly to moderately abnormal lipid profiles. Numerous references and resources are available reviewing different aspects of the primary prevention of CHD by lipid modification. Controversy exists concerning several aspects, such as cost effectiveness, whether to treat, which subgroups to treat, which lipid parameter should guide therapy, at what level to initiate therapy, and what the target level for therapy should be. For the aviator population, there are also the considerations of short- and long-term safety profiles of medications and subtle performance decrements due to medications. The AME/FS has to walk the line between providing the best care for the aviator versus the acceptable use of medications in various aviation environments.

All of these issues are beyond the scope of this work. Guidelines for therapy of aviators should be derived from the standards recommended and published by national and international medical societies dealing with cardiovascular and preventive medicine. For example, a report of lipid-lowering therapy in military aviators included a review of lipid-lowering drugs from an aeromedical perspective, and suggested treatment initiation and target lipid levels adopted from published guidelines.[63] Though directed at military aviators, it is a useful discussion for all aviation environments.

Other informative resources are a recent review of available drug therapies for lipid disorders and an excellent, concise review of early and recent CHD primary prevention trials, including the issue of cost effectiveness of lipid-lowering therapy and the public health implications of the most recent statin primary prevention trials.[64,65] Others discuss the aeromedical issues of lipid screening and lipid-lowering therapy in the first and second European workshops in aviation cardiology.[66,67] Suffice it to say that recent primary prevention trials using effective drug therapy have demonstrated relative risk reductions of approximately 30%-35% for CHD and a variety of other cardiovascular and cerebrovascular events. Primary prevention of CHD is definitely effective in reducing CHD deaths and other events.

Several practical points deserve emphasis. It is often simpler and quicker for the practitioner to prescribe lipid-lowering medications than it is to properly counsel, encourage, and periodically reassess nonpharmacologic measures, and it also requires much less effort on the part of the patient. In spite of this, in the medical community we do not treat patients eligible for such treatment according to published guidelines, even for secondary prevention of CHD. It is estimated that only 6.6% of Americans eligible for lipid-lowering therapy under the guidelines of the National Cholesterol Education Panel (NCEP) are receiving such therapy, including only 14% of secondary prevention eligible patients and only 4% of primary prevention eligible patients.[65] Further, 65% of those who are eligible for diet or drug therapy are not receiving any therapy at all. Similarly discouraging statistics have been reported in Europe. While debating the various issues regarding primary (and secondary) prevention, we fail to appropriately treat even those we already know are most likely to benefit from such therapy. In the case of the aviator, if nonflying observation periods are required prior to special certification to fly on an approved lipid-lowering medication, the AME/FS and aviator may both be reluctant to initiate medical therapy. Consequently, aviators may be even more poorly treated than their nonaviator counterparts.

It is often said that the lifestyles of commercial airline and military aviators are conducive to poor diet and other bad health habits. Although this seems sensible, it is not necessarily true. Aviators, especially commercial airline pilots and military aviators, tend to be from middle to upper socioeconomic classes, are better educated and more health-oriented, and typically are more compliant and motivated about health issues such as cardiac risk factor modification. Most current emphasis is on drug therapy with dietary restriction, smoking cessation, and control of hypertension. Formal diet, weight loss, and exercise counseling with periodic reassessment are not emphasized as strongly.

An organized exercise and diet program was recently proposed as the primary means for preventing CHD in aviators.[68] The proponents reviewed intervention trials consisting of diet alone, exercise alone, and exercise plus diet as the intervention. They concluded that the combination of formal exercise and diet programs had the most favorable effect on lipid profile by lowering total and LDL cholesterol, while raising HDL cholesterol and thereby improving (lowering) the ratio of total cholesterol to HDL cholesterol. A survey of United States Air Force flight surgeons supported this position as an initial primary preventive effort. The survey also called for more primary preventive training in medical school, graduate medical education, and flight surgeon training courses.

Similar findings were reported by others.[69] In a 1-year study, 377 middle-aged men and postmenopausal women with low HDL and elevated LDL cholesterol levels were randomly assigned to control, diet only, exercise only, or diet plus exercise groups. The diet plus exercise group had the most beneficial lipid modification, with mean LDL cholesterol reduction of 14.5 mg/dL (women) and 20.0 mg/dL (men). Others have used a model of the U.S. adult population to assess the population-wide effect of full implementation of the most recent NCEP guidelines.[70] They reported that all benefits of the NCEP "screen and treat" primary prevention guidelines could be achieved by a population-wide reduction of LDL cholesterol of 11 mg/dL (8%) in persons without known CHD. This goal appears attainable in many cases through a formal diet and exercise program alone. Formal programs for diet and exercise prescription and follow-up are available in the civilian sector. Similar facilities are often available to military aviators on their military installations. But both populations seem to use these options rarely, especially for primary prevention.

This very brief mention of primary prevention of CHD is offered primarily to encourage all aeromedical practitioners to become better educated and more actively involved in CHD primary preventive efforts with our aviators. The nuisance of acquiring special issuance for flying on lipid-lowering medications should not deter their use. Aviators deserve the best care that we can provide, but too often, especially in the area of CHD prevention, they receive less than the best. If formal diet and exercise programs are readily available, their use should be strongly encouraged. As with medication use, periodic follow-up of the aviator's diet and exercise participation should be conducted by the AME/FS to ensure compliance. These programs should be recommended even more strongly as secondary preventive efforts for aviators with documented CHD. Lipid-lowering medications are discussed further in a later section of this chapter.

Valvular Heart Diseases

Bicuspid Aortic Valve

Clinical Features

Bicuspid aortic valve (BAV) is the most common congenital heart disease, occurring in an estimated 1%-2% of the general population. BAV was reported in 0.5% (5/1036 and 15/3335) of screening echocardiograms performed on United States Air Force pilot training candidates,[71,72] and in 0.9% (14/1476) of Canadian Forces pilot training candidates.[12] These figures may underestimate prevalence because these pilot training candidates had already passed a preliminary examination that likely eliminated some with BAV. In another study, routine echocardiography was performed on 543 experienced pilots from 13 NATO countries who had no known heart disease.[73] BAV was found in only 0.4% (2/543).

BAV may be diagnosed by physical examination and by echocardiography. The typical physical finding is an aortic ejection sound, a high-frequency early systolic clicking sound heard best with the stethoscope's diaphragm at the upper right sternal border and at the apex. There may be a midsystolic diamond-shaped murmur due to distorted aortic outflow, even in the absence of aortic stenosis. And, if aortic insufficiency is present, there may be a diastolic blowing decrescendo murmur along the left sternal border. Echocardiography is the gold standard for diagnosing BAV and for identifying and grading the severity of associated valvular stenosis and insufficiency. There are no specific therapies for BAV per se other than infective endocarditis prophylaxis per established recommendations. Periodic reassessment by examination and echocardiography should be performed to follow possible progression. Therapeutic measures are directed toward the two primary consequences of BAV, development of aortic stenosis and/or aortic insufficiency, which are discussed separately below.

Natural History and Aeromedical Considerations

Adequate natural history data, with studies of large numbers of subjects with long-term follow-up, examining development and progression rates of valvular aortic stenosis (AS) and aortic insufficiency (AI) in BAV are sorely lacking. An estimated 30%-40% of subjects with BAV will require surgery for aortic valve replacement between the ages of 20 and 60. From a review of pertinent literature, it is estimated that the annual incidence of aortic valve surgery for BAV in the United States is 1.2% per year. However, this surgery is predominantly performed in patients over 40-45 years of age. Uncomplicated BAV in an aviator candidate is an investment issue rather than an immediate flight safety issue. Aviator candidates with BAV who are trained at a young age will be at risk of possible disqualification from flight duty predominantly when they are older, more experienced, and for military aviators, in prominent command positions. Loss of an aviator at this stage may be more costly than loss at an earlier age or rejection from initial flight training.

Aeromedical concerns regarding BAV include development of AS and/or AI, progression of AS or AI to a severe grade, requirement for medical therapy for severe AI, requirement for surgical valve replacement, and infective endocarditis. There really are no suddenly incapacitating events of concern associated with BAV except in the presence of associated significant AS or AI. These are discussed below in the more general discussions of AS and AI. Therefore, policies regarding the return to flying of a trained aviator with a new diagnosis of BAV should be determined by the presence and severity of associated AS and AI. Policies regarding entry into flight training should also consider the presence and severity of AS/AI, but should also take into account the potential loss of the aviator late in his or her career due to associated significant AS or AI or valve surgery. One might think that a candidate aged 20-25 presenting with BAV and associated mild AS or AI has a more aggressive process and would be more likely to progress than a candidate with BAV but no AS or AI. However, there are no data to support this suggestion.

Aortic Stenosis

Clinical Features

Aortic stenosis (AS) usually occurs at the aortic valve. Supravalvular and discrete subvalvular forms exist, but are congenital and unlikely to be a new diagnosis in an adult aviator, so they will not be discussed. Hypertrophic cardiomyopathy, which may cause subvalvular stenosis, is discussed in the cardiomyopathy section. Valvular AS has several etiologies. In industrialized countries, the most common cause in older adults is senile AS, a degenerative-calcifying process, and in younger adults it is bicuspid aortic valve. Rheumatic heart disease remains a frequent etiology of AS in countries where rheumatic fever is still a health problem. There is usually other evidence of rheumatic heart involvement, especially of the mitral valve. Other etiologies include severe atherosclerosis, rheumatoid disease, and end-stage renal disease.

The AS murmur is a classic midsystolic, crescendo-decrescendo outflow murmur usually heard best at the upper sternal borders and radiating into the neck. It may also be heard at the apex. An early systolic ejection sound may also be present. Other features of physical examination that may help determine severity of AS include duration and peak of the murmur, effects on heart sounds S_1 and S_2, palpable and audible S_4, and effect on the carotid pulse contour.

Medical therapy is limited to endocarditis prophylaxis per recommendations, and treatment of consequences of moderate to severe AS, such as heart failure or tachyarrhythmias. The treatment of choice for symptomatic moderate to severe AS is surgical valve replacement. Discussion of the indications for surgery is beyond the scope of this work. Valve repair and catheter balloon valvuloplasty are not clinically acceptable options at this time in adults with stenotic, calcified aortic valves. One exception is balloon valvuloplasty for severe AS patients who are not surgical candidates due to other comorbidities.

Natural History

Excellent reviews of the natural history of AS and recommendations for the management of aortic valvular disease have been published.[74,75] The hemodynamic burden in AS is obstruction to left ventricular outflow with a subsequent left ventricular pressure overload and left ventricular hypertrophy. Progressive stenosis and pressure overload may lead to left ventricular diastolic and later systolic dysfunction, left ventricular dilation, and symptoms. The clinical determinants of prognosis are development of severe AS and AS-related symptoms. Angina may occur even in the absence of atherosclerotic coronary heart disease. The classic symptom triad is syncope, angina, and dyspnea. These three symptoms may present in moderate or severe AS and should prompt valve surgery as soon as possible. Unless valve replacement is performed, the average time to AS-related death is 5, 3, and 2 years, respectively, after onset of the three symptoms. Sudden death due to AS is reported in as many as 3%-5% of asymptomatic patients with moderate to severe AS, but it is usually preceded by the onset of one or more of the above three symptoms. However, sudden death may follow symptom onset by as little as 3 months. Many of these AS-related deaths occur during exertion.

AS is typically graded as mild, moderate, and severe, usually by echocardiography, or by cardiac catheterization. Unfortunately, the cardiac literature offers grading of AS by different parameters including mean pressure gradient across the stenotic valve, calculated aortic valve area and, more recently, maximum velocity of systolic flow through the stenotic valve. Although promising as a means of following progression, maximum velocity is a newer parameter with fewer available data on outcomes and is therefore untested for aeromedical purposes. Additionally, various authors use different ranges of values of these parameters to classify a stenotic aortic valve as mild, moderate, or severe. This makes it difficult to compare different reports from the literature and determine annual rates of defined aeromedical events because clinical event rates are related to the severity of the stenosis.

The best grading criteria using mean pressure gradient come from recommendations for competitive athletes and are: mild AS, mean gradient ≤20 mm Hg; moderate AS, mean gradient 21-39 mm Hg; and severe AS, mean gradient ≥40 mm Hg.[76]

Grading criteria using valve area vary considerably in the literature. Recommended valve area criteria come from published guidelines for the management of valvular heart disease.[75] On the basis of a variety of hemodynamic and natural history data, this expert panel defined these parameters: mild AS, valve area >1.5 cm²; moderate AS, valve area 1.1-1.5 cm²; and severe AS, valve area ≤1.0 cm².

Events considered in the following discussions of mild, moderate, and severe AS are AS-related death, development of AS-related symptoms, progression to severe AS, and aortic valve replacement.

Mild AS. Once mild AS has developed, valve area decreases at a mean rate of 0.12 cm² per year and mean pressure gradient increases by 7 mm Hg per year,[74,75] but not all cases of mild AS progress beyond the mild stage. Unfortunately, there are no known criteria that predict which AS patients will progress. One can only follow all

AS patients for progression. There seem to be three subsets of patients: nonprogressors, slow progressors, and rapid progressors.

In a study of 142 patients with mild AS (valve area >1.5 cm^2) followed for over 25 years, 38% remained mild, 25% progressed to moderate AS, and 35% had valve replacement for severe AS and/or symptom development.[77] Clinical outcomes were quite favorable; only 12% of these 142 mild AS patients had clinical progression in the first 10 years of follow-up. In a contrasting study of 123 AS patients, those with mild AS by maximum velocity criteria (<3 m/sec) had an event rate of 8% per year during only 2 years of follow-up.[78]

Moderate and Severe AS. In a cohort of 42 patients with moderate or severe AS who were followed for a mean of 20 months, 50% developed AS-related symptoms necessitating valve surgery, and there were no clinical predictors for this event.[79] A recent literature review disclosed event rates of at least 5% per year over 5 years of follow-up in asymptomatic or mildly symptomatic moderate to severe AS.[74] Another study of 66 patients with moderate AS reported an event rate of approximately 5% per year at 2 and 4 years of follow-up in the asymptomatic subset.[80] Probability of AS-related death at 3 years was 4% for asymptomatic moderate AS and 23% for symptomatic moderate AS.

From these and similar results found in the literature, it is clear that outcome rates depend on presence or absence of symptoms, rate of progression of AS in an individual patient, severity of valvular stenosis, and the definitions used for mild, moderate, and severe AS. Event rates are more favorable using 1.5 cm^2 as a cutoff point between mild and moderate AS compared to 1.2 cm^2. Also, using 0.7 cm^2 as a lower limit of moderate AS gives that category a very broad definition (from 0.7 to 1.2 or 1.5 cm^2). Many of the events likely occur at the lower range of this moderate valve area definition, and many cardiologists would consider valve areas ≤1.0 cm^2 to be severe.

Aeromedical Considerations

Before considering aeromedical disposition, it may be helpful to briefly review published recommendations for competitive athletes with AS. Athletes with mild AS are recommended for unlimited athletic competition, using the above mean pressure gradient criterion (mean gradient ≤20 mm Hg). Athletes with mild to moderate AS should only participate in selected low to moderate intensity static (isometric) and dynamic (aerobic) competitive sports. Avoidance of all competitive sports is recommended for athletes with severe AS or symptomatic moderate AS.[76]

The suggested method of aeromedical disposition combines the above mean pressure gradient and valve area grading criteria. Mild AS is defined as a mean gradient ≤20 mm Hg and valve area >1.5 cm^2. Moderate AS is defined as a mean gradient of 21-39 mm Hg and valve area 1.1-1.5 cm^2. Severe AS is defined as a mean gradient

≥40 mm Hg and a valve area ≤1.0 cm². Incorporating both valve area and mean gradient as criteria obviously leaves room for overlap. A category of mild-moderate AS is also proposed—the mean gradient criterion remains ≤20 mm Hg, but the valve area criterion is 1.1-1.5 cm². This classification is admittedly imperfect and will undoubtedly evolve as our ability to assess and stratify risk of this disease evolves.

This distinction of mild versus mild-moderate AS is important when considering return to high-performance aerobatic or military flying. As discussed above, there are very different event rates in the literature, partly because of the different definitions of mild and moderate AS. The fixed obstruction to left ventricular outflow may limit ability to increase cardiac output during exertion. And, depending on the severity of AS, cardiac output may be very preload dependent. These considerations make the high-performance environment a definite concern. Allowing high-performance flying for mild-moderate AS seems unwise. Moderate AS has an overall event rate of 10% per year or higher; the subset of asymptomatic moderate AS has an event rate of about 5% per year. Yet mild AS, and probably the lesser degrees of moderate AS, seem to have normal or near normal prognosis for at least 5 years. Future changes in prognosis would be related to progression of AS, a relatively slow process that can readily be followed by examination and echocardiography.

Given all these considerations, return to high-performance flying is recommended only for mild AS as defined above. Restriction to low-performance flying may be recommended for most cases of asymptomatic mild-moderate AS. A return to military flying is not recommended for asymptomatic moderate or severe AS. Licensing agencies considering a possible return to civilian commercial or private flying for asymptomatic moderate and severe AS must carefully consider the above event rates. Return to any kind of flying should be prohibited for symptomatic moderate or severe AS; these patients should be considered for surgical valve replacement. Annual reevaluation should include careful questioning about symptom development, and echocardiography to follow valve area and mean pressure gradient changes.

Aortic Insufficiency

Clinical Features

Aortic insufficiency (AI) has many etiologies including idiopathic AI, dilation of the aortic root, hypertension, connective tissue disorders, bicuspid aortic valve, endocarditis, aortitis, and rheumatic heart disease. According to standard literature, in clinical U.S. populations idiopathic dilation of the aortic root and hypertension are the most common causes of AI. However, in the healthy aviator population, idiopathic AI without root dilation is likely most common, followed by bicuspid aortic valve and AI with idiopathic root dilation. The insufficient aortic valve presents a volume overload to the left ventricle. If the AI becomes significant, the volume overload leads to left ventricular dilation with proportional left ventricular hypertrophy. Left ventricular contractility remains normal, or may even increase, until late in the process when the left ventricle decompensates under the chronic volume overload and left ventricular failure ensues with a dilated and hypocontractile ventricle.

The patient generally remains asymptomatic until late in the process, when left ventricular function begins to fail, usually in the fourth or fifth decade. Symptoms seen are those associated with the dilated and hypocontractile left ventricle, ie, congestive symptoms such as exertional dyspnea, reduced exercise tolerance, fatigability, orthopnea, and paroxysmal nocturnal dyspnea. Syncope is rare and angina is unusual in the absence of coronary heart disease.

The murmur of AI is a soft, high frequency diastolic decrescendo blowing murmur along the left sternal border. Maneuvers which may help the examiner better appreciate an AI murmur include leaning forward, breath held at end expiration, squatting, and hand grip. As the severity of AI worsens, the murmur becomes longer in duration. A systolic ejection murmur due to the increased stroke volume is often present and more easily heard than the diastolic AI murmur itself. An aortic ejection sound due to bicuspid valve or abrupt distension of the aorta due to the increased stroke volume is commonly heard. Soft S_1, soft or absent S_2, an S_3, and diffuse, displaced hyperdynamic apical impulse are typical of chronic severe AI. Several peripheral signs of chronic severe AI are described, such as widened pulse pressure and waterhammer pulses.

Echocardiography with Doppler imaging diagnoses and quantifies the severity of AI. Severity is typically graded as trace, mild, moderate, and severe, primarily by color Doppler imaging. Echocardiographic parameters of primary concern include AI severity, left ventricular end diastolic and end systolic diameters, left ventricular systolic function, and aortic root dimension.

Natural History and Aeromedical Considerations

In the aviator population, AI will most likely present as an asymptomatic systolic or diastolic murmur on routine examination, or an incidental finding on echocardiography. Progression rates of AI severity after development of mild AI are not well established, especially for the normal, 3-leaflet aortic valve. Most literature focuses on the natural history of chronic severe AI and the proper timing of valve replacement. In one study, 190 adults with AS or AI of varying severity were followed for over 10 years for the endpoints of death or aortic valve replacement.[81] At 1 year, endpoints occurred in 4% of cases of severe AI, but in no cases of moderate or mild AI. After 10 years, endpoints had occurred in 83% of severe AI patients, 78% of moderate AI patients, and 25% of mild AI patients. At 2 years the mortality for severe AI was 6%, but there were no deaths among the moderate or mild AI cases. Another study followed 246 patients with moderately severe or severe AI.[82] At 10 years, 75% had died or had valve surgery, and 83% had experienced cardiovascular events.

Progression rates were reported in 127 AI patients with at least 6 months of echocardiographic follow-up.[83] AI progressed in 25%, 44%, and 50% of mild, moderate, and severe AI patients, respectively. Another study followed 104 asymptomatic patients with severe AI but normal left ventricular function at rest.[84] During a mean follow-up of 8 years, about 4% per year developed symptoms or evidence of left ventricular dysfunction on noninvasive testing. There were also 2 sudden cardiac deaths. A similar cohort of 104 patients was followed for a mean 7.3 years.[85] The event rate was 6% per year for sudden death (4 cases), operable symptoms, or subnormal left ventricular performance. Several clinical parameters stratified the cohort into a lowest risk tertile (2% per year) and highest risk tertile (13% per year).

The sudden death rate for severe AI appears then to be less than 0.5% per year and the annual rate of significant events (operable symptoms and/or left ventricular dysfunction) is about 5% per year. What about the prognosis of trace AI? Trace and mild regurgitation of the other 3 cardiac valves (mitral, pulmonary, and tricuspid) are common findings in many echocardiographic studies of normal subjects and are felt to be physiologic occurrences. But trace AI with a 3-leaflet valve is relatively uncommon, raising the question of whether it should be considered physiologic. Twenty-seven patients with trace AI were followed for 3-5 years.[86] All 8 patients with normal leaflet morphology remained unchanged (trace AI). Of 19 with multiple leaflet thickening or calcification without stenosis, 13 progressed to mild AI and 4 progressed to moderate AI; only 2/19 remained trace AI. More information is needed to address this question, but these data suggest that trace AI with a thickened or calcified 3-leaflet valve is not normal and should be followed for progression. Trace AI with a normal 3-leaflet valve is reasonably considered a normal variant.

Suddenly incapacitating events are not likely to be associated with AI, even with severe AI, and therefore are not a significant aeromedical concern. Aeromedical issues are related to the degree of AI and the progression from mild and moderate to severe AI. These concerns involve questions of restricted versus unrestricted flying duties, medical therapy of severe AI and the ensuing aeromedical impact, and potential future loss of the aviator due to severe AI, symptoms, left ventricular dysfunction, or surgical valve replacement.

Theoretical concerns exist regarding the combination of AI and high-performance flight (aerobatic and military fighter aircraft). The combination of the hemodynamic effects of high $+G_z$, the anti-G straining maneuver, G-suits, and in some aircraft, positive pressure breathing, may transiently worsen the degree of AI in an aviator with preexisting AI. The real question is whether such transient effects, repeated over time, would have chronic persistent effects, and thereby hasten the progression of AI and the need for surgical valve replacement. These concerns are also reflected in guidelines for athletes with AI who participate in high intensity isometric competitive sports.[76] Earlier guidelines had excluded moderate or high intensity isometric sports for asymptomatic mild or worse AI. In the absence of data to confirm or refute these concerns, the more recent guidelines only limit isometric sports competition for athletes with asymptomatic mild or moderate AI associated with moderate but stable left ventricular dilation.

A study compared echocardiograms of 289 experienced and active high-performance military pilots to those of 254 low-performance pilots to assess for significant cardiac effects of high-performance flying.[73] Findings of significant valvular regurgitation were too few for statistical calculations, but there were no cases of significant AI in the high-performance group compared to 4 cases of significant AI in the low-performance group. In another study, a small cohort of 16 high-performance pilots and 16 age-matched low-performance pilots with mild AI were followed for a mean of 5 years while on active flight duty.[87] There was no change in chamber dimensions or left ventricular function in either group. AI severity increased in only 1 high-performance pilot and 5 low-performance pilots.

Medical therapy of severe AI is also a pertinent aeromedical issue. Good evidence exists in the literature that treatment of severe AI with vasodilators such as hydralazine, ACE inhibitors, and nifedipine, has favorable hemodynamic effects such as decreased left ventricular size and mass, and improved function. In one study, nifedipine was shown to extend these hemodynamic effects into clinical benefits by delaying the need for aortic valve surgery and improving operative survival.[88] This clinical benefit is so widely accepted that many, if not most, cardiologists would consider vasodilator therapy to be the standard of care for severe AI.

Due to the theoretical concerns discussed above, high-performance flying (military and aerobatic) is recommended only for mild AI. Asymptomatic mild and moderate AI with normal cardiac chamber sizes and ventricular function are acceptable for return to low-performance flying. Disqualification from military flying is recommended for severe AI. Aviators with severe AI probably should not be allowed to return to civilian commercial flying unless the licensing authority considers vasodilator therapy acceptable in that setting. Reevaluation is recommended at 1-3 year intervals, depending on the severity of AI and the status of left ventricular size and function. Echocardiography should be performed to monitor AI severity, cardiac chamber sizes, and left ventricular function. Graded exercise testing may be useful to document and follow exercise tolerance for moderate and severe AI.

Mitral Valve Prolapse

Clinical Features

Prevalence. Mitral valve prolapse (MVP) may be a primary valvular disorder or associated with a large number of acquired or inherited disorders. Primary MVP may be inherited in an autosomal dominant pattern and is the type most likely to be encountered in an aviator or aviator candidate. This discussion will consider only primary MVP, which is said to be the most common valvular disorder in adults. Prevalence in the general population has been reported as high as 35%, but most recent publications report a much lower prevalence, in the range of 5% or less. The previous impression of a higher prevalence was due to tertiary referral bias and older M-mode and two-dimensional echocardiographic criteria that over-diagnosed MVP.

MVP was reported in 0.6% (6/1036) and 0.5% (15/3335) of screening echocardio-grams performed on United States Air Force pilot training candidates,[71,72] and in 4.0% (59/1476) of Canadian Forces pilot training candidates.[12] A report of echocardio-graphic findings of 543 experienced NATO pilots found MVP in 0.9% (5/543), equally distributed between high- and low-performance pilots.[73] Again, these figures are underestimates, reflecting a type of survivor referral bias—the pilot candidates and pilots had no suspected organic heart disease after routine and periodic screening physical examinations. Echocardiograms performed on 3491 participants in the fifth examination Framingham Heart Study offspring cohort revealed MVP in 2.4%.[89] Because the cohort was older (mean age 54.7 years), a survivor bias also affects this figure. Nevertheless, the prevalence of MVP does appear to be much less than previously believed.

History and Physical Examination. The vast majority of MVP patients are asymptomatic. However, many different symptom complexes have been ascribed to MVP, including syncope, presyncope, chest discomfort, palpitations, dyspnea, fatigability, postural orthostasis and neuropsychiatric complaints. Whether these symptoms are actually related to MVP is unclear. However, recent studies with age- and gender-matched controls have shown no increased prevalence of many of these symptoms in MVP subjects.

Classic findings on cardiac examination are one or multiple midsystolic clicks and a late systolic murmur. The murmur becomes longer and more holosystolic as mitral regurgitation progresses from mild to moderate and severe. Dynamic auscultation characterizes these findings. Maneuvers that decrease left ventricular volume or increase its contractility will augment prolapse and cause the clicks and murmur to occur earlier in systole. Maneuvers that increase left ventricular volume or decrease contractility will delay prolapse and cause the clicks and murmur to occur later in systole.

Natural History and Aeromedical Considerations

Several risk factors for MVP-related events have been repeatedly demonstrated. Demographic and clinical factors include male gender, age older than 40–45 years, and a mitral regurgitation murmur. Echocardiographic parameters include severe mitral regurgitation, dilated left ventricle or left atrium (≥60 mm and ≥40 mm, respectively), and mitral leaflet thickening. Reported annual event rates are in the range of 1%-5% per year, depending on the characteristics of the study population. In a cross-sectional study of 84 MVP subjects from the Framingham Heart Study, 5 of the 84 (6%) had a history of atrial fibrillation, cerebrovascular disease, or syncope, the same rate as that of a control population without MVP.[89] However, 7% of subjects with classic prolapse had severe mitral regurgitation, compared to 0% with nonclassic MVP, and only 0.5% of a control group without MVP. This was a cross-sectional study without follow-up; annual event rates were not available.

Another cross-sectional study identified high- and low-risk MVP subsets.[90] In the high-risk subset (echocardiographic MVP with leaflet thickening and redundancy), 22.1% reported infective endocarditis, moderate to severe mitral regurgitation, or mitral valve surgery, compared to only 0.7% of the low-risk subset (MVP without thickening or redundancy). However, stroke occurrence was similar in the high- and low-risk groups, at 7.5% and 5.8%, respectively. Similar findings were reported in an M-mode echocardiographic study of 237 MVP patients followed for a mean of 6.2 years.[91] Of 97 subjects with redundant (thickened) leaflets on echocardiography, 10.3% experienced sudden death, infective endocarditis, or a cerebral ischemic episode, whereas only 0.7% of 140 MVP subjects without redundant leaflets had such events. Seventeen, or 7.2%, of the entire group of 237 developed progressive mitral regurgitation requiring surgery; initial left ventricular diastolic size was the only echocardiographic predictor. Other researchers reported an annual event rate of 1.0% per year for 316 MVP subjects followed for a mean of 8.5 years.[92] These events included 0.2% per year cardiac death, 0.3% per year cerebral ischemic episodes, 0.1% per year infective endocarditis, and 0.4% per year mitral valve surgery.

Possible suddenly incapacitating events associated with MVP include sudden death, syncope/presyncope, and cerebral ischemic episodes. An annual event rate of 0.3% for these events was found in 404 military aviators with MVP followed for a mean of 8.6 years.[93] Other reported events of aeromedical concern included sustained supraventricular and ventricular tachyarrhythmias, progression to severe mitral regurgitation, and requirement for mitral valve surgery. These additional events occurred at a rate of 1.1% per year. In this same group of 404 military aviators with MVP,[94] predictors of events were age >45 years, mitral leaflet thickening, and left ventricular or left atrial dilation (>60 mm and >40 mm, respectively). Gender was not a factor; 98% of this military aviator cohort was male.

Stroke has frequently been reported to be associated with MVP and young patients with stroke have been reported to have an increased prevalence of underlying MVP. However, this association may be exaggerated due to use of older, less specific echocardiographic criteria. As noted above, two studies found no difference in stroke or cerebral ischemic events in high- and low-risk MVP subsets.[90,91] And in the Framingham Heart Study, 1.2% of MVP subjects reported cerebral ischemic events compared to 1.5% of a control group without MVP.[89] Finally, 213 patients aged 45 years or younger with documented stroke or transient ischemic attack were compared to a control group of 263 without known cardiovascular disease.[95] Prevalence of MVP in the two groups was 1.9% and 2.7%, respectively. Only 2.8% of subjects with an otherwise unexplained cerebral event had MVP. None of the MVP subjects in either group had high-risk MVP characteristics. These studies suggest that there may not be a significant occurrence of stroke or cerebral ischemic events associated with MVP.

An intriguing study evaluated 94 MVP subjects without mitral regurgitation (MR) at rest by performing supine bicycle stress echocardiography.[96] Thirty patients (30/94, 32%) developed MR during stress (21 mild MR, 5 moderate MR, and 4 severe MR). During a mean follow-up of 38 months, the group with exercise-induced MR had significantly more syncope, congestive failure, and progressive MR requiring surgery. These findings warrant further investigation because of the possible implications for risk stratification and exercise prescription in MVP subjects.

Both supraventricular and ventricular arrhythmias are reported associated with MVP, however the strength of these associations is difficult to determine. Some investigators have documented increased supraventricular ectopy compared to controls. Others have shown apparently frequent supraventricular ectopy in MVP subjects, but this was not significantly different from the frequency of ectopy in controls. The severity of associated mitral regurgitation is important in a consideration of ventricular ectopy and MVP. It may be that ventricular arrhythmias are primarily related to severe mitral regurgitation regardless of cause.

Aeromedical disposition policies regarding MVP must take into account the above information. Newer, more specific echocardiographic criteria have resulted in lower reported rates of MVP. Older reports regarding MVP outcomes suffer from tertiary center referral bias and overestimate annual event rates. Recent community-based studies are more applicable to the aviator population and present a more benign, favorable outlook. Aeromedical disposition policies should consider the well-documented high-risk characteristics of MVP—male gender, age >45 years, mitral valve thickening, severity of mitral regurgitation, and dilation of the left ventricle and atrium.

Return to unrestricted flying can usually be recommended if mitral regurgitation is no worse than moderate and cardiac chamber sizes and ventricular function are normal. Periodic reassessment at 1-3 year intervals is recommended to track presence and severity of mitral regurgitation and cardiac size and function. Presence of high-risk characteristics should prompt more careful follow-up. One might consider disallowing high-performance military and aerobatic flying for MVP with myxomatous, thickened, and redundant mitral leaflets or chordae due to a theoretical concern about high $+G_z$ forces and integrity of the leaflets and chordae, but no data support this. See the following discussion of mitral regurgitation for further recommendations.

Mitral Regurgitation

Clinical Features

Abnormalities of the mitral valve annulus, the leaflets, the chordae tendinae, or the papillary muscles can cause mitral regurgitation (MR). There are various causes for pure or isolated MR. In the United States and much of the Western world, the most common cause is mitral valve prolapse, accounting for as much as one-half to two-thirds of MR cases. Other causes include ischemic heart disease, dilated cardiomyopathy, endocarditis, collagen vascular disease, and rheumatic heart disease. In developing countries rheumatic disease remains a common cause of MR. Natural history and aeromedical disposition of secondary MR depend on the underlying etiology. Many of the considerations were discussed above in the section on mitral valve prolapse. This discussion will deal with primary MR (primary disorders of the valve apparatus) rather than secondary MR (eg, MR due to ischemic disease or cardiomyopathy). Also, discussion will be limited to chronic MR and will not include acute MR.

Symptoms are contingent on the underlying etiology and the severity of the MR. Symptoms due to chronic MR are related to progressive severity of the volume overload with resultant pulmonary congestion and left ventricular dysfunction. They include dyspnea, chronic weakness, fatigability, and decreased exercise tolerance. However, patients may be asymptomatic with severe MR, even with associated left ventricular dysfunction. Symptom onset may be quite insidious and not appreciated by the patient; careful history taking is important to elicit subtle symptoms or lifestyle changes due to the patient "slowing down" as a result of progressive MR.

Auscultation reveals a harsh, high-pitched holosystolic murmur heard best at the apex and just medial to the apex, often radiating to the left axilla and back. Intensity of the murmur correlates only weakly if at all to severity of MR. Other findings, such as an S_3 and an enlarged and displaced apical impulse may also be present. Echocardiography is vital for confirming and assessing the severity of MR, as well as evaluating chamber sizes and ventricular function.

Natural History and Aeromedical Concerns

The natural history is determined by the underlying etiology, the severity of MR, and the status of left ventricular function. A review of MR estimated a 5-year mortality rate of 20% and a 10-year mortality rate of 40% for medically treated chronic MR of all causes; 5-year mortality for symptomatic MR was about 50%.[97] Another report studied 229 patients with MR due to flail leaflet; the MR was moderate to severe in most patients.[98] Of those initially treated medically, the annual mortality rate was 6.3% per year; in those with no or minimal symptoms, mortality was still 4.1% per year. These event rates were seen at 5 and 10 years of follow-up: cardiac death, 21% and 33%; congestive heart failure, 30% and 63%; chronic atrial fibrillation, 8% and 30%; thromboembolism, 12% and 12%; endocarditis, 5% and 8%; and mitral valve surgery, 57% and 82%.

Suddenly incapacitating aeromedical endpoints include sudden cardiac death, ventricular tachycardia, and thromboembolic events. Less obvious events of aeromedical concern include acute congestive symptoms during stress and reduced exercise tolerance. Other aeromedical endpoints are atrial fibrillation, progression to severe MR, and mitral valve surgery. Aeromedical disposition should consider underlying etiology, the presence of symptoms, severity of MR, status of left ventricular function, left atrial and ventricular size, and presence of significant arrhythmias. Compatibility of warfarin therapy with flight duties is another possible concern.

Medications to reduce afterload, such as ACE inhibitors, have documented clinical benefit in acute MR and chronic aortic insufficiency, but no studies have shown such a clinical benefit for chronic MR. Although some studies have shown hemodynamic improvement and relief of symptoms, this has not been shown to delay the need for surgery or improve surgical outcome, as is the case for severe aortic insufficiency. Use of these medications in asymptomatic MR may or may not be beneficial, but is probably common clinical practice. Use in symptomatic MR is appropriate, but at that stage the aviator should be disqualified; aeromedical disposition should be secondary to consideration of proper timing of valve surgery.

Return to unrestricted flying is recommended for asymptomatic primary MR of mild or moderate degree with normal cardiac chamber sizes, left ventricular function, and sinus rhythm. A return to aerobatic or military flying is not recommended for severe MR or for moderate MR with chamber dilation or left ventricular dysfunction. A cautious return to civilian multipilot flying may be permissible for asymptomatic moderate and severe MR with only mild ventricular dilation, normal left ventricular function, and normal sinus rhythm. Symptomatic MR merits disqualification from all flying. Periodic review at 1- to 3-year intervals is recommended, depending primarily on the severity of the MR and the status of left cardiac chamber sizes and left ventricular function. Echocardiography and 24-hour monitoring are appropriate. Graded exercise testing may be useful for moderate and severe MR, to document and follow exercise tolerance and exercise-induced arrhythmias.

Other Valvular Diseases

Mitral Stenosis

Clinical Features. Congenital mitral stenosis (MS) is rare and presents in infancy or childhood. The etiology of acquired MS is rheumatic, even in industrialized countries. Isolated MS occurs in about 40% of cases of rheumatic heart disease, and about 60% of patients with isolated MS have a history of rheumatic fever. The rheumatic process causes a progressive thickening and calcification of the mitral leaflets and fusion of the commissures and chords, resulting in a funnel-shaped valve orifice that becomes progressively more stenotic. Flow across the mitral valve then depends on an elevated pressure gradient. The result is elevated left atrial and pulmonary pressures; exercise often causes marked elevation of the latter.

Exercise, febrile illness, or other stress often induces the first symptoms of dyspnea and fatigability. As the stenosis increases, cardiac output becomes subnormal at rest and does not increase significantly with exertion. Symptoms worsen, including fatigue, dyspnea, orthopnea, and paroxysmal nocturnal dyspnea. Atrial fibrillation is common and thromboembolism is a threat, even in normal sinus rhythm. There is a long latent period after initial infection before the onset of symptoms, followed by a slowly progressive course over about 10 years before symptoms become significant or disabling. Classically, MS presents with significant symptoms in patients in their 30s and 40s. In North America and Europe the course has become milder and more delayed, such that presentation is now in the 40s and 50s, and many patients undergoing valvotomy are over age 65.

The classic findings on examination are an opening snap and a low-pitched diastolic rumble (murmur) at the apex heard best with the stethoscope's bell, with duration of the murmur related to severity of the stenosis. S_1 is accentuated if the valve is still mobile and reduces as the leaflets become less mobile. P_2 is accentuated as pulmonary pressures increase. Echocardiography is diagnostic and assesses severity of the stenosis and subsequent hemodynamic changes. Medical therapy is nonspecific and directed at controlling symptoms and atrial fibrillation and preventing thromboembolism.

Natural History and Aeromedical Considerations. Atrial fibrillation occurs in 30%-40% of symptomatic MS patients. Systemic thromboembolism occurs in 10%-20% and is related primarily to patient age and presence of atrial fibrillation, not MS severity, left atrial size, or presence of symptoms. Risk of repeat thromboembolism is extremely high, with up to 15-40 recurrent events per 100 patient months.[75] All patients with significant MS should undergo surgical or catheter-based correction unless contraindicated by other conditions.

The aeromedical disposition of MS must take into account the features listed above. The risks of atrial fibrillation and thromboembolism, reduced cardiac output and increased pulmonary pressures in response to stress, elevated pulmonary pressures upon exposure to a hypoxic environment, and the potential for dyspneic symptoms during stress weigh heavily against continuation of flight duties. Civilian aerobatic and all military flying are not recommended for any degree of MS. Asymptomatic mild to moderate MS with normal sinus rhythm and normal or only mildly elevated pulmonary artery systolic pressure may be considered for civilian commercial flying limited to multipilot operations and with annual review.

Surgical commissurotomy improves symptoms, lessens severity of stenosis, and improves prognosis. However, it is basically palliative and causes the disease process to revert to an earlier, more mild to moderate stage from which point it again slowly progresses. With open commissurotomy, the 5-year reoperation rate is 4%-7%, and the 5-year complication-free survival rate is 80%-90%.[75] Outcomes for mitral valve balloon valvuloplasty for MS are similar to those for surgical open commissurotomy. Aeromedical disposition is the same as recommended above in the preceding paragraph, depending on the degree of postoperative residual mitral stenosis.

Tricuspid Valve Disease

Tricuspid Stenosis. Tricuspid stenosis is most commonly rheumatic in origin, and is rarely associated with congenital or carcinoid etiologies. Rheumatic tricuspid disease usually causes both stenosis and regurgitation; involvement of other valves, especially the mitral valve, is the rule. Multivalvular rheumatic disease would likely be a cause for permanent disqualification, at least from military and commercial flying, due to the complexities of multiple valve disease.

Tricuspid Regurgitation. Trace and mild tricuspid regurgitation (TR) as isolated findings on echocardiography may be normal physiologic variants. Pathologic TR is usually caused by right ventricular dilation and failure due to pulmonary or right ventricular hypertension from a variety of pulmonary and cardiac causes. Left sided or diffuse cardiac disease such as significant mitral regurgitation and car-diomyopathy are examples. TR is rarely a primary finding due to such diverse etiolo-gies as rheumatic disease, trauma, infective endocarditis, and carcinoid.

A lower left sternal border decrescendo or holosystolic murmur that increases with respiration is usually heard. A right sided S_3, systolic hepatic pulsations, and dis-tended neck veins may also be present if TR is significant. Echocardiography grades the severity of TR, allows estimation of right ventricular systolic pressure, evaluates right chamber sizes and right ventricular function, and assesses for concomitant heart disease. The clinical approach as well as aeromedical disposition are deter-mined by severity of TR and its underlying etiology. The same considerations as those discussed above for mitral regurgitation would generally apply. Because of the likely association with concomitant pathology, flight duties will generally be con-traindicated. Exceptions might be TR due to prolapse and traumatic TR that is stable and not hemodynamically significant.

Pulmonary Valve Disease

Pulmonic Stenosis. Pulmonic stenosis (PS) presenting in the adult aviator will almost certainly be congenital in origin and is usually mild in severity. Such cases usually have a cone-shaped pulmonary valve with fused leaflets. Physical examina-tion reveals a harsh systolic crescendo-decrescendo murmur similar to aortic steno-sis, but loudest at the left upper sternal border and with inspiratory accentuation. An early systolic pulmonary ejection sound that decreases with inspiration is often pres-ent. Doppler echocardiography confirms the diagnosis and grades its severity. Most PS presenting in adulthood is mild as graded by transvalvular gradient with Doppler echocardiography. Such mild cases are asymptomatic, have a normal prognosis, and rarely progress. Endocarditis prophylaxis is recommended, although the risk of infective endocarditis is low.

Mild PS should pose no aeromedical concern, and flight duties are unrestricted with periodic reevaluation for the rare case with progression and/or development of symptoms. Moderate or severe PS is more likely to progress or cause symptoms such as exertional dyspnea and fatigue due to inability to adequately increase cardiac out-put during exercise. Exertional syncope or presyncope can occur, but sudden death is very unusual. Untreated severe PS will eventually lead to right ventricular hyper-trophy followed by right ventricular failure. Return to restricted flight duties for avia-tors with greater than mild PS may be considered if there are no symptoms (including during maximal graded exercise testing), exercise tolerance is normal, and there are no secondary effects such as right ventricular hypertrophy or dysfunc-tion. These patients should be followed more closely than cases of mild PS for pro-gression or symptom development.

Previously, the treatment of choice for significant PS was surgical valvotomy. However, balloon valvuloplasty is currently the preferred treatment and this procedure is extremely successful. Only 4% of surgically repaired PS required a repeat procedure over 25 years of follow-up, and balloon valvuloplasty appears to be equally successful.[75] Aeromedical disposition of PS corrected by surgical valvotomy or balloon valvuloplasty should be based on excellent hemodynamic results and no significant residua or complications. Nearly all corrected cases will have some degree of pulmonary insufficiency, usually mild.

Pulmonic Insufficiency. Trace and mild pulmonary insufficiency (PI) as isolated findings on echocardiography may be normal physiologic variants. Like PS, primary PI presenting in the adult is congenital in origin, most likely mild and unlikely to progress. It is often associated with and caused by idiopathic dilation of the pulmonic root. Physical examination reveals a soft blowing diastolic murmur at the upper left sternal border that sounds similar to aortic insufficiency, but PI increases in intensity with inspiration. An early systolic pulmonic ejection sound may be present, especially with idiopathic dilated pulmonic root. Infective endocarditis prophylaxis is recommended.

As with mild PS, mild primary PI should pose no aeromedical concern for unrestricted flight duties with only periodic reevaluation for the very rare case of progression and/or development of symptoms. More severe PI should be judged on a case-by-case basis, considering the particular aviation environment, severity of PI, presence of symptoms, and secondary effects such as right ventricular dilation and dysfunction and secondary tricuspid regurgitation.

In the adult, significant PI is more often secondary to pulmonary hypertension of various causes. Because of the variability in clinical course based on underlying etiology, aeromedical disposition should be individualized, but if pulmonary hypertension is present, return to flight duties is probably not wise, because the hypertension would likely be associated with significant underlying cardiac or pulmonary disease. Also, exposure to a hypoxic environment would further increase pulmonary pressures via pulmonary vasoconstriction, acutely increasing the burden on the right heart, and possibly precipitating symptoms such as dyspnea, fatigue, and even syncope.

Prosthetic Valves

Prosthetic valves are of two basic types—mechanical and biological. Biological prosthetic valves may be animal (porcine, bovine) or human tissue valves. Prosthetic valves do not cure the patient. Rather, it is more appropriate to consider that the patient has exchanged one disease for another. Based on a favorable risk/benefit ratio, the patient has traded significant valvular disease for the potentially trouble-some prosthetic valve and its attendant need for careful follow-up and the possibility of long-term complications, including late reoperation. Prosthetic valves are pre-dominantly placed in the aortic and mitral positions in adults.

Mechanical Prostheses and Nonhuman Bioprostheses

Although randomized trials of prosthetic valves are few and usually of small size, published guidelines for the management of valvular disease summarize the poten-tial complications very well.[75] In one study comparing mechanical and animal valve prostheses, 12-year survival without reoperation was 75% for mechanical valves and 42%-55% for animal valves. In another trial, 11-year actuarial survival was 53%-64% for mechanical valves versus 59%-67% for biological valves. Most patients are improved by valve replacement and many become asymptomatic, but total mortality is nevertheless increased compared to the general population.

Valve-related complications occurred in 62%-71% of mechanical valves and in 64%-79% of biological valves over 11-12 years. The risk of thromboembolism was 1%-2% per year for mechanical valves on anticoagulation, and the risk for biological (animal) valves in sinus rhythm without anticoagulation was about 0.7% per year. Late reoperation may be required due to structural failure or deterioration of the prosthesis over time, and is more likely in the mitral versus the aortic position, and with biological versus mechanical valves. Reoperation rates at about 10 years range from approximately 10%-45%, depending on valve type and position. Because endocarditis occurs in about 5%-15% of prosthetic valves, all require infective endo-carditis prophylaxis.[75]

Other considerations include the status of the underlying cardiac disease (espe-cially left ventricular function), arrhythmias, exercise tolerance, and the risk of major hemorrhage if on anticoagulation. All mechanical prosthetic valves require chronic warfarin anticoagulation, whereas tissue valves generally do not. Aspirin antiplatelet therapy, if prescribed for tissue valves, is not associated with a medically or aeromedically increased risk and is acceptable for all flying. Also, mechanical and biological valves are inherently stenotic, causing a transvalvular pressure gradient of varying degree at rest in most patients. Hemodynamics, including cardiac output, may be within the range of normal at rest, but may respond abnormally to exercise.

Aerobatic and military flying are not recommended for aviators with mechanical or biological prosthetic valves. The armed forces of many countries consider a pros-thetic valve, with or without chronic warfarin anticoagulation, to be unacceptable for any military service. Recommendations for civilian flying are more problematic. A conservative approach would be to prohibit such patients from all civilian avia-tion, or at from least commercial flying. Another approach is a cautious return to general, private flying and multipilot commercial flying for low-risk aviators. These include individuals with a good hemodynamic result, including a mild pressure gradient across the prosthetic valve, normal or near normal cardiac chamber sizes, normal ventricular function, and normal sinus rhythm without significant arrhythmias. If chronic warfarin anticoagulation is allowed, an observation period of at least 6 months on a stable dose is recommended. Monthly INR checks should be required and should document stability without hemorrhagic complications for at least 6 months. Return to any flying should require at least a 6-month period of nonflying observation after surgery. Thorough annual review is recommended, including echocardiography, 24-hour ambulatory monitoring, and graded exercise testing (for exercise tolerance and induced arrhythmias).

Human Homograft and Autograft Valve Replacements

More promising possibilities are offered by aortic homograft and pulmonary autograft valves presently available for aortic valve replacement. An autograft is other valve tissue from the patient, a homograft is valve tissue from the same species (ie, human), and a heterograft is valve tissue from a different species (eg, porcine). The human tissue options have very low thromboembolic rates without anticoagulation, but structural integrity 20 years into the future is uncertain.

Pulmonary autograft (Ross procedure) involves transplanting the patient's own pulmonary valve (autograft) to the aortic position, then replacing the pulmonary valve with a homograft or heterograft valve. This requires a double valve replacement, with the possibility of complications occurring in either location.

Aortic homograft (replacing the patient's aortic valve with another human aortic valve) is considered by many to be the surgery of choice for younger patients because it has a low incidence of thromboembolism and achieves a very good hemodynamic result. Three techniques are used, so aeromedical consideration must include awareness of the surgical technique used in a given case. One technique involves replacing only the valve itself. Another involves placing the donor valve with a small segment of attached aortic root into the recipient's aortic root below the coronary artery ostia. The third involves aortic root replacement, requiring reimplantation of the right and left coronary arteries. This third option is least appealing aeromedically because of concern, at least theoretically, about the long-term results of the coronary arteries and the aortic root segment. Another consideration is the type of preservation used for the grafted tissue; cryopreservation seems to have the best success.

A literature review of homograft aortic valve replacement indicated a thromboembolic rate of 0.1% per year or less, an endocarditis rate less than 1% per year, no acute valve failures reported using cryopreservation, and a low rate of slow valve deterioration that can easily be diagnosed with regular follow-up.[99] In a report of 117 patients receiving aortic homograft with cryopreservation techniques, freedom from valve-related mortality was 93% at 10 years, and freedom from reoperation for homograft-related causes was 92%.[100] Freedom from thromboembolism was 100% and from endocarditis 98%. Long-term durability is not yet well known; a major consideration is possible degeneration of the prosthetic valve over time, requiring future reoperation.

Aeromedical disposition of pulmonary autograft or aortic homograft patients should include a 6- to 12-month period of observation after surgery, to assess the short-term hemodynamic result and left ventricular size and function, and to detect any residua such as aortic insufficiency. If results are good, with no more than trace or mild aortic insufficiency, left ventricular size and function are normal at rest (and perhaps during exercise), and there are no associated arrhythmias, then return to military or civilian multipilot low-performance flight duties is feasible. Thorough and regular review for continued recertification would be essential. The United States Air Force has returned one pilot to restricted multipilot low-performance flight duties 4 years after homograft replacement of the aortic valve for severe aortic insufficiency caused by endocarditis of a bicuspid aortic valve.[99] After reviewing this topic, the second United Kingdom workshop in aviation cardiology recommended that recertification to fly as or with copilot could be extended to low-risk patients with a normally functioning aortic homograft 1 year after surgery.[101]

Another aortic valve replacement procedure that holds future aeromedical promise is aortic valve replacement with a stentless porcine prosthesis. Early reports demonstrate hemodynamic and clinical outcomes similar to homografts, but with significantly less aortic insufficiency. This procedure may become similarly acceptable for low-performance flying when reports of long-term outcomes are available.

Mitral Valve Repair

Mitral valve repair is another surgical valve procedure with aeromedical promise. In most situations, mitral valve repair is currently considered the surgery of choice for isolated mitral regurgitation (MR), especially for nonrheumatic, nonischemic MR. The outlook for flight certification in repaired ischemic MR is poor due to the underlying ischemic cardiac disease. Mitral valve repair of rheumatic MR also has an unacceptable rate of repair-related complications of about 4% per year.[102] This discussion will therefore focus on mitral repair of degenerative, myxomatous MR.

Repair of isolated MR due to degenerative (myxomatous) mitral valve disease has potential to allow certification for some categories of flying. Experienced surgeons can successfully repair about 90% of such valves. The mitral leaflets and chordae are primarily repaired as needed. Usually a prosthetic ring is sutured to the mitral annulus to resize and reshape it. This ring is endothelialized within several weeks and essentially becomes the new mitral annulus. The repair thus preserves the native mitral valve apparatus, resulting in better postoperative left ventricular function and increased survival. The absence of a valve prosthesis results in low thromboembolic rates and obviates the need for chronic warfarin anticoagulation unless atrial fibrillation is present.

Preoperative atrial fibrillation does not seem to affect outcome, but postoperative atrial fibrillation has been associated with reduced survival out to 4 years. Other predictors of less favorable outcome include age greater than 60-70 years, residual reduced left ventricular function, residual left atrial and ventricular dilation, and residual significant MR.

The rate of late reoperation due to deterioration of the repair is low, as are rates of thromboembolism and endocarditis. In a report on 195 patients with mitral valve repair, operative mortality for patients younger than 75 years was 1.3%.[103] At 10 years, late deaths occurred in 31%, but this rate was no different from expected deaths. In another report of 62 patients with mitral valve repair followed for a mean of 5 years, operative mortality was 1.6%, overall death rate was 4.8%, reoperation was performed in 6.5%, and there was no endocarditis or thromboembolism.[104] A third study reported on the durability of mitral valve repair in 1062 patients. At 10 years, freedom from reoperation was 93%. However, 53% (16/30) of reoperations were thought to be due to progressive degeneration of the valve itself, not the repair.[105]

From the available literature, it seems reasonable to return a low-risk aviator to multipilot low-performance aircraft flying 6-12 months after successful mitral valve repair for degenerative MR. Low-risk predictors include age less than 60, no postoperative atrial fibrillation or other significant arrhythmias, normal or near normal left ventricular and atrial dimensions, normal left ventricular function at rest (and perhaps during stress), and no residual MR greater than trace to mild. Return to high-performance flying is not recommended for aviators with degenerative valves that develop severe MR, often with associated with chordal rupture. As noted above, half of late reoperations are due to progressive degeneration of the valve. Thorough annual noninvasive reevaluation is recommended.

Tachyarrhythmias, Preexcitation, and Radiofrequency Ablation

Supraventricular Tachycardia

Clinical Features

For the purpose of this discussion supraventricular tachycardia (SVT) is classically defined as three or more consecutive supraventricular beats at a rate of 100 beats per minute or faster. However, clinically-sustained SVT is usually faster, in the range of 140-250 beats per minute. Discussions of SVT usually consider only clinical, sustained rhythms, but this discussion will also consider nonsustained SVT. There are no widely accepted definitions of sustained and nonsustained SVT. However, clinically-sustained SVT typically lasts at least several minutes and often up to one or more hours, whereas nonsustained SVT is usually only several supraventricular beats in a row or less than a minute in duration.

Prevalence. SVT prevalence in apparently healthy individuals is reported as about 0.02% on electrocardiography, 0.6% on graded exercise testing, and up to 5.0% on ambulatory monitoring.[10] In a population-based study comprising about 50,000 residents, the estimated prevalence of clinical, sustained SVT was about 0.2%, and the incidence of new cases was 36/100,000 persons per year in the United States.[106]

History. SVT typically occurs suddenly and unexpectedly. Depending on the rate and other factors, presentation ranges from asymptomatic or palpitations and a sensation of rapid heartbeat, to serious hemodynamic symptoms including presyncope, syncope, and even sudden cardiac death. Intermediate symptoms include dyspnea, anxiety, chest discomfort, and lightheadedness. When eliciting a history of palpitations, the examining AME/FS should carefully attempt, without influencing the aviator, to differentiate between palpitations due to isolated ectopy versus a racing heartbeat suggesting a tachyarrhythmia.

When discussing SVT, one often thinks of relatively young and otherwise healthy individuals. However, there are two basic subsets of patients with SVT in the clinical population: 1) a group with associated coronary, myocardial, or valvular heart disease who tend to be older and male, and 2) a group without underlying heart disease who tend to be younger and female. When SVT is associated with underlying heart disease it is difficult to differentiate prognosis of SVT from that of the associated disease. From an aeromedical perspective, the associated heart disease could be quite significant. SVT in the presence of underlying disease such as coronary artery disease or aortic stenosis might be more likely to cause symptoms that could affect performance of flight duties, such as angina, dyspnea, or presyncope. Therefore, although there may not be a causative relationship between SVT and underlying disease, the additive effect that may produce hemodynamic symptoms should prompt an evaluation for associated heart disease in an aviator with SVT.

Medical therapy to suppress SVT is generally indicated when symptoms occur frequently or interfere with quality of life, including participating in certain occupations such as flying or participating in competitive sports. Curative therapy by radiofrequency ablation should be considered for significant hemodynamic symptoms or for lifestyle considerations.

Natural History and Aeromedical Considerations

A review of SVT recurrence rates from tertiary centers reveals one group that had an average recurrence rate of 71% within 3 months, whereas in their own population-based study, the recurrence rate of sustained SVT was only 6% at 3 months and 20% at 2 years.[106] This discrepancy represents a significant tertiary center referral bias. Tertiary referral bias also significantly affects reported syncope due to SVT. In a review of private and public safety issues related to arrhythmias and private and commercial driving and flying, it was reported that about 25% of SVT referrals for electrophysiologic studies have a history of at least one episode of syncope.[107] Another study found that 90 (15%) of 589 patients receiving radiofrequency ablation for symptomatic SVT had a history of syncope or near syncope.[108] Similarly, syncope occurred in 33 (20%) of 167 consecutive patients receiving ablation for SVT.[109] Finally, a report described 290 patients receiving electrophysiologic studies for aborted sudden death; in 13 (4.5%) of these patients the initiating mechanism of cardiac arrest was SVT.[110] These studies found no cofactors predictive of recurrent SVT or associated hemodynamic symptoms.

The above data are not intended to alarm the AME/FS who is evaluating an aviator with SVT for possible return to flight duty. Instead, this information is shared to emphasize two points. First, SVT is not always benign; serious hemodynamic symptoms and even sudden death may occur. Second, a significant tertiary referral bias may be encountered in the clinical literature. The above figures probably seem high to the community level practitioner. In the above cited population-based study, only sustained SVT causing symptoms or requiring medical therapy was included.[106] Even so, of 33 new incident cases of SVT, only 2/33 (6%) presented with hemodynamic instability (hypotension, cardiovascular collapse, or syncope).

Another aeromedical problem is the appropriate disposition of asymptomatic nonsustained episodes of SVT. Is nonsustained SVT predictive of sustained SVT? Is it predictive of SVT-associated hemodynamic symptoms. These are the pertinent aeromedical concerns regarding SVT, including nonsustained SVT: What is the likelihood of future episodes of sustained SVT and SVT-associated hemodynamic symptoms? Surprisingly, the literature contains little useful information to help answer these questions, especially for nonsustained SVT.

These issues were addressed in a review of 430 military aviators with sustained or nonsustained SVT followed for a mean of 11.4 years.[17] In this study 42 of 430 (10%) had associated hemodynamic symptoms; there were no instances of sudden death but there were 5 episodes of syncope. Of those initially presenting with asymptomatic nonsustained SVT, only 0.9% experienced sustained SVT during the follow-up period, and none of these subjects had hemodynamic symptoms. Of those initially presenting with asymptomatic sustained SVT, the rate of recurrence was about 1% per year for initial presentation with a single sustained SVT episode, and about 2% per year for initial presentation with recurrent episodes of sustained SVT. Approximately 8% of these recurrences were associated with hemodynamic symptoms. Frequent and paired premature atrial beats and nonsustained SVT were not predictive of sustained SVT episodes or of hemodynamic symptoms. Use of caffeine, nicotine, or alcohol was also not predictive. Only initial presentation with sustained SVT and initial presentation with hemodynamic symptoms imposed an increased relative risk for these aeromedical endpoints.

This study does suffer from a bias as well, a survival bias, in that aviators with more significant SVT and symptomatology were likely not referred for evaluation but were permanently disqualified locally. Also, there may be a reporting bias involved with aviator populations. Nevertheless, this aviator cohort and the general population study provide more applicable data for the AME/FS evaluating military or civilian aviators than does the standard cardiac literature.[17,106]

Unrestricted flying is recommended for nonsustained SVT without associated hemodynamic symptoms. Any duration of SVT causing hemodynamic symptoms is reasonably considered disqualifying for all flying in the absence of aeromedically acceptable therapy.

Clearly, sustained SVT may cause hemodynamic symptoms that could adversely affect flying performance. With recurrence rates of at least 1%-2% per year (military aviators) and up to 10% per year (general population), the aeromedical disposition of single and recurrent sustained episodes of SVT without hemodynamic symptoms is debatable.[17,106] It is suggested that recurrent sustained SVT without aeromedically acceptable therapy should be disqualifying, at least for military and civilian commercial aviation. It may be acceptable to recommend return to restricted, or even unrestricted, flying for a single, asymptomatic episode of sustained SVT, especially if there is no recurrence during a nonflying observation period of 3-6 months. Alternatively, one might consider the above recurrence rates unacceptable for even a single episode of sustained SVT, especially for certain types of aviation, such as military, high-performance (aerobatic, jet fighters), or any single pilot aircraft.

The use of medications to suppress clinically significant SVT (hemodynamic symptoms or sustained SVT) may itself be cause for disqualification, especially for military aviators. (Medications are discussed below and in a later section of this chapter.) Recurrent SVT in spite of the use of prescribed medication is a possibility that must always be considered. Consequently, published guidelines for competitive athletes recommend no restrictions for medically controlled SVT that is asymptomatic, but a return to only low-intensity sports for medically treated SVT that previously caused significant hemodynamic symptoms.[111] Therapy would, of course, be limited to those medications considered acceptable by the licensing authority. If medically treated SVT is considered for return to flying, this should probably be limited to low-performance and multipilot aircraft.

Any consideration of a special issuance to return an aviator with SVT to unrestricted or restricted flying duties, with or without antiarrhythmic therapy, should incorporate appropriate testing to document control of SVT. Such testing should include graded exercise testing and 24-72 hour ambulatory monitoring during routine activities. Graded exercise testing also serves to exclude underlying significant coronary heart disease. Echocardiography to exclude structural disease is prudent. Electrocardiographic monitoring during performance of actual or simulated flight is advisable, as is monitoring during altitude chamber or centrifuge testing for appropriate types of aircraft.

Preexcitation

Clinical Features

Conditions of preexcitation have a bypass tract or accessory pathway of conduction from atrium to ventricle (and ventricle to atrium). The classic preexcitation condition is Wolff-Parkinson-White (WPW), having the diagnostic electrocardiographic pattern of a short PR interval and delta wave. The WPW electrocardiographic pattern may be only intermittently present in some patients, and at times the electrocardiogram is normal. Other types of accessory pathways also exist, having variable electrocardiographic findings including a normal electrocardiogram. When the electrocardiogram is normal in the presence of an accessory pathway, the pathway is said to be **concealed** because it does not appear on the surface electrocardiogram. Such patients would likely only be diagnosed by electrophysiologic testing performed after clinically manifest supraventricular tachycardia.

The incidence of the WPW electrocardiographic pattern is reported as 0.1-3.0/1000 (average, 1.5/1000) in the general population.[112] The prevalence in military aviators is about 1-1.5/1000, comparable to that of the general population.[5,113] These two reports in military aviators appeared shortly after the use of screening electro-cardiograms in those aviator populations became routine. Screening electrocardiography is now commonly performed in military and civilian aviators and flight training candidates. If WPW is considered unacceptable for entry into flight training, then the prevalence of WPW in a trained aviator population would obviously be lower than the figures reported above.

Natural History and Aeromedical Considerations

The clinical and aeromedical concerns regarding preexcitation are risks of sudden cardiac death and sustained supraventricular tachycardia (SVT). The literature on accessory pathways is mostly concerned with sudden cardiac death. This event reportedly occurs in 0%-6.0% of WPW individuals over 10 years or 0.0%-0.6% per year; the average in all WPW patients is 0.1%-0.15% per year.[114] Invasive and noninvasive tests have a poor positive predictive value to detect individuals at risk for sudden cardiac death. However, the greater aeromedical concern is probably the risk for SVT, simply because it occurs more frequently, occurs suddenly and unexpectedly, and certainly could affect an aviator's safe performance of flight duties.

The reported incidence of SVT associated with WPW varies widely, from 12%-80%.[114] The most accurate figure may be that reported in a population-based study from the Mayo Clinic.[115] The risk of SVT was 3% per year for 10 years after diagnosis of the WPW electrocardiographic pattern. In military aviators, the prevalence of SVT in WPW has been reported to be 12%-16%.[5,113,116] In a report on 430 military aviators with sustained or nonsustained SVT, the presence of preexcitation was predictive of an approximately 4- to 5-fold increased risk of hemodynamic symptoms or recurrent sustained SVT.[17] Nine of 18 (50%) aviators with WPW and any degree of SVT had either hemodynamic symptoms or asymptomatic episodes of recurrent sustained SVT. Surprisingly, there are few published data regarding the predictive value of frequent and/or complex supraventricular ectopy (atrial pairing and nonsustained SVT) as predictors of sudden cardiac death or sustained SVT in preexcitation subjects.

WPW pattern is the electrocardiographic finding only, without prior documented SVT or symptoms suggesting sustained SVT. Consideration of entry into flight training or a return to flying with WPW pattern must take into account the above-mentioned slight risk of sudden arrhythmic death and the 3%-per-year risk of SVT. Also, therapeutic options and their aeromedical impact must be considered, especially because curative therapy of accessory pathways by radiofrequency ablation is available. Discussion and recommendations regarding ablation appear at the end of this section. Initial entry into military aviator training is not recommended. A new diagnosis of WPW pattern in an older aviator may not contraindicate return to flying, even unrestricted flying, if there is no SVT by careful history and noninvasive testing, and especially if review of all electrocardiograms shows the pattern to be only intermittently present. A more cautious approach, especially for younger aviators, would be electrophysiologic testing that may detect individuals at higher risk of sudden death, and can assess for inducibility of SVT, although this does not completely exclude later spontaneous occurrence of clinical SVT.

Aviators with accessory pathways with associated SVT by history or electrocardiographic documentation are not recommended for military flying, even with apparently successful medical suppression; SVT may still occur under different autonomic and other conditions. A wide variety of antiarrhythmic medications may be used to suppress tachyarrhythmias associated with accessory pathways; the agents most commonly used are calcium channel antagonists and beta-blockers. Disqualification from civilian flying is a disposition option. Alternatively, electrophysiologic testing may be used to exclude individuals at higher risk of sudden death and to assess apparently-successful medical suppression of SVT. Recommendation for return to general, private flying and/or multipilot commercial flying might then be permissible.

Atrial Fibrillation and Atrial Flutter

Lone Atrial Fibrillation

The aeromedical disposition of atrial fibrillation (AFib) associated with underlying disease should be guided by policies for the underlying disease, with the AFib considered a complication or endpoint. This discussion will be limited to lone AFib, usually defined as paroxysmal or chronic AFib without underlying structural heart disease, hypertension, or hyperthyroidism. Many sources also add age <60 years to the criteria. Using this definition and a thorough noninvasive evaluation to exclude underlying disease, lone AFib has a low rate of morbid events, including stroke. It may occur as a single, isolated episode, as recurrent paroxysmal events, or as persistent, chronic AFib. Lone AFib comprises only about 5%-10% of all cases of AFib, depending partly on the age of the subjects studied. Of 3632 patients with AFib, only 97 (2.7%) had lone AFib, including subjects aged <60 years.[117] And in a randomly selected population of 9067 individuals aged 32-64 years, only 25 (0.3%) had chronic AFib and only 8 of these 25 had lone AFib.[118]

Natural History and Aeromedical Considerations

Aeromedical concerns are thromboembolism, warfarin anticoagulation, medications to control ventricular rate and/or maintain sinus rhythm, and symptoms related to the AFib itself, especially if the ventricular rate is rapid. Stroke is the most common thromboembolic event; practitioners are well aware of the risk of stroke associated with AFib and the possibility of reducing that risk with anticoagulation. However, the risk of stroke is less than 1% per year in lone AFib without anticoagulation. (Medications are discussed below and in a later section of this chapter.)

Of 97 lone AFib cases (mean age, 44 years) followed for a mean of 14.8 years, 20 (21%) had an isolated episode of AFib, 56 (58%) had paroxysmal AFib, and 21 (22%) had chronic AFib.[117] Only 8 of the 97 were treated with warfarin; indications were deep venous thrombosis in 3, left ventricular thrombus in 1, and prophylaxis in 4. There were a total of 4 embolic strokes. On a cumulative actuarial basis, 1.3% had suffered a stroke at 15 years and the probability of survival was 94%. There was no difference in survival among the 3 types of AFib. Stroke risk was 0.55% per year and was no different from that of an age- and gender-matched control population. In a review of electrocardiograms from 13,037 aviators, only 8 had AFib; 2 of the 8 had an isolated AFib episode, and 3 each had paroxysmal and chronic AFib.[119] During 13.6 years mean follow-up, one aviator had a systemic embolism to the leg. And in the Framingham Heart Study, lone AFib accounted for 11.4% of all AFib; the risk of stroke during 30 years follow-up was 28%, compared to 7% in controls without AFib.[120] However, hypertension was included in the Framingham definition of lone AFib, and most lone AFib subjects were over age 60 years.

An excellent aeromedical review of lone AFib also concluded that with age 60 years or younger, lone AFib has a low risk of stroke, comparable to that of controls.[121] However, the author also raised some concerns regarding total mortality with lone AFib, citing a report of insurance applicants in whom mortality was normal for paroxysmal lone AFib, but increased 2.6-fold for chronic lone AFib with or without associated disease. He also cited his own work that demonstrated 39% mortality in 46 patients with lone AFib during 77 months mean follow-up, compared to 13% mortality in 46 controls. In contrast, follow-up of 97 lone AFib patients demonstrated a 15-year probability of death of only 6%, comparable to that of a normal population.[117]

Two more recent reports add to this concern regarding lone AFib. The Framingham Heart Study examined mortality in the 621 subjects who developed AFib over 40 years of follow-up.[122] After adjusting for age, hypertension, smoking, diabetes, left ventricular hypertrophy, myocardial infarction, congestive heart failure, valvular heart disease, and stroke or transient ischemic attack, AFib was associated with an increased mortality with an odds ratio of 1.5 for men and 1.9 for women. This population was older than the aviator population, with a mean age of 75 years (range, 55-94 years). In another study, 145 lone AFib subjects aged 50 years or younger were followed for a mean 10 years; 96 had paroxysmal lone AFib and 49 had chronic lone AFib.[123] In the paroxysmal group, 1 had a stroke, 2 had a transient ischemic attack, and 1 had a myocardial infarction. In the chronic AFib group, 8 embolic events occurred in 7 patients (16.3%), 2 died suddenly (6.1%), 1 had a transient ischemic attack, 1 had heart failure, and 2 had a myocardial infarction. The authors concluded that paroxysmal lone AFib had a benign prognosis, whereas chronic lone AFib had an increased risk of embolic events and mortality.

The 3 types of lone AFib (a single episode without recurrence, paroxysmal, and chronic persistent types) are usually mixed together in one cohort. The above studies suggest that the prognosis of the 3 types of lone AFib may differ significantly. In the natural history study of 97 patients noted above, stroke occurring in paroxysmal lone AFib subjects did so only after they had "progressed" to chronic AFib.[117] However, others have noted stroke associated with paroxysmal lone AFib, so it does occur in these subjects. There is a large proportion of isolated and paroxysmal lone AFib subjects in these studies. If the risk of mortality and embolic events is largely associated with the chronic persistent type, this might be underappreciated because of the larger numbers of subjects with the other 2 types of lone AFib.

An interesting study suggested myocarditis as an etiology for at least some cases of lone AFib.[124] Atrial and ventricular myocardial biopsies were performed on 12 patients with paroxysmal lone AFib and 11 controls. All biopsy specimens from the controls were normal, whereas the atrial biopsies from all 12 lone AFib patients were abnormal; in addition, 3 had similar abnormal findings on ventricular specimens. Thus, all cases of lone AFib might not be idiopathic. Perhaps apparently lone AFib should periodically be reevaluated for underlying disease.

Impaired cardiac performance may occur due to the loss of atrial contribution, loss of atrioventricular synchrony, and rapid ventricular rate at rest and/or during exercise. This is particularly troubling with regard to physiologic responses to the high $+G_z$ environment of aerobatic and high-performance military flight. While not necessarily a risk for sudden incapacitation, this is an operational consideration, especially for military aviators who are expected to meet physical as well as medical standards, and are more likely to be exposed to harsh conditions. This concern applies to both paroxysmal and chronic AFib. In fact, one could argue that paroxysmal AFib might be more of a concern due to its unexpected, sudden onset and immediate change from normal conditions, whereas chronic AFib is persistent, prompting adaptive changes. And with chronic AFib, rate response to exertion and effect on exercise tolerance can be assessed by methods such as graded exercise testing, actual and simulated flight, altitude chamber exposure, and centrifuge testing.

All of these various issues plus the issue of medication use must be considered by licensing authorities in establishing aeromedical disposition policies for lone

AFib, and it may be reasonable to consider the 3 types of lone AFib separately and handle them differently. At present, pending review of its experience with AFib in military aviators, the United States Air Force essentially treats lone AFib and atrial flutter like SVT. An aviator with a single episode without associated hemodynamic symptoms is eligible for return to unrestricted military flying after thorough evaluation. Permanent disqualification for any military flying is recommended for any AFib with associated hemodynamic symptoms and for paroxysmal or chronic AFib, with or without medical therapy.

Similarly, an aeromedical review regarding civilian licensure recommended return to full flight duties for a single episode of AFib after thorough noninvasive evaluation and a nonflying observation period of 6 months to ensure a lack of recurrence and exclude underlying disease.[121] Permanent disqualification was suggested for paroxysmal AFib due to the possibility of aeromedically relevant symptoms, including subtle effects. Another option that was offered was certification for restricted flying duties after 6 months if one or more medications controlled the rhythm and/or symptoms without side effects, and if the medications were acceptable to the licensing authority. As discussed above, these authors also made the point that hemodynamic and symptomatic stability and normal performance are more readily established for chronic AFib simply because the rhythm is persistent. Thus, the recommended option for chronic lone AFib was return to restricted multicrew operations after documentation of adequate ventricular rate control, including during exercise and simulated flight conditions. This assumes a low mortality and stroke risk for chronic lone AFib. As discussed above, chronic lone AFib may not be as benign as previously thought.[122,123]

Atrial Flutter

Atrial flutter occurs much less frequently than AFib, and often coexists with or degenerates into AFib. As an isolated rhythm it is uncommon. It is generally felt that pure atrial flutter is a lower risk than AFib, because it has a more regular and organized atrial rhythm and contraction. However, in the relatively healthy, young aviator, ventricular rate response in the absence of controlling medication would certainly be a concern. Expected atrioventricular conduction would be 2:1, yielding a ventricular response of about 150 beats per minute; 1:1 conduction with a ventricular rate of about 300 beats per minute would also be possible. Medication to block atrioventricular conduction and control ventricular rate is indicated for atrial flutter. (Medications are discussed below and in a later section of this chapter.)

For aeromedical disposition, atrial flutter could be handled using the same guidelines as for AFib or SVT. As with AFib, this would involve only "lone atrial flutter." Atrial flutter associated with AFib may best be handled within AFib policies. On the other hand, licensing authorities might choose to disqualify atrial flutter altogether due to the undefined risk of 1:1 conduction and a very rapid ventricular rate. For example, one aeromedical review addressing civilian aviation issues recommended that atrial flutter be permanently disqualifying for civilian flying.[121] The recommendation is disqualification for aerobatic, military, and civilian commercial aviation. Selected cases that are well controlled by medication might be certified for general, private aviation after an observation period.

Medical Therapy of SVT, AFib, and Atrial Flutter

General considerations for medication use in aviators that were briefly discussed earlier certainly apply to antiarrhythmic agents. Warfarin is generally not indicated for lone AFib, lone atrial flutter, or the other arrhythmias discussed above. Aspirin antiplatelet therapy is acceptable; there is a slight risk of hemorrhagic events, but there is no increase compared to placebo in many trials. No anticoagulation is currently recommended for lone AFib patients younger than 60 years of age; however, some practitioners might prefer aspirin therapy for additional protection, particularly for chronic lone AFib.

Approval of antiarrhythmic medication in an aviator will depend on both the type of arrhythmia and the medication used, as well as symptoms previously experienced during the arrhythmia. Maintenance of sinus rhythm versus controlling ventricular rate are the uses for medication for AFib and atrial flutter, whereas preventing the arrhythmia is the treatment goal for SVT. Before initiating long-term antiarrhythmic therapy, the physician and patient must consider the risk of the arrhythmia versus the risk of medical therapy, the frequency of the arrhythmia, and the severity of associated symptoms. Side effect and safety profiles of the medications are certainly of aeromedical concern. Perfect control with medication is often not achieved with tolerable side effects, and one must accept that the arrhythmia may "break through" and recur. Another clinical and aeromedical concern is the proarrhythmic effect of many antiarrhythmics. In other words, some antiarrhythmics also cause arrhythmias, usually ventricular. A final issue is compliance of the aviator in taking the medication.

For some licensing authorities and aviation environments, these concerns may preclude the use of any antiarrhythmic medications. One aeromedical review discussed the medication issue thoroughly, concluding that antiarrhythmic medication may be acceptable in civilian aviators without underlying disease if the arrhythmia has been well tolerated on a physical, mental, and performance basis.[125] In addition, the medication selected must have documented efficacy without proarrhythmic effects or significant side effects and the aviator must be compliant. These are rather significant restrictions; it was recommended that only hydrophilic beta-blockers, calcium channel antagonists, and digitalis meet these requirements. (Further discussion of cardiac medications appears in a later section of this chapter.)

Return to military flying is not recommended for any antiarrhythmic therapy. Return to commercial multipilot or general, private flying may be considered for selected cases, especially if there are no hemodynamic symptoms associated with the supraventricular tachyarrhythmia. The above restrictions are then recommended, including a nonflying observation period of at least 6 months.

Ventricular Tachycardia

Clinical Features

Ventricular tachycardia (VT) is defined as three or more consecutive ventricular beats at a rate of 100 beats per minute or faster, although some sources use the criterion of 120 beats per minute. The rate of clinically sustained VT is usually in the range of 140-200 beats per minute. In the electrophysiology literature, sustained VT is usually defined as lasting 30 seconds or longer, and this definition will be used for this discussion. The spectrum of VT may then range anywhere from a 3-beat run that is asymptomatic and unnoticed by the patient to a sustained run with hemodynamic collapse.

Natural History and Aeromedical Considerations

In the absence of aeromedically acceptable therapy, any VT associated with hemodynamic symptoms should likely be permanently disqualified for all types of flying, as should asymptomatic sustained VT. Even nonsustained VT, which is associated with some underlying heart diseases (eg, coronary artery disease and cardiomyopathy), is known to have an unfavorable prognosis, and this combination should also be disqualifying. Indeed, the underlying disease itself may often merit disqualification. On the other hand, VT may be associated with other underlying cardiac diagnoses that are not known to have an unfavorable prognosis when combined with VT (eg, mild aortic insufficiency or bicuspid aortic valve). These diagnoses should be considered separately for aeromedical disposition.

Idiopathic VT is that which occurs in the absence of underlying disease. This discussion will focus on the appropriate disposition of nonsustained and hemodynamically asymptomatic idiopathic VT. This will most likely be detected on ambulatory monitoring or graded exercise testing performed for a variety of indications. The cardiac literature is often said to demonstrate a benign prognosis for nonsustained idiopathic VT. However, the literature is often concerned only with risk of sudden death, and not other aeromedically pertinent events such as syncope and lightheadedness.

There is little guidance regarding how many episodes and what duration of nonsustained VT is benign and therefore acceptable.

Another consideration is what testing is required to document VT as idiopathic. Coronary heart disease, hypertrophic and other cardiomyopathies, right ventricular dysplasia, and long QT syndrome must be reasonably excluded. Ambulatory monitoring to assess for repetitive events is warranted. Echocardiography and graded exercise testing are also recommended. At age >35-40 years, exercise radionuclide myocardial imaging and screening for coronary artery calcification should also be considered. Performance of coronary angiography to definitely exclude coronary heart disease is also an option. Some literature on idiopathic VT even recommends myocardial biopsy, although this seems extreme for routine evaluation of the asymptomatic aviator.

A review of the aeromedical disposition of ventricular arrhythmias for purposes of civilian commercial and private aviation suggested an algorithm for the aeromedical disposition of VT.[126] Permanent disqualification was recommended for VT associated with underlying heart disease. Disqualification was also recommended for idiopathic VT with a duration of 10 beats or longer, or for VT of shorter duration if associated with hemodynamic symptoms. For asymptomatic idiopathic VT of less than 10 beats duration, special issuance for a restricted license was recommended without comment on the number of episodes of VT.

Published guidelines regarding competitive athletes with VT take a similar stance and may be of some use in developing aeromedical disposition policies.[111] Regardless of treatment, a thorough evaluation and no competitive sports for 6 months after the VT episode were recommended. If structural heart disease is present, possible return only to low-intensity competitive sports was recommended, even if the VT was suppressed by medication. For idiopathic VT, return to all competitive sports was recommended if there is no clinical recurrence of VT, and if exercise and electrophysiologic testing do not induce VT. Finally, return to all competitive sports was recommended for asymptomatic idiopathic VT of short duration (8-10 beats) with rates generally less than 150 beats per minute, if exercise does not significantly worsen the baseline arrhythmia. These individuals were not felt to be at increased risk for sudden death. Again, no mention was made regarding number of runs of VT allowed.

A policy very similar to the above recommendations has been implemented for some military aviators. A recent report followed 193 military aviators with nonsustained VT for a mean of 10.6 years.[18] Idiopathic VT was present in 103 of the 193. No endpoints occurred during follow-up in the 99 of 103 presenting initially with asymptomatic idiopathic nonsustained VT; 4 of 103 initially presented with hemodynamic symptoms. Based on 95% confidence limits and Poisson distribution, the maximum expected annual event rate during follow-up was 0.33% per year for the endpoints of documented sustained VT, sudden death, syncope, and presyncope. Most of the nonsustained idiopathic VT (81%) was only 3-4 beats in duration, and 69% had only 1 run of nonsustained VT by 24-hour ambulatory monitor or graded exercise test. Idiopathic VT longer than 11 beats in duration occurred in only 2%, and only 10% had more than 4 episodes of nonsustained VT by 24-hour ambulatory monitoring or graded exercise test. The authors recommended return to low-performance multipilot flying for asymptomatic idiopathic VT with duration of 11 beats or less and frequency of 4 runs or less per 24-hour monitoring period. Return to unrestricted flying was recommended for a single, isolated occurrence of asymptomatic idiopathic VT of duration of 11 beats or less without associated frequent ventricular ectopy or any ventricular pairing. Return to flying·is not recommended for ventricular tachycardia treated with antiarrhythmics.

Radiofrequency Ablation of Tachyarrhythmias

Supraventricular Tachycardia

The most common cause of SVT (about 60% of cases) is a reentry circuit within the atrioventricular (AV) node, and is termed **AV node reentrant tachycardia** (AVNRT) by cardiologists. The next most common cause of SVT (about 30%) is a macroreentrant circuit involving an accessory pathway called **AV reentrant tachycardia** (AVRT). WPW syndrome discussed above is the classic AVRT. The remaining small percentage (10% or less) of SVTs are atrial tachycardias due to an automatic focus in one of the atria or other relatively unusual mechanisms.

Radiofrequency ablation is a potentially curative treatment for SVT. Ablation has previously been performed by surgery and by catheter techniques using DC current. However, radiofrequency ablation has emerged in recent years as the ablative technique of choice, with a high success rate and low complication rate. The immediate complication and success rates are in a sense irrelevant, because only those aviators with a successful procedure without significant complications are likely to be considered for return to flight duty. However, the aeromedical specialist needs to be aware of this information to properly counsel the aviator considering ablation primarily for occupational rather than clinical indications. Aeromedical considerations of successful ablation include the long-term success rate of ablation, late complications of ablation, and what studies are necessary to document a successful ablation. A recent general review of radiofrequency ablation of tachyarrhythmias and a recent single-center experience with 1136 ablations in 1050 patients with different SVT mechanisms are excellent general references for this topic.[127,128]

Radiofrequency Ablation of AVRT. The initial research with radiofrequency ablation was for the treatment of AVRT, therefore this application has the largest reported experience. The immediate success rate is 90% or more in experienced electrophysiologic laboratories, with a complication rate of less than 5%, most of which are minor. However, one very significant complication is complete heart block requiring permanent pacemaker implantation. This occurs in approximately 0.5% of all accessory pathway ablations, but the actual risk is limited to a small number of accessory pathways in a critical location. About 5%-10% of accessory pathways are located adjacent to the anterior surface of the AV node. Pathways in this location have a 5%-10% risk of developing complete heart block as a complication of ablation. Accessory pathways located away from the AV node are not at risk for complete heart block.

Recurrence of a functioning accessory pathway occurs in 5%-10% of cases, with most recurrences appearing within 2-4 months after ablation. However, post-ablation electrophysiologic testing is not routinely performed clinically; reported recurrence is the clinical event of return of a WPW electrocardiographic pattern (short PR interval and delta wave), or recurrence of SVT. The recurrence rate might be somewhat higher if determined by routine post-ablation electrophysiologic testing.

Special catheters similar to temporary transvenous pacing catheters are used to deliver radiofrequency current anywhere along the circuit of reentrant tachycardias, or at or near the arrhythmogenic focus for automatic tachycardias. The heat injures the myocardial tissue, interrupting the reentrant circuit or eliminating the arrhythmogenic focus. The radiofrequency ablation site is therefore an area of myocardial injury, and theoretically might itself be arrhythmogenic. Some approaches are from the ventricular side of the atrioventricular plane, raising concern about resultant ventricular arrhythmias. This theoretical concern has not been substantiated in the literature, however, nor have any other significant long-term complications been reported.

A final issue is the extent of testing required to document a successful ablation for aeromedical disposition. In the absence of symptoms suggesting sustained SVT, routine 24-hour ambulatory monitoring is unlikely to reveal SVT but should nevertheless be performed. Treadmill testing might be useful, especially if SVT was induced by exercise prior to ablation. In WPW patients, intermittent appearance of the short PR and delta wave may be demonstrated on ambulatory monitoring or during the recovery phase of exercise testing. Clinically, one would generally only observe the patient for return of the WPW electrocardiographic pattern or return of symptoms suggesting SVT. Electrophysiologic testing post-ablation would not routinely be performed unless clinical SVT had recurred or unless pre-ablation SVT had been associated with very significant hemodynamic symptoms.

However, performance of electrophysiologic testing post-ablation is reasonable for occupational reasons to document successful ablation and support return of the aviator to flying. It must be noted that during the development of radiofrequency ablation, investigating centers routinely performed electrophysiologic testing at varying intervals post-ablation. No false negative studies were reported if electrophysiologic testing was performed at least 30 days after ablation. Negative electrophysiologic tests performed earlier than 30 days post-ablation were at times associated with later clinical recurrence of SVT or the WPW electrocardiographic pattern. Based on this experience and the fact that most recurrences appear 2-4 months after the procedure, routine electrophysiologic testing should be performed 3-6 months after ablation.

An additional consideration favors routine post-ablation electrophysiologic testing, at least for some types of flying. Like a wire, accessory pathways can conduct impulses in both directions. Unlike a wire, accessory pathways may have very different conduction properties in one direction versus the other, both before and after ablation. Antegrade conduction down the accessory pathway from atrium to ventricle may be ablated such that the 12-lead electrocardiogram is normal (normal PR, no delta wave). This should preclude risk of sudden death, which is thought to be due to very rapid antegrade conduction of atrial fibrillation down the accessory pathway. However, ablation may fail to eliminate retrograde conduction up the accessory pathway from ventricle to atrium. This would not be apparent on the 12-lead electrocardiogram, but it may maintain an SVT because the direction of travel for most AVRTs is down the normal AV nodal pathway into the ventricles, then retrograde up the accessory pathway back into the atrium. As discussed earlier, SVT may be a greater aeromedical concern than sudden death because of its greater frequency. Electrophysiologic testing could document successful elimination of conduction in both directions through the accessory pathway and allow quicker aeromedical disposition. If only noninvasive testing is performed after ablation, then a nonflying observation period of at least 6 months, and possibly up to 12 months, would be prudent to exclude the vast majority of recurrences. An excellent overview of AVRT radiofrequency ablation can be found in the references.[129]

The high success rate of AVRT ablation, the scarcity of late problems, and the ability to clearly document successful ablation by electrophysiologic testing support a return to unrestricted flying, including single seat high-performance aircraft. Routine post-ablation electrophysiologic testing is recommended for aerobatic and for all military flying. Noninvasive testing alone may be sufficient for general, private aviation and for commercial multipilot flying, if the SVT was not associated with serious hemodynamic symptoms. However, routine electrophysiologic testing should be considered for SVT associated with significant hemodynamic symptoms, especially for return to commercial flying. Isolated reports of very late recurrence do exist, so noninvasive reevaluation at 1-3 year intervals is appropriate. Subsequent electrophysiologic testing should probably only be performed for documented or suspected late recurrence.

Radiofrequency Ablation of AVNRT. Only a few comments need be made about ablation of AVNRT. This rhythm is caused by a reentry circuit within the AV node and was the second application of radiofrequency ablation research. Because AVNRT is the most common type of SVT, the published experience for ablation of AVNRT is comparable to that of AVRT discussed above. The immediate success rate, recurrence rate, scarcity of late complications, and ability to document success by electrophysiologic testing are essentially identical to those of AVRT. Complete heart block occurs as a complication in about 1% of AVNRT ablations. This initially seems surprising because ablation of accessory pathways on the anterior surface of the AV node has a 5%-10% risk of complete heart block. Indeed, initial efforts at AVNRT ablation were performed at an anterior location on the AV node and had a higher risk of complete heart block. However, an approach from the posterior surface of the AV node was developed which yielded the much safer rate of about 1%. The above discussion and aeromedical recommendations regarding AVRT ablation apply to AVNRT ablation as well. A general review of AVNRT ablation and a review of AVNRT from an aeromedical perspective are recommended reading.[130,131]

Radiofrequency Ablation of Other Atrial Tachycardias. As noted earlier, AVRT and AVNRT comprise about 90% of all SVTs. The other 10% are a variety of different atrial, junctional, and even sinus node tachycardias of different mechanisms, including reentrant pathways and automatic foci. Published reports of radiofrequency ablation for these SVTs are obviously limited in number. Options for aeromedical disposition are to either disqualify all of them due to lack of data or to consider them on a case-by-case basis for restricted flying at minimum, considering the above experience with AVRT and AVNRT and the limited data available for the particular rhythm disturbance. A source for a good review of ablation of these uncommon atrial tachycardias is provided in the references.[132]

Radiofrequency Ablation of Atrial Flutter. Atrial flutter is an uncommon rhythm and there is therefore little reported experience regarding ablation of this rhythm disturbance. Atrial flutter is due to a localized reentrant circuit in the right atrium involving a critical isthmus of myocardium between the tricuspid annulus and the insertion of the inferior vena cava. This localized circuit makes curative radiofrequency ablation very feasible with success and recurrence rates similar to those of AVRT and AVNRT. Documentation of cure by post-ablation electrophysiologic testing is possible; one must demonstrate bidirectional conduction block through the isthmus to be assured of success. Without demonstration of bidirectional block, recurrence is much more likely. As a precautionary note, if atrial flutter does recur post-ablation, it could do so at a lower atrial rate of about 250 beats per minute rather than the typical 300 beats per minute. This could easily be conducted 1:1 through the AV node, resulting in a rapid ventricular rate and high likelihood of significant impairment. Because of this possibility, post-ablation electrophysiologic testing is encouraged prior to a certification of return to flying. Atrial flutter ablation is promising for return to flight duty. If considered, restriction to low-performance, multicrew aircraft is recommended pending more published experience and longer follow-up data.

One very important clinical and aeromedical consideration, however, is that of associated AFib. Atrial flutter is not common as a pure rhythm disturbance, but is often associated with AFib. Paroxysmal or chronic AFib might be a residual rhythm disturbance after successful ablation of the atrial flutter circuit. This is more likely if AFib was present before ablation. Aeromedical disposition policies for paroxysmal or chronic AFib should then direct the final disposition. The aviator should be counseled regarding these several aeromedical ramifications prior to consenting to ablation of atrial flutter for occupational indications. Various aspects of ablative therapy of atrial flutter have been reviewed.[133,134]

Radiofrequency Ablation of Atrial Fibrillation. Keep in mind that this discussion considers only lone AFib. The perception is that paroxysmal AFib usually progresses over time to become a chronic, persistent arrhythmia. Multiple reentrant wavelets or circuits within the atria characterize and perpetuate the arrhythmia. Electrophysiologists have recently appreciated the existence of focal AFib, in which the rhythm is initiated and maintained by a more focal arrhythmogenic site or sites within the atria, often near or within the orifice of one or more pulmonary veins. Ablation of these more focal origins of AFib has curative potential. As a precautionary note, pulmonary vein stenosis has been reported as a complication of ablation in or adjacent to the pulmonary vein orifices. The clinical and aeromedical importance of this complication is not yet well defined.

It may be that focal AFib is more typical early in the course of this process when the arrhythmia is only paroxysmal and atrial dimensions are normal. As AFib persists and becomes chronic, atrial remodeling and dilation may occur, accompanied by the more diffuse multiple reentrant wavelets required to maintain chronic AFib. Ablation of the focal process has the clinical potential of sparing some patients from a lifetime of chronic AFib. More complicated and extensive ablative techniques for chronic AFib are being developed. At the present time and for aeromedical disposition purposes, these procedures should probably all be considered investigational. Consideration of return to some types of flight duty should await large series with long-term follow-up. Ablation of AFib and all aspects of the treatment of AFib have been reviewed in detail.[134,135]

Radiofrequency Ablation of Ventricular Tachycardia. This is a more difficult question than ablation of SVT, and discussion is limited to idiopathic VT (ie, there is no evidence of underlying heart disease after thorough evaluation). The tendency may be to equate the success of VT ablation to that of SVT ablation and press for a special issuance. But there are other considerations, not the least of which is the underlying rhythm. VT ablation is usually performed for sustained or hemodynamically symptomatic VT, not for asymptomatic episodes of nonsustained VT. Often ablation is performed only after failure of one or several antiarrhythmic medications. Recurrence of the arrhythmia post-ablation is thus more likely to be associated with significant hemodynamic consequences.

There are several mechanisms and locations of VT genesis, and they have different prognoses and responses to radiofrequency ablation. VT may originate from one of several sites within the right or left ventricle, or may involve a reentrant circuit within the His bundle and bundle branches. Bundle branch reentry VT is not acceptable for any flight certification after ablation because there is usually associated conduction system disease within the AV node or His/bundle branch system. This diseased conduction system creates the reentrant circuit. A permanent pacemaker is a common requirement after ablation of bundle branch reentry VT.

VT originating from the right ventricular outflow tract (RVOT-VT) seems to be the more common and most "benign" idiopathic VT, followed by left ventricular VT. RVOT-VT generally occurs in one of two presentations; as very frequent short runs of VT with a background of frequent ventricular ectopy and pairing, or as runs of sustained VT with much less background ectopy. Either form can be induced by exertion and both can precipitate hemodynamic symptoms.

Ablation of VT, especially RVOT-VT, is promising as a potential cure and for future consideration of at least restricted flying. But at present the published experience is quite meager compared to ablation of AVRT and AVNRT. Available reports generally have small numbers of patients, relatively short follow-ups, and outcomes that are not very detailed except for sudden death. Also, electrophysiologic testing is not as helpful as with SVT. Sustained VT cannot always be induced, even in patients with documented spontaneous sustained VT. Also it is not as reliable as a method of documenting success post-ablation. Published series therefore often define a cure as no recurrence of symptoms or clinical VT or as no recurrence on electrocardiographic monitoring. Recurrence rates vary from 0% up to as much as 30% within 1-2 years. In some series "cure" is maintained with antiarrhythmic medications, and some patients continue to have recurrent episodes of nonsustained VT.

A recent study reported experience from a single center with its first 1022 radiofrequency ablation patients from October 1991 through December 1999.[136] There were 480 patients with AVNRT and 429 with AVRT, but only 14 with RVOT-VT and 22 with idiopathic left ventricular VT. This case distribution clearly illustrates the vast difference in published experience with ablation of AVNRT and AVRT compared to VT. Although this procedure holds promise for future aeromedical disposition policies, more information is needed about long-term success, long-term outcomes, recurrence rates, and late adverse consequences. A general overview of ablative therapy for ventricular arrhythmias is listed in the references.[137]

Pacemakers and Other Implantable Antiarrhythmic Devices

Pacemakers

This portion of the discussion covers cardiac pacing for bradyarrhythmias. Brief sections covering cardioverter-defibrillators and anti-tachycardia pacing devices follows. A superb and thorough discussion of the aviation considerations and available supporting data on cardiac pacing can be found in the first European workshop in aviation cardiology.[138] The reader is referred to this excellent review for a more detailed discussion. The intent of permanent cardiac pacing for a bradyarrhythmia is to duplicate normal physiology as much as possible with a paced rhythm. This would include normal atrioventricular synchrony and a chronotropic or rate-adaptive response, as needed by the patient. Considerations for aeromedical disposition include the presence and severity of hemodynamic symptoms due to the bradyarrhythmia prior to pacing, the degree of pacemaker dependence, the possibility of pacemaker failure, and the risk of electromagnetic interference with the pacemaker.

Hemodynamic symptoms, especially syncope/presyncope, due to the bradyarrhythmia prior to pacemaker implantation are aeromedically very important. Such history at minimum warrants a cautious policy for return to flight duty, if certification is granted at all. In the unlikely event that pacemaker failure should occur, the possibility of recurring hemodynamic symptoms is a compelling obstacle.

Pacemaker dependence is a reliance on the pacemaker for a supportive rhythm. In other words, in the event of pacemaker failure, the patient who is totally pacemaker-dependent does not have an adequate intrinsic escape rhythm, and very likely will become hemodynamically symptomatic.

Pacemaker failure may involve the pacemaker itself, the pacing wire or electrode, the connections between the two, or the interface of the electrode and cardiac tissue. Although some lead systems have had unacceptable failure rates, more recent data have documented failure rates of less than 1% per year.[138] Unipolar leads are less likely to fracture or develop insulation problems compared to bipolar leads, but they are also more susceptible to interference from extracardiac sources such as myopotentials and electromagnetic waves. In the past, insulation breaks due to long-term wear have occurred more often with polyurethane than with silicone insulation.[139]

In recent years, several sources of electromagnetic interference with pacemakers have been reported, including cellular phones and anti-theft electronic surveillance systems used in many retail stores. Radar, radio communication systems, and other microwave sources are also potential causes of electromagnetic interference. Unipolar lead pacing systems have been shown to be susceptible to interference from field strengths comparable to those seen under normal aircraft operating conditions, but bipolar pacing systems were unaffected.[138] Other clinical experience has also shown that bipolar lead systems are less affected than unipolar lead systems. So it seems prudent to consider only bipolar lead systems for return to flight duty. Pacemaker patients are typically provided with and instructed to always carry a card that identifies all components of their pacemaker system and the manufacturers' names and telephone numbers. Any questions should be easily resolved by calling the attending cardiologist or the manufacturer.

The above referenced aeromedical review of cardiac pacing concludes with a thorough, although somewhat complicated and technical aeromedical recommendation.[138] The authors recommend against unrestricted flight duties due to the unlikely yet real and unpredictable risk of pacemaker failure and electromagnetic interference. Restricted flying duties are recommended under certain conditions, including 3 months observation after pacemaker implantation and with a bipolar lead system, especially in pacemaker-dependent patients. In a recent review of private and public safety issues of arrhythmias that might affect consciousness, the authors presented a similar but much briefer discussion of pacemakers.[107] They advised that the probability of sudden pacemaker failure is remote and made the excellent point that recurrent hemodynamic symptoms in a pacemaker patient are unlikely to be due to pacemaker failure; more often a tachyarrhythmia is the cause. Safety is related to the presence or absence of syncope prior to pacemaker implantation, reliability of the pacing system, and underlying cardiac pathology. In summary, they recommended a return to commercial driving and flying with a 4-week observation period after pacemaker implantation. Because pacemaker patients often have associated underlying cardiac pathology, any aeromedical disposition considerations would also involve the type and severity of associated disease.

From the above expert references, it seems reasonable to recommend a return to private and commercial flight duties, especially in multipilot aircraft, after an observation period of 1-3 months, with bipolar lead systems highly preferred. Severity of symptoms prior to pacemaker implantation, degree of pacemaker dependence, and presence and severity of underlying disease should be considered in the aeromedical disposition. In addition, regular and sophisticated pacemaker follow-up must be performed at intervals of 6 months or less. This requirement alone may mitigate against return to military flying duties. Such follow-up requires medical personnel expert in dealing with the problems of pacemakers, and special equipment including pacemaker interrogative equipment and ambulatory electrocardiographic monitoring. The requirement for a military aviator to deploy to field conditions in remote areas makes proper pacemaker follow-up difficult. Return to military flying is not recommended. However, it deserves mentioning that the Royal Air Force returned a nonaviator aircrew member to restricted flight duties after pacemaker implantation for recurrent episodes of syncope due to documented episodes of asystole.[140]

Implantable Cardioverter-Defibrillators (ICDs)

ICDs are implanted devices similar to pacemakers. They alleviate potentially lethal or unstable tachyarrhythmias by delivering intracardiac defibrillation shocks after a preset monitoring interval. Some experts recommend against return to commercial driving or commercial and military flight duties after implantation of an ICD for ventricular tachycardia or ventricular fibrillation.[138,139] Several clinical and aeromedical considerations are operative in these cases. First, there is often underlying cardiac pathology of relatively poor prognosis which itself may warrant permanent disqualification from flying. Ischemic and other forms of cardiomyopathy are the most common underlying conditions. Second, the underlying rhythm disturbance is expected to recur unpredictably and may cause hemodynamic symptoms, including syncope, prior to ICD discharge. Third, the ICD discharge itself may cause discomfort sufficient to lead to loss of control of the vehicle or aircraft, or at least a performance decrement. Fourth, ICDs, like pacemakers, are susceptible to electromagnetic interference. Among other induced malfunctions, the interference may inappropriately be sensed as ventricular fibrillation and cause the device to discharge a shock.[141]

The overall prognosis in individuals with ICD devices depends on the underlying cardiac diagnosis, but the death rate alone is usually significantly greater than 1% per year. Not all ICD discharges are appropriate, but reported discharge rates are up to 20% per year in low-risk ICD patients and up to 50% per year in high-risk subjects. Syncope prior to ICD discharge is reported in up to 20% of patients, and presyncope prior to device discharge is also common.[138,139] Also, many patients with an ICD are continued on antiarrhythmic therapy to reduce the incidence of tachyarrhythmias and hence reduce the need for ICD shocks. Side effects of such antiarrhythmic medications are therefore also a matter of concern.

Anti-Tachycardia Devices

Anti-tachycardia devices are also implanted devices similar to pacemakers. They sense supraventricular or ventricular tachycardias and use various pacing patterns that terminate the tachycardia by taking over control of the cardiac rhythm rather than by intracardiac defibrillation. As with ICDs, the tachyarrhythmia is not prevented, but is converted after it occurs. Therefore the subject would be expected to experience recurrences of the tachyarrhythmia, possibly with hemodynamic symptoms that might impair flight performance.

These devices no longer have a prominent role in the treatment of tachycardias. They are almost never indicated as the only treatment for ventricular tachycardia; they are used in combination with an ICD in case the anti-tachycardia component fails to convert the ventricular arrhythmia. Concerns regarding ICDs would therefore also apply to patients with anti-tachycardia devices. And given the availability and effectiveness of radiofrequency ablation, these devices are not likely to be used for supraventricular tachyarrhythmias. They would only be used if ablation was inappropriate or unsuccessful, and if medical therapy failed to control the supraventricular tachyarrhythmia. Because these devices are so infrequently used for supraventricular tachyarrhythmias, only a few tertiary referral centers have proper experience with follow-up and programming and reprogramming of these devices.[139]

The above aeromedical concerns inherent in the use of ICDs and anti-tachycardia devices would seem to dictate a contraindication to return to any flying, commercial or military.

Pericarditis and Myocarditis

Pericarditis

Clinical Features

Although there are many underlying causes of pericarditis, the etiology in the healthy and relatively young aviator population is usually idiopathic or viral. And most community-acquired idiopathic pericarditis is probably due to an undocumented viral infection.

Chest pain, pericardial friction rub, and serial ST-T wave changes on ECG characterize acute viral or idiopathic pericarditis. Onset is usually within 2 weeks of a presumed viral illness, and is characterized by fever, mild to moderate constitutional symptoms, and precordial pain. The pain is typically positional and often pleuritic, aggravated by lying and respiratory movements, and abated by sitting or standing. A pericardial friction rub is usually present but may be quite transient. Diffuse ST-T wave changes are characteristic. Therapy is nonspecific, including bedrest until symptoms and fever have resolved and nonsteroidal antiinflammatory agents. Steroids are rarely required for control of symptoms. Baseline echocardiography is prudent to assess for the presence and volume of pericardial effusion, signs of cardiac tamponade, and depressed myocardial systolic function due to associated myocarditis. Small pericardial effusions are common, but large effusions and tamponade are unusual. Echocardiography is often normal in the acute phase.

Natural History and Aeromedical Considerations

The natural history has been well described.[142,143] Viral/idiopathic pericarditis is generally self-limited, with resolution of all symptoms and signs within 2-6 weeks. Pericardial pain may recur in about 25% of patients and is usually responsive to repeat nonsteroidal antiinflammatory therapy or colchicine. Rarely, recurrent symptoms are resistant to therapy. It is unclear whether the recurrent symptoms are due to an immunologic response to the initial viral infection, relapsing chronic infection, or recurrent infection. Other complications (chronic pericardial constriction, late pericardial effusion, and late cardiac tamponade) are uncommon.

Aeromedical concerns include recurrence of symptoms, late pericardial effusion, development of constrictive pericarditis, and arrhythmias, particularly supraventricular tachyarrhythmias. The aeromedical disposition of pericarditis from etiologies other than viral or idiopathic should be determined on a case-by-case basis according to the prognosis of the underlying process (eg, other infectious agents, myocardial infarction, uremia, cancer, and autoimmune disorders).

Suggested aeromedical disposition policy is to perform an evaluation a minimum of 2 months after symptoms have resolved and a minimum of 1 month after discontinuation of antiinflammatory medications. The evaluation should consist of echocardiography and a 24-hour ambulatory monitor. Some might consider graded exercise testing to document normal exercise tolerance and absence of exercise-induced arrhythmias. However, this seems unnecessary in the absence of associated myocarditis or arrhythmias presenting clinically or on ambulatory monitoring. Also, the ST-T wave changes secondary to pericarditis evolve over weeks to months and might reasonably be expected to cause "false positive" ST segment changes during exercise testing. If coronary artery disease is otherwise suspected in an individual aviator, a more specific and targeted evaluation should be performed. Some might also consider late follow-up echocardiography to exclude developing chronic constrictive pericardial disease, but this is an uncommon occurrence, and routine follow-up echocardiography is unlikely to be positive in the absence of symptoms or signs. Thus, there seems to be no benefit to routine follow-up other than by history and physical examination during routine periodic flight physicals. If the viral or idiopathic pericarditis is clinically resolved, the echocardiogram is normal, and the ambulatory monitor is aeromedically acceptable, a return to unrestricted flying is recommended without requirement for routine periodic reevaluation.

Myocarditis

Clinical Features

As with pericarditis, most cases of myocarditis in this population are due to viral infection. The clinical presentation ranges from asymptomatic to fulminant congestive heart failure which is rapidly fatal. In fact, some cases of idiopathic dilated cardiomyopathy are probably due to unrecognized or subclinical myocarditis. Myocarditis is often associated with or a complication of acute viral or idiopathic pericarditis, although the seasonal peak incidence of pericarditis is in the spring and fall, whereas the peak incidence of myocarditis with clinical heart failure is in late winter. Coxsackie and echoviruses are common etiologies for both pericarditis and myocarditis.

The clinical presentation of acute myocarditis is similar to that of pericarditis; myocardial involvement is inferred or diagnosed by symptoms, electrocardiographic changes, elevation of myocardial enzymes, and evidence of left ventricular dysfunction. Dyspnea, palpitations, and chest discomfort are common. Fever and constitutional symptoms may also be present. Examination may include a soft S_1, an S_3, and a mitral regurgitation murmur, as well as signs of pulmonary congestion. Pericardial friction rub may also be present.

Therapy is nonspecific, supportive, and directed at the clinical manifestations of the process. Some animal and human studies suggest that exercise is potentially harmful until the process resolves, so bedrest during the initial acute phase and restricted activity later are considered advisable. The clinical scenario has been well summarized by others.[143,144]

Natural History and Aeromedical Concerns

Acute viral myocarditis may result in cardiomegaly, depressed ventricular systolic function, congestive heart failure, arrhythmias, and conduction disturbances. Although the process usually resolves completely, it may lead to a dilated cardiomyopathy during the acute phase of the illness or later after a latent period. Symptomatic recovery usually occurs within a few weeks, but cardiac chamber sizes and ventricular function as assessed by echocardiography may not return to normal for several months.

Published recommendations for competitive athletes with acute viral myocarditis may provide guidance for disposition. Appropriate clinical management and convalescence is advised for about 6 months.[145] Return to full activities and competition is advised after ventricular function and cardiac chamber sizes have returned to normal and there are no clinically significant arrhythmias (sustained supraventricular tachycardia or any ventricular tachycardia) by 24-hour ambulatory monitoring and graded exercise testing. Recommended evaluation includes assessment of ventricular function at rest and with exercise by echocardiography or radionuclide ventriculography.

The aeromedical concerns are similar, requiring resolution of the myocarditis process and full recovery of cardiac size and function with no significant arrhythmias. The aviator should be grounded for a period of observation (6 months is suggested) and treated as clinically appropriate. Subsequent evaluation for return to flying should include graded exercise testing, 24-hour ambulatory monitoring, rest echocardiography, and assessment of left ventricular function during exercise (stress echocardiography or radionuclide ventriculography). Cardiac chamber sizes and ventricular function should have returned to normal and there should be no disqualifying arrhythmias. If the evaluation is acceptable, unrestricted return to flying may be recommended. The risk of later decompensation and development of chronic dilated cardiomyopathy is unknown. Therefore, in contrast to uncomplicated pericarditis, future reassessment for continued normal cardiac function is advised. An assessment consisting at minimum of repeat history, physical examination, electrocardiography, and resting echocardiography at 1-3 year intervals seems appropriate. Ambulatory monitoring and repeat assessment of ventricular function response to exercise are also considerations.

Cardiomyopathies

Introduction

The cardiomyopathies are primary disorders of myocardium of unknown etiology. Diseases such as atherosclerotic coronary artery disease, hypertensive heart disease, and Chagas' disease cause secondary cardiomyopathies; most of these have a dilated pattern. This section deals only with the primary cardiomyopathies; these have traditionally been divided into 3 categories—dilated, hypertrophic, and restrictive. A fourth category, arrhythmogenic right ventricular cardiomyopathy or dysplasia, is added to this classification by some sources, most notably the World Health Organization. Ventricular dilation, systolic dysfunction, and congestive heart failure typify dilated cardiomyopathy and most secondary cardiomyopathies. Hypertrophic cardiomyopathy is characterized by left ventricular hypertrophy, often asymmetric, with normal to increased systolic function, but diastolic dysfunction. Restrictive cardiomyopathy causes impaired diastolic filling and diastolic dysfunction. An excellent overview of cardiomyopathies is listed in the references.[144]

Dilated Cardiomyopathy

Epidemiologic and Clinical Features

Left ventricular dilation, systolic contractile dysfunction, and congestive failure characterize dilated cardiomyopathy (DCM); the right ventricle may be similarly involved. Although the etiology is by definition unknown, DCM probably represents the clinical expression and common endpoint of multiple causative factors. Some cases are undoubtedly due to previously unrecognized viral or other myocarditis. The estimated incidence is 5-10/100,000 person-years, however the incidence is probably considerably higher due to a lack of detection of mild asymptomatic cases.[144] A population-based study reported an incidence of 6/10,000 person-years and an overall prevalence of 36.5/100,000 population.[146] Men are affected more often than women and blacks more often than whites.

Symptoms associated with left and right ventricular congestive failure, such as dyspnea, orthopnea, fatigability, and decreased exercise tolerance, develop gradually. Angina may occur, even in the absence of coronary heart disease. Some patients with mild DCM may remain asymptomatic for months or even years.

Physical examination reveals evidence of ventricular dilation and failure, such as a displaced apical impulse, right ventricular heave, an S_3, murmurs of mitral or tricuspid regurgitation, basilar rales, distended neck veins, and peripheral edema. The electrocardiogram may have several nonspecific findings, such as ST-T wave changes, low voltage, supraventricular or ventricular ectopy, intraventricular and other conduction defects, and left atrial abnormality. Echocardiography is diagnostic, usually revealing four-chamber enlargement, diffusely reduced left or biventricular contractility, and mitral and tricuspid regurgitation. Left ventricular thrombus may be detected in up to 40% of cases with significant left ventricular dysfunction.

Therapy is the same as for heart failure of any etiology, and includes sodium restriction, diuretics, ACE inhibitors, hydralazine plus isosorbide, digitalis, and beta-blockers. Anticoagulation with warfarin is indicated in selected subsets of cases. Thromboembolic events were reported in 18% of DCM patients not on anticoagulation, compared to no events in anticoagulated patients.[147] Thromboembolism occurred in 33% of patients with atrial fibrillation and 14% of patients in sinus rhythm. However, the presence of left ventricular thrombus by echocardiography does not correlate well with clinical events. The ultimate therapeutic option for severe DCM is cardiac transplantation.

Natural History and Aeromedical Considerations

The usual expected course of symptomatic DCM is progressive deterioration with recurrent hospitalizations and finally death due to pump failure, or sudden cardiac death due to arrhythmia. Ventricular arrhythmias are common; the combination of complex ventricular arrhythmias and reduced left ventricular ejection fraction creates a high risk of sudden death. It has been reported that 25% of newly diagnosed cases of DCM referred to major medical centers for therapy are dead within 1 year and 50% are dead within 5 years.[144] As many as 25% may show immediate or delayed improvement in chamber dilation, ventricular function, and symptomatology, but complete recovery is rare. Individuals with no or mild symptoms and only mildly dilated cardiac chambers and reduced function have a better prognosis, but still have a 5-year fatality rate of 20%. Another review found that the prognosis of DCM is poor, with the majority of related deaths occurring within 2-3 years of diagnosis.[147] Annual mortality is 10%-20% per year and 25%-40% of deaths are sudden. However, 20%-30% do improve or stabilize regarding symptoms and left ventricular function.

A third review of DCM reported annual incidence figures of 5-8/100,000 and prevalence in the United States of 36/100,000 population with 10,000 deaths annually.[148] The reviewers cited earlier tertiary referral studies with 1- and 5-year mortalities of approximately 25% and 50%, respectively, but more recent studies found 5-year mortality averaging 20%. Another study compared survival rates for 2 groups of DCM patients, one a population-based sample and the other a tertiary referral center sample.[149] Survival at 1 year was 95% and 69%, and at 5 years 80% and 36%, respectively.

The placebo arms of recent heart failure drug trials also define the natural history of DCM. In a recent review, 6 major trials reported mortality rates ranging from 6.7% at 6.5 months follow-up to 46.0% at 2.3 years follow-up in the placebo arms of non-ischemic heart failure (DCM) subsets.[150] In contrast, a cohort of 32 asymptomatic DCM patients diagnosed by evaluation of palpitations or by abnormal chest x-ray or electrocardiogram had an excellent 2-year survival of 100%, but 5- and 7-year survival was poor, at 78% and 53%, respectively.[151] These survival figures were not significantly different from those of a group of 54 DCM patients who had a prior history of congestive symptoms, but were asymptomatic at the beginning of the study. These more recent and clinically more favorable figures probably reflect an emphasis on population-based studies, better medical therapy, and earlier diagnosis of some cases.

Aeromedical concerns for suddenly incapacitating events obviously include sudden cardiac death, complex ventricular arrhythmias with hemodynamic symptoms, and thromboembolism. Less obvious events, such as acute exacerbation of dyspnea and other congestive symptoms, and atrial arrhythmias, especially atrial fibrillation, might also compromise flying performance. The likelihood of non-sudden death related to heart failure within 5 years and hospitalizations for exacerbation of congestive symptoms are also a concern. Annual event rates for these acute occurrences are not readily available, but the survival statistics alone indicate denial of certification for return to military or civilian commercial flying, even in the more recent studies with clinically improved profiles. Return to general, private aviation with annual reevaluation might be considered only for mild, asymptomatic cases.

Hypertrophic Cardiomyopathy

Epidemiologic and Clinical Features

Excellent reviews of hypertrophic cardiomyopathy (HCM) have been published in recent years,[144,152,153] including some with an aeromedical perspective.[154,155] HCM is characterized by inappropriate left ventricular hypertrophy in the absence of any apparent cause (such as hypertension) and the etiology is unknown. The hypertrophy is classically asymmetric, predominantly involving the interventricular septum. The stiff, noncompliant left ventricle causes diastolic dysfunction with impaired left ventricular filling, but the chamber size is normal and systolic function is normal or hypercontractile. HCM may be classified as obstructive or nonobstructive. Hypertrophy involving the ventricular septum may cause a partial obstruction to left ventricular outflow, resulting in a pressure gradient at rest and/or with provocative maneuvers, such as Valsalva or inhalation of amyl nitrite—termed **obstructive HCM.** Nonobstructive HCM has no resting or inducible pressure gradient across the left ventricular outflow tract.

Spontaneous cases are common, but about one-half are inherited in an autosomal dominant pattern with variable penetrance and clinical expression. About 60% of families with one index case of HCM will have at least one primary relative with HCM. Affected relatives are usually asymptomatic with only mild echocardiographic features of the disease. Although the classic term of earlier days for this condition was ***idiopathic hypertrophic subaortic stenosis***, only about one-fourth of cases have a dynamic subaortic obstruction or pressure gradient (ie, obstructive HCM).

Prevalence is estimated at 0.02%-0.2% of the population. A population-based study reported an incidence of new cases of 2.5/100,000 person-years and a prevalence of 19.7/100,000 U.S. population.[146] Screening echocardiograms performed in 3335 United States Air Force pilot candidates revealed no cases of HCM and screening echocardiograms in 1476 Canadian Forces pilot applicants revealed two cases (0.14%) of asymmetric septal hypertrophy.[12,71] These are biased studies, however; these military pilot applicants had already passed initial screening physical examinations, possibly eliminating more obvious cases prior to the echocardiographic screening.

HCM brings to mind images of a terrible malady primarily affecting young people, with severe symptoms and a high risk of sudden death. In fact, the majority of patients are asymptomatic or mildly symptomatic, although symptoms can be severe and the first manifestation of the disease may be sudden cardiac death. Symptoms are often exertion-related and may include dyspnea, anginal or atypical chest pain, fatigue, palpitations, lightheadedness, postural symptoms, and presyncope/syncope. Most sudden death occurs at rest or with mild exertion, but about one-third occurs during or just after vigorous activity. Strenuous exercise is usually therefore proscribed for HCM patients; HCM is one of the recognized causes of sudden death in athletes.

Classic physical examination findings are seen in the obstructive form of HCM, while nonobstructive HCM may have an unremarkable examination except for an S_4 and a left ventricular lift. Obstructive HCM often has a bifid carotid pulse with a brisk upstroke. Apical impulse is forceful, enlarged, and displaced leftward, and is often a double or even triple impulse due to a presystolic impulse (palpable S_4) plus a single or double systolic impulse. An S_4 is typical and an S_3 is common. The hallmark is a harsh crescendo-decrescendo systolic murmur between the apex and left sternal border that radiates widely across the precordium, but not into the neck. The murmur has a characteristic response to maneuvers, increasing with Valsalva, standing, and amyl nitrite, and decreasing with squatting, handgrip, supine position, and passive leg raising.

The electrocardiogram is abnormal in the vast majority of cases, but no pattern is diagnostic. Usual abnormalities are increased left ventricular voltage, ST-T wave changes, prominent septal Q waves inferolaterally, and left atrial abnormality. Diagnosis is made or confirmed by echocardiography, which demonstrates various patterns of left ventricular hypertrophy, usually asymmetric septal hypertrophy, with normal left ventricular dimensions and normal to exaggerated contractility. Associated findings that may be seen are left atrial enlargement, mitral valve thickening and regurgitation, systolic anterior motion of the mitral valve, diastolic dysfunction, and a resting or inducible gradient across the left ventricular outflow tract.

Medical therapy is primarily for symptomatic relief; it does not prevent sudden death or cause regression of the left ventricular hypertrophy. Therapies include beta-blockers, calcium channel antagonists, and disopyramide. The entire spectrum of antiarrhythmics has been used in HCM, and infective endocarditis prophylaxis is often recommended. One study of 810 HCM patients evaluated and followed for infective endocarditis found a prevalence of 3.7 per 1000 patients and an incidence of 1.4 per 1000 person-years.[156] All patients with infective endocarditis had a left ventricular outflow tract gradient/obstruction and most also had left atrial enlargement. The investigators concluded that infective endocarditis prophylaxis is indicated only in the obstructive variety of HCM. Nonpharmacologic treatments include dual chamber permanent pacing, mitral valve replacement, and septal myectomy by surgery, ablation, or other techniques.

Natural History and Aeromedical Considerations

Annual mortality is reported as 2%-6% per year in adults at tertiary medical centers, but 1% or less per year is reported in more recent studies involving outpatient, community hospital, elderly, and asymptomatic populations.[153] Sudden death most commonly occurs in children and young adults up to age 35 years. However, sudden death is reported in middle-aged adults, even without prior symptoms. Clinical progression is otherwise slow and 10%-15% of symptomatic patients progress to an end-stage dilated cardiomyopathy, while 10% experience atrial fibrillation. Syncope and sudden death may be caused by atrial and ventricular tachyarrhythmias, bradyarrhythmias, heart block, ischemia, left ventricular outflow tract obstruction, and activation of ventricular baroreflexes resulting in hypotension with or without bradycardia. Predictors of sudden death include young age at diagnosis, history of syncope, and family history of HCM with sudden death. Other possible predictors are certain genetic abnormalities or markers, severe hypertrophy, and nonsustained ventricular tachycardia on ambulatory electrocardiographic monitoring. The presence and severity of left ventricular outflow tract obstruction are not related to sudden death or to symptoms in general. In some studies development of atrial fibrillation has been associated with a worse prognosis.

An aeromedical review of HCM recommended risk stratification as follows.[154] Mortality risk less than 1% per year is indicated by no ventricular tachycardia on 48-hour ambulatory monitoring, normal blood pressure response on graded exercise testing, and no history of syncope. Mortality risk greater than 1% per year is predicted by nonsustained ventricular tachycardia on ambulatory monitoring, hypotension during graded exercise test, or a history of syncope. A restricted commercial license with annual review was recommended for the low-risk group and permanent disqualification for the high-risk group. This may be reasonable for some categories of flying, but it does not consider nonfatal but potentially incapacitating events, such as presyncope, lightheadedness, atrial fibrillation, chest pain, dyspnea, and reduced exercise tolerance.

Use of medications for control of symptoms again must be considered in aeromedical dispositions. In a report on 58 asymptomatic HCM patients followed for a mean of 11 years, annual cardiac and sudden death mortality rates were 0.9% and 0.1% per year, respectively.[157] However, 36% were symptomatic at last evaluation and 60% of the initial cohort were on cardiac medications at the beginning of the study; they did not report how many were on medication at the time of last evaluation. Four subjects developed chronic or paroxysmal atrial fibrillation.

A population-based cohort of 202 HCM patients (mean age, 41 years; range, 1-74 years) was followed for a mean of 10 years.[158] At the end of the study, 76% were asymptomatic or mildly symptomatic, but most were on medications and 24% had symptomatically deteriorated, had significant functional impairment, or had died. Annual cardiac and sudden death mortality rates were 0.6% and 0.1% per year, respectively. Atrial fibrillation developed in 28% and syncope occurred in 16%. The annual cardiac event rate was 6% per year. These events included atrial fibrillation, peripheral embolization, abrupt worsening of congestive symptoms, requirement for permanent pacemaker, endocarditis, and syncope, nearly all potentially incapacitating events. Most (91%) of those experiencing syncope had this event occur after age 25. In another study, 29 middle-aged HCM subjects who were essentially asymptomatic and 35-55 years old at the time of initial diagnosis were followed for a mean of 8 years.[159] Significant symptoms or sudden death occurred in 24% and the annual mortality rate was 1.7% per year.

These and other studies on lower-risk subsets of HCM patients do document much more favorable outcome rates than earlier studies from tertiary referral centers. Annual mortality rates of 1.0%-1.5% per year or less and symptom development in 25% represents a tremendous clinical "improvement" over annual mortality rates of about 5% per year and significant symptoms in up to 50% of patients. But is this acceptable for return to flying? Most studies focus on rates of total cardiac death, heart failure death, and sudden death, and do not emphasize nonfatal symptoms and events that can be aeromedically quite important. As discussed, these other events are still significant clinical problems. And, as noted, many of these lower-risk subjects are clinically stable and often asymptomatic or only mildly symptomatic on medication. Return to military, civilian commercial, or aerobatic flying is not recommended. As with DCM, return to general, private aviation might be considered for the above noted low-risk subset, with annual cardiologic review to include 24-48-hour ambulatory monitoring, graded exercise testing, and echocardiography.

A common dilemma in aviators is differentiation of physiologic hypertrophy, or athlete's heart, from HCM. This is discussed earlier in this chapter under left ventricular hypertrophy (LVH) in the section on electrocardiographic abnormalities.

Apical Hypertrophic Cardiomyopathy

Apical HCM is a form of HCM that is not usually seen outside of Japan. In Japan about 25% of HCM cases are apical HCM, whereas outside Japan only 1%-2% are apical. The inappropriate left ventricular hypertrophy is confined to the apex. Apical HCM is characterized by increased QRS voltage on electrocardiogram with giant negative T waves in the mid-precordial leads. Prognosis is more favorable than for typical HCM, and sudden death, syncope, presyncope, and arrhythmias are rare. However, angina and atypical chest pain, exertional dyspnea, and fatigue are common. Apical myocardial infarction can occur in the absence of atherosclerotic coronary artery disease. Diastolic function is abnormal as in typical HCM. Treatment is generally for symptoms, using beta-blockers and calcium channel antagonists. Return to military or aerobatic flying is not recommended. Return to civilian flying may be permissible in patients with no or minimal symptoms, again with annual review.

Restrictive Cardiomyopathy

Clinical Features

In Western countries restrictive cardiomyopathy (RCM) is the least frequently encountered of the three classic cardiomyopathies (dilated, hypertrophic, and restrictive). It may be idiopathic or secondary to a systemic disorder with an infiltrative or scarring process that involves the myocardium. Examples of secondary causes include amyloidosis, hemochromatosis (however, this usually causes dilated cardiomyopathy), carcinoid, scleroderma, and sarcoidosis. Secondary causes such as hypereosinophilic syndrome and endomyocardial fibrosis are common causes of RCM in certain geographic areas such as equatorial Africa and South America.

Stiffening of the ventricular walls due to myocardial scarring, fibrosis, and/or infiltration causes abnormal diastolic function; systolic contractile function is usually not impaired even in advanced disease. Reduced exercise tolerance is prominent because the impaired diastolic filling results in decreased cardiac output, especially inability to normally augment cardiac output during exertion. Symptoms and signs are due to pulmonary and systemic venous congestion. Common symptoms include exercise intolerance, dyspnea, fatigability, and weakness. Chest discomfort is not a typical feature. Elevated jugular venous pressure, soft heart sounds, S_3, peripheral edema, congested liver, and ascites typify the examination. Electrocardiogram may show low QRS voltage and nonspecific ST-T wave changes. Routine noninvasive studies may help with diagnosis, but cardiac catheterization with myocardial biopsy is generally recommended to confirm the diagnosis and establish etiology. Chronic constrictive pericarditis has a similar presentation and must be differentiated from RCM because constrictive pericarditis is treatable by surgery.

Natural History and Aeromedical Considerations

The prognosis of RCM is variable but is usually progressive with a high mortality rate. Hemochromatosis may be improved by removal of iron overload; otherwise there is no specific therapy and treatment is symptomatic. Diuretics must be used cautiously in order to avoid reducing filling pressures too much, which causes a decreased cardiac output. Calcium channel antagonists may provide some symptomatic relief. Specific outcomes data are lacking for this uncommon condition and patients usually present because of symptoms. A recommendation against return to flying seems to be the most prudent disposition.

Arrhythmogenic Right Ventricular Cardiomyopathy (Dysplasia)

Clinical Features

Awareness of arrhythmogenic right ventricular dysplasia (ARVD) has been heightened in recent years because of its association with ventricular tachycardia and sudden death, especially in young subjects, and the advent of radiofrequency ablation of ventricular tachycardia. ARVD involves variable replacement of predominantly the right ventricular free wall with adipose and fibrous tissue. Etiology is unknown, but many cases are inherited in an autosomal dominant pattern with variable penetrance. Clinical presentation is usually with nonsustained or sustained ventricular tachycardia, often exercise-induced, in males younger than age 40. Involvement has been said to be limited to the right ventricle, especially the free wall, with sparing of the interventricular septum and a resultant dilated and hypocontractile right ventricle, but a relatively normal-sized and normally-functioning left ventricle. However, several studies have demonstrated that ARVD is progressive in those who survive to adulthood and middle age, with more diffuse involvement of the right and left ventricles. Such "end-stage" ARVD may be difficult to differentiate clinically from idiopathic dilated cardiomyopathy. Also, it is possible that some cases of idiopathic ventricular tachycardia, especially in young patients, are actually mild or undiagnosed ARVD.

Physical examination is not revealing. Characteristic electrocardiographic changes including QRS prolongation and inverted T waves in the right precordial leads have been noted. The ventricular tachycardia associated with ARVD has a left bundle branch block, superior axis configuration, whereas the more common ventricular tachycardia of right ventricular outflow tract origin has a left bundle branch block, inferior axis configuration. Diagnosis is made by the total clinical picture. Echocardiography, magnetic resonance imaging, gated blood pool radionuclide scanning, right ventricular angiography, and myocardial biopsy demonstrate various features of ARVD. Although the clinical arrhythmia is often exercise-induced, it is often not precipitated by graded exercise testing. Beta-blocker therapy is often useful to suppress the ventricular tachycardia, but other antiarrhythmics may be required. The role of radiofrequency ablation for the ventricular tachycardia associated with this disorder is not yet determined.

Natural History and Aeromedical Considerations

The natural history is not well defined, partly due to the infrequency of the diagnosis, especially prior to clinical presentation with ventricular tachycardia. But the risks of sudden death and sustained ventricular tachycardia appear to be too high to consider return to any type of flight duty. Supraventricular tachycardias (SVT) have also been associated with ARVD. In a report on 47 patients with ARVD, 8 had a history of spontaneous SVT and 2 others later developed SVT (10/47, 21%).[160] At electrophysiologic testing, 72% (34/47) had inducible SVT, compared to only 5.5% (2/36) of controls.

In another study, two groups of ARVD subjects were followed for a mean of 7 years.[161] One group comprised 15 young subjects with a mean age of 15 years and the other group was 19 adults with a mean age of 38 years. During follow-up, 2 of the young subjects died suddenly, 2 survived ventricular fibrillation, 3 had multiple episodes of sustained ventricular tachycardia, and 4 subjects experienced syncope. The adult group experienced no syncope, sudden death, or resuscitated ventricular fibrillation, but 9 had one or more episodes of sustained ventricular tachycardia. Five subjects were younger than age 30 when their ventricular tachycardia occurred and 4 were older than age 30. Many subjects in both groups were on beta-blockers and/or other antiarrhythmics. Return to any type of flying is not recommended.

Common Congenital Heart Diseases

Introduction

Bicuspid aortic valve is the most common congenital heart disease, occurring in an estimated 1%-2% of the general population. Its primary consequences, aortic stenosis and aortic insufficiency, emerge as clinical problems primarily in the middle-aged adult. This entity is discussed in detail in the valvular heart disease section, as are congenital pulmonary valve stenosis and insufficiency. This section will deal with other common congenital conditions such as atrial and ventricular septal defects, patent ductus arteriosus and aortic coarctation, including some considerations of the postsurgical repair state.

Congenital heart disease in the adult population is a complicated topic, involving both common and uncommon defects, with or without surgical or catheter-based repair. Repair may be corrective or only palliative. Natural history and clinical information in the literature are generally limited to life expectancy and functional ability or quality-of-life considerations. Tremendous advances in surgical repair have resulted in good survival rates and reasonable quality of life in many instances of even complex congenital disease, but these are purely clinical considerations.

Consideration of aeromedical certification would demand a near normal cardiovascular status with an aeromedically acceptable low risk of suddenly incapacitating events and no significant residual disability or dysfunction. The required periodic reassessment should be reasonable, not requiring testing that is excessively frequent, exotic, or invasive. Detailed data for all aeromedical considerations are extremely difficult to extract. Consideration of special issuance for continued flying or entry into initial flight training seems permissible only for common, simple congenital defects that are either hemodynamically insignificant with essentially normal expected outcome, or simple defects that have been repaired and have no residua and again no aeromedically significant expected outcomes. To produce aeromedically acceptable results after repair, surgical or other correction must usually have been done early (ie, in childhood). Correction later in life generally results in decreased survival rates and/or increased event rates due to chronic and persistent effects of the defect prior to repair. More complex or hemodynamically significant lesions, with or without repair, are unlikely to be considered acceptable for continued flying or entry into training due to the many concerns regarding late outcome, residual dysfunction, and the relative lack of helpful literature.

For now, catheter-based closures of shunt lesions should probably be considered experimental procedures from the standpoint of aeromedical disposition. Long-term results of new minisurgical procedures are not yet available; one should not necessarily assume that they would be as good as or better than standard surgical techniques for which long-term outcomes are better documented. Catheter-based corrective procedures are not specifically discussed; the outcomes concerns for these procedures will, for the most part, be identical to those for surgical repair. Most of the concerns relate to consequences of residual abnormalities, and in that sense are somewhat independent of the type of reparative procedure, although exceptions to this certainly may exist. Congenital defects, uncorrected or corrected, may require infective endocarditis prophylaxis, for which current recommended guidelines should be consulted.

As a practical reminder, for patients with these defects surgical repair has usually been done in early childhood, and they therefore would not be considered for flight training, especially military or commercial training, for several years (ie, until early adulthood or 1-2 decades after repair). Thus, individual cases often will have had a considerable period of time for documentation of stability or clinical deterioration. On the other hand, some late complications and consequences of repaired complex congenital defects may not become apparent for 10, 20, or even 30 years. The potential physical demands and the possibility of worldwide deployment and combat missions for military aviators mandate more conservative aeromedical disposition than civilian aviators.

Because of the rigorous physical screening done prior to aviation training, especially for commercial and military aviators, aeromedical considerations of congenital heart defects will mostly be for hemodynamically and structurally insignificant lesions, or significant lesions successfully repaired during early childhood with good results, minimal residua, and relatively good expected outcomes. As surgical and catheter-based reparative techniques continue to be developed and perfected, more complex defects will be repaired at earlier ages with better clinical results versus the unrepaired natural course of these defects. The AME/FS should use caution in aeromedical disposition of these cases, with licensing authorities insisting on favorable long-term results before flight certification is granted.

Atrial Septal Defect

Atrial septal defect (ASD) is the second most common congenital heart defect found in adults after bicuspid aortic valve. Left-to-right shunting at the atrial level and subsequent right ventricular volume overload are the primary consequences. Of the 3 types of ASD, ostium secundum ASD comprises about 75% of cases, ostium primum 20%, and sinus venosus defect 5%.

Ostium Secundum ASD

Secundum ASD involves the mid-atrial septum at the fossa ovalis. Survival into adulthood without surgical correction is expected for significant ASDs, although life expectancy is shortened. Without surgical correction, about 50% of patients die before age 40-50, with a death rate of about 6% per year thereafter. Most patients older than age 50 are symptomatic due to increased left-to-right shunting caused by age-related left ventricular noncompliance. Patients may also develop symptoms due to mild to moderate pulmonary hypertension, atrial tachyarrhythmias, and progressive mitral regurgitation.[162] Middle-aged or older adults with uncorrected hemo-dynamically significant ASDs typically develop mild to moderate pulmonary hypertension and right ventricular volume and pressure overload, leading to right heart failure and atrial tachyarrhythmias, especially atrial fibrillation. Ultimately, Eisenmenger's complex may develop with right-to-left shunting.

The presence and time course of symptom development depends on the magnitude of the left-to-right shunt. Significant shunts may cause fatigability, exertional dyspnea, and eventually right heart failure. Symptoms may also be due to associated atrial tachyarrhythmias. Adults with unrepaired secundum ASD may be asymptomatic, with the defect found incidentally on examination or after presenting with atrial fibrillation or other atrial tachyarrhythmia. The expected course of significant but unrepaired ASD is atrial fibrillation and right heart failure presenting in the fourth to fifth decade or later.

Physical examination findings include a normal or split S_1, a pulmonary midsystolic ejection murmur due to increased outflow, a prominent right ventricular impulse along the mid-left sternal border, and wide, usually fixed splitting of S_2. A large shunt may also have a mid-diastolic murmur due to increased forward flow through the tricuspid valve. The classic electrocardiographic finding is right axis deviation and rSR′ pattern or incomplete right bundle branch block in the anterior precordial leads (V_1/V_2). Echocardiography has replaced cardiac catheterization for definitive and preoperative assessment. Mitral valve prolapse is present in 10%-20% of secundum ASDs and may be appreciated by examination or echocardiography.

Surgical repair is usually recommended for all significant shunts (greater than 1.5/1.0 pulmonary to systemic flow ratio). Ideally, this should be performed during early childhood because closure of significant ASDs in adulthood is associated with a residual risk of atrial tachyarrhythmias, especially atrial fibrillation, with its ensuing risk for stroke and need for chronic warfarin anticoagulation. Surgical repair is not generally recommended for insignificant shunts, although opinions may vary, especially as transcatheter and minisurgical repair techniques become perfected. One study reported 27-32 years of follow-up of 123 patients with surgical repair of secundum ASD at varying ages.[163] Late survival and outcome were essentially normal for ASD repair performed at age 11 or younger and age 12-24 years (the two younger age quartiles). However, late survival and outcome were significantly reduced for surgery at age 25-41, and poor for surgery performed after age 41. Morbidity and mortality for surgical repair in older patients was commonly due to atrial fibrillation, stroke, and late heart failure.

Special issuance for unrestricted flying or entry into flight training for unrepaired but hemodynamically insignificant ASD may be considered. Such special issuance may also be granted for repaired ASD after a nonflying observation period of at least

6 months, and subsequent demonstration of no residual shunt, chamber dilation, ventricular dysfunction, or significant arrhythmias. Noninvasive evaluation with echocardiography, 24-hour ambulatory monitoring, and possibly graded exercise testing should usually be sufficient. Licensing authorities may also wish to consider age at operation in the aeromedical disposition or in the timing of periodic reassessment. Periodic review at 1-3 year intervals should be considered for relicensure; this may not be necessary for very insignificant ASDs because they are unlikely to progress and have essentially normal long-term outcomes.

Ostium Primum ASD

Ostium primum ASD is a feature of partial atrioventricular canal defect and is thus a more complex lesion than secundum ASD. The mitral and tricuspid valves are therefore also involved with some degree of regurgitation, and residual regurgitation may be present postoperatively as well. Conduction system abnormalities before and after surgery are also a possibility. Physical examination findings are similar to those of secundum ASD, with the addition of murmurs of mitral and/or tricuspid regurgitation. The electrocardiogram typically demonstrates left axis deviation, right bundle branch block, and often first degree AV block

Repair performed early in childhood may have a good prognosis. One study reported up to 14 years of follow-up on 38 patients repaired at 5 years of age or younger.[164] Late mitral regurgitation was present in 0.9% and there was one late reoperation. Eighty-seven percent were asymptomatic at follow-up. In contrast, another study reported on 31 patients repaired at age 40 or older.[165] Late follow-up was available for only 19 of the 31 subjects, but was notable for significant events such as atrial fibrillation in 6, permanent pacemaker in 5, moderate to severe mitral regurgitation in 6, functional class II-III in 12, and reoperation for mitral or tricuspid valve replacement in 4.

The outcome for ostium primum ASD repair in adults does not appear to be favorable for aeromedical consideration. Successful repair performed during childhood with no or minimal residual valvular regurgitation, no atrial level shunt, normal cardiac chamber sizes and function, normal hemodynamics, and no arrhythmias or conduction disturbances might be considered for some categories of restricted flying. However, careful and frequent follow-up should be required for possible development of future valvular regurgitation, arrhythmias, and conduction disturbances. These concerns would seem to preclude return to most if not all types of flying.

Sinus Venosus Defect

Sinus venosus ASD is rare, comprising only about 5% of ASDs. This atrial septal defect involves the superior atrial septum and is usually associated with anomalous pulmonary venous return, typically the right upper pulmonary vein. An aeromedical review of adult congenital heart disease recommended that repaired sinus venosus ASD should probably be treated like ostium secundum ASD.[166] However, the reviewer also indicated that some evidence suggests that surgical repair does not decrease risk of atrial arrhythmia, and may even increase that risk. Outcome is otherwise good and comparable to that of secundum ASD. Therefore, initial and periodic repeat assessment for atrial arrhythmias (24-hour ambulatory monitor and possibly graded exercise test) should definitely be performed if return to flight status or entry into initial flight training is contemplated for patients with repaired sinus venosus ASD.

Ventricular Septal Defect

Ventricular septal defect (VSD) is common in children but seldom seen in adults. Defects that are significant from birth are usually surgically repaired during childhood. Insignificant defects usually close spontaneously by early adulthood; spontaneous closure after age 20 is unusual. Occasionally, some may only partially close, leaving a small hemodynamically insignificant VSD in an adult patient. Infective endocarditis is a risk regardless of shunt size.

As with ASDs, the presence of symptomatology is related to the size of the defect. Insignificant VSDs typically cause no symptoms and do not progress. Physical examination findings are limited to the characteristic VSD murmur, a harsh holosystolic murmur heard best along the mid-left sternal border and radiating across the precordium. This murmur results from flow left to right through the defect and is often loudest (grade 3-4/6) in small, hemodynamically insignificant VSDs.

Significant shunts may cause fatigability and reduced exercise tolerance. Patients with significant VSDs that are not surgically repaired will generally survive into adulthood, but with pulmonary hypertension and Eisenmenger's complex (right to left shunting, cyanosis). Additional features of examination include a forceful left ventricular impulse and left parasternal thrill, S_3, a mid-diastolic mitral murmur due to increased flow, and a midsystolic pulmonary flow murmur.

Flying should only be considered for unrepaired but hemodynamically insignificant VSDs or for successfully repaired VSDs without residua. A return to unrestricted flying or entry into flight training is acceptable for unrepaired but hemodynamically insignificant VSDs. A small VSD with normal heart size and normal pulmonary vascular resistance poses no increased risk of sudden death or disability. Repaired significant VSDs may be quite a different matter. One review of 145 patients with surgically repaired VSDs demonstrated a decreased 30-year survival of 82% versus

97% in age- and gender-matched controls.[166] For patients having surgical repair at age 2 years or younger, 30-year survival was 88%. Late survival depended on age at surgery and presence of pulmonary vascular occlusive changes. Two sources reported a late risk of sudden death after surgical repair of 0.1%-0.2% per year.[166] The mechanism is unclear, but intraventricular conduction defects and ventricular arrhythmias may well be causative factors.

Nevertheless, special issuance may be considered for repaired VSD without sequelae—no residual shunt, normal pulmonary vascular resistance and pulmonary artery pressure, an otherwise normal echocardiogram, no significant arrhythmias, and no significant conduction defects. Because of the above concerns about late outcome, licensing authorities may choose to limit special issuance to flying as or with copilot. However, if the surgical repair was performed during infancy or early childhood and there are no residua as described, unrestricted licensure seems reasonable. In either case, periodic review is warranted to document continued stability of the repair and verify that there are no arrhythmias or conduction disturbances. Serial echocardiography, routine 12-lead electrocardiography, and 24-hour ambulatory monitoring are considered standard; graded exercise testing is also an option, especially for unrestricted licensure.

Patent Ductus Arteriosus

In utero, the ductus arteriosus connects the pulmonary artery trunk and the descending aorta, diverting blood flow away from the high-resistance pulmonary circuit into the aorta. Failure of the ductus arteriosus to close postnatally results in an abnormal communication between the aorta and pulmonary trunk (persistent or patent ductus arteriosus) with resultant left-to-right shunting. A significant patent ductus arteriosus (PDA) generally presents clinically in infancy. In the absence of severe pulmonary vascular disease and Eisenmenger's complex, the presence of any PDA in an infant or child is usually considered a surgical indication, because surgical ligation via thoracotomy is a very low-risk procedure and is curative. Transcatheter closure devices are currently being investigated, but adequate long-term follow-up data are not yet available. Smaller PDAs are initially asymptomatic, but if the shunt is hemodynamically significant, heart failure develops beginning in the third decade. Patients with significant shunts usually do not reach adulthood without intervention or development of elevated pulmonary resistance and subsequent shunt reversal. Therefore, PDA in an adult is also usually considered a surgical indication because of the significant risk of infective endocarditis and left heart failure. In addition, surgical repair in the adult is more complicated than it is in children due to calcification, friability, and aneurysmal dilation of the ductus itself.

PDA is in essence an arteriovenous fistula and therefore produces bounding pulses and a prominent left ventricular impulse. The classic feature on physical examination is described as a continuous, machinery murmur located at the second left intercostal space.

Adults with an uncorrected PDA should not be recommended for any flying due to the considerations noted above; they should be referred for surgical repair. Successfully repaired PDA is acceptable for unrestricted special issuance for training and continued flying after evaluation demonstrates no residual shunt, no ventricular dysfunction or dilation, and normal pulmonary artery systolic pressure and pulmonary vascular resistance. Periodic reassessment is probably not necessary beyond about 5 years after successful repair and initial certification.

Coarctation of the Aorta

Coarctation is a discrete narrowing of the aorta usually located just distal to the left subclavian artery at the level of the ductus/ligamentous arteriosus. This causes partial obstruction to flow, resulting in elevated blood pressure in the upper limbs, with normal or low pressure in the lower limbs. Associated abnormalities include bicuspid aortic valve (25%-33% of coarctations), congenital aneurysms of the circle of Willis (may present with rupture), and aortic aneurysms (may dissect or rupture). Aortic aneurysms are typically in the proximal ascending aorta or just distal to the coarctation. The risk of rupture of aneurysms in the circle of Willis is not defined, but rupture has even been reported in normotensive coarctation patients late after surgical repair.

Coarctation is usually diagnosed in childhood, but up to 20% may not be identified until adolescence or adulthood. Patients may present with symptoms, but are often diagnosed during an evaluation for a murmur or hypertension. Depending on the severity of the obstruction, onset of symptoms may occur in infancy or not until early adulthood. Presenting symptoms may include headache, cold extremities, and claudication. Cardiac examination demonstrates upper limb hypertension and a lag or delay between simultaneously palpated brachial and femoral artery pulses. A systolic murmur across the coarctation may be present, but auscultatory findings are more likely to be those of an associated bicuspid aortic valve—early systolic ejection sound, midsystolic aortic outflow murmur, and possibly an aortic insufficiency murmur. As a consequence of hypertension an S_4 may be present, and the electrocardiogram may show changes of left ventricular hypertrophy.

Unrepaired coarctation with a resting gradient ≥20 mm Hg between upper and lower extremities carries an increased risk for progressive left ventricular hypertrophy and subsequent left ventricular dysfunction, persistent systolic hypertension, and premature atherosclerotic cerebrovascular and coronary heart disease. For unrepaired significant coarctation, the average age at death is in the mid 30s.[162] Death is due to coexisting acquired and congenital heart disease and acquired cerebrovascular disease, complications of hypertension, ruptured cerebral aneurysm, and dissection or rupture of aortic aneurysm. Repair is therefore recommended for coarctation with a significant gradient. The natural history of insignificant coarctation (gradient <20 mm Hg) is not known; these individuals are probably often not detected. After repair the aorta is still abnormal, with a late risk of aneurysmal formation, dissection, and rupture. Other postoperative sequelae include the consequences of associated bicuspid aortic valve, persistent hypertension, and recurrence of coarctation in 10%-20%, depending on surgical technique. Recurrence of coarctation is lowest, 10% or less, with end-to-end anastomosis.

The prognosis after coarctation repair is strongly related to age at time of repair. In a long-term follow-up study of 646 patients with repaired coarctation, age at time of repair was the strongest predictor of late survival, with optimal age for repair 9 years or younger.[167] Twenty-year survival was 91% for repair at age 14 or younger, but only 79% for repair after age 14. Age at the time of repair was also the strongest predictor of chronic postoperative hypertension. Twenty-five percent had persistent hypertension and the higher the persistent systolic blood pressure, the higher the probability of death. Mean age at death was 38 years, and the most common causes of death were coronary heart disease, sudden death, heart failure, cerebrovascular accident, and ruptured aortic aneurysm. In another study of 226 cases of coarctation repair, long-term survival was normal in those repaired earlier than age 20, but reduced in those repaired after age 20 compared to appropriate population statistics.[168] Two-thirds developed late hypertension, often later than 10 years postoperatively. In addition, a hypertensive response to exercise has been noted in repaired coarctations.

As with ASD, VSD, and PDA, it seems reasonable to allow return to at least some categories of flying for repaired coarctation if there is no evidence of residual coarctation, blood pressure is normal at rest and during graded exercise testing, and cardiac status is normal. Coexisting bicuspid aortic valve must also be addressed as a separate aeromedical issue. Again, licensing authorities may wish to consider age at repair in the aeromedical disposition. Careful periodic reassessment is mandatory for all patients to screen for recoarctation, development of hypertension, and premature coronary heart disease. Given the more stringent requirements for military service and aviation, these concerns weigh heavily against acceptance for military flight duties. Return to high-performance military and aerobatic flying is not recommended because of the aortic surgery itself and the risk of dissection or rupture of aortic aneurysm.

Tetralogy of Fallot

Tetralogy of Fallot (TOF) is the most common cyanotic heart disease seen in adults. Features of TOF include a large subaortic VSD, right ventricular outflow tract obstruction (usually at the infundibulum but also often at the pulmonary valve), aorta overriding the VSD, and right ventricular hypertrophy. Right and left ventricular pressures are essentially equal due to the VSD, but right-to-left shunting occurs due to the right ventricular outflow obstruction. Infundibular hypertrophy is progressive, so the shunt and cyanosis may worsen over time. Nearly half of TOF patients have other anomalies, including anomalous coronary arteries. Patients are usually cyanotic at birth or become cyanotic within the first year of life.

If not repaired, TOF is nearly 100% fatal by age 40. Without surgery, survival is only 11% at age 20, 6% at age 30, and 3% at age 40.[162] There should be no consideration for certifying any flying for unrepaired TOF.

Surgical repair involves closing the VSD and relieving the right ventricular outflow obstruction. Any consideration of licensing for flying should include detailed knowledge of the location(s) of right ventricular outflow tract obstruction and the reparative procedure used (eg, infundibular resection, infundibular patch, pulmonary valvotomy, pulmonary valve excision, and placement of a prosthetic conduit from the right ventricle to the pulmonary artery).

Late concerns after surgical repair include residual structural, functional, and hemodynamic abnormalities, as well as sudden death (due predominantly to ventricular arrhythmias), supraventricular arrhythmias, and sinus node dysfunction. Reported arrhythmic complications include 10% for supraventricular tachycardia or atrial flutter, 10%-15% for ventricular tachycardia, and 2%-5% for sudden death.[169] Residual pulmonary insufficiency is common; its long-term consequences are not well defined, but it may cause or contribute to right ventricular failure and require valvular repair.

Risk factors for poor late outcome following surgical repair include increased age at time of repair, preoperative heart failure, persistent right ventricular systolic hypertension, residual right ventricular dysfunction, and residual VSD. The sudden death rate is about 0.5% per year and caused by ventricular arrhythmias, but the predisposing factors for sudden death are not well elucidated.[166] Advanced age at repair, residual right ventricular volume and/or pressure overload, right ventricular dysfunction, and pulmonary insufficiency seem to be related to sudden death risk. Ambulatory monitoring demonstrates ventricular ectopy in up to 50% of repaired TOF, but it is not clear if this ectopy is a predictor of sudden death. In the absence of significant structural and hemodynamic residua, survival is very good but still significantly worse than that of age- and gender-matched normal populations.

Because of these very significant late consequences of repaired TOF, military flying is not recommended for any aircraft type, nor are aerobatic and commercial airline flying. However, in an aeromedical review of congenital heart disease, one author concluded that restricted (multicrew) civilian certification might be allowed for selected low-risk cases.[166] Recommended criteria included repair at an early age, absence of symptoms, no significant hemodynamic residua (eg, normal right and left ventricular size and function, no significant residual right ventricular outflow tract obstruction, and mild or no pulmonary insufficiency), and no frequent or complex ventricular ectopy. If any special issuance is granted, annual review should be performed, including echocardiography, 24-hour ambulatory monitoring, and graded exercise testing.

Hypertension

Epidemiologic and Clinical Features

Hypertension is a significant risk factor for cardiovascular and cerebrovascular disease as well as renal disease, and is therefore a major health problem. Although the focus has traditionally been on elevated diastolic blood pressure, comparable risks associated with systolic hypertension have been well established. Clinical trials and population studies demonstrate that both systolic and diastolic blood pressure have continuous, independent relationships with cardiovascular diseases and events, stroke, renal disease, cardiovascular mortality, and total mortality. This has been demonstrated across a wide range of blood pressures with no demonstrated threshold effect. Furthermore, this effect is present regardless of age, gender, and ethnic origin.

Blood pressure control has been clearly shown to significantly reduce these events, although the benefit is greater for stroke than for cardiac events. This may be due to the confounding influence of other cardiac risk factors in hypertensive subjects. The risk reduction benefit is greater in absolute terms for higher risk groups such as those with more severe hypertension, advanced age, and hypertension with target organ effects, and is therefore more cost-effective in these groups over relatively short time periods. However, lower risk subsets such as those of younger age and with milder hypertension also benefit to the same relative degree, with approximately 15%-35% reduction depending on endpoint. In the longer term of reducing disease expression, morbidity, and target organ damage, treatment of lower risk hypertensives would seem to be more effective preventive medicine.

A recent "call to action" for physicians reported that hypertension affects about 25% of the adult population of the United States.[170] The authors emphasized that although great strides have been made over the years in identification and treatment of hypertension, recent reports suggest that this progress has leveled off in the past few years, and that only about 25% of hypertensive adults in the United States are currently controlled. In association with this, reductions in national mortality for stroke and heart disease also seem to have leveled off.

The Joint National Committee on Prevention, Detection, Evaluation and Treatment of High Blood Pressure published its most recent recommendations (JNC VI) in 1997.[171] JNC VI defined hypertension as systolic blood pressure ≥140 mm Hg, diastolic pressure ≥90 mm Hg, or the current use of medication for hypertension control. Control is then defined as maintaining blood pressure below 140/90 mm Hg, except for certain high-risk groups for whom lower levels are recommended. JNC VI also recognized an intermediate or borderline risk pressure of 130-139/85-89 mm Hg for whom nonpharmacologic therapy is recommended to help prevent future development of hypertension. As a new feature, JNC VI also included treatment guidelines based on the presence of other risk factors in addition to the blood pressure level. Higher risk groups with additional risk factors, target organ damage (eg, left ventricular hypertrophy), or coexisting cardiovascular disease are recommended for lower medication treatment thresholds and lower target blood pressures. The JNC VI report contains valuable guidelines for any practitioner likely to deal with hypertensive patients, including the AME/FS. Applying these guidelines to the hypertensive aviator is recommended, within the confines of medication use considered acceptable by the appropriate licensing authority.

Routine laboratory evaluation for newly diagnosed essential hypertension should include urinalysis, electrolytes, BUN and creatinine, fasting glucose, lipid panel, 12-lead electrocardiogram, and possibly chest X-ray. Other testing may be indicated in selected patients to further assess cardiovascular status, target organ effects, or correctable causes of hypertension.

Aeromedical Considerations

The medical benefits of diagnosing and treating hypertension appear to be irrefutable. Hypertension in an aviator should be treated by lifestyle modification and medication as discussed below. Other aeromedical concerns include a consideration of white coat hypertension, the disposition of left ventricular hypertrophy, and antihypertensive medication allowance by licensing authorities.

Aeromedical Recommendations

Nonpharmacologic therapy or lifestyle modifications are recommended for initial treatment of hypertension in the range of systolic 140-159 and/or diastolic 90-99 mm

Hg. These modalities include weight reduction if overweight, limiting alcohol ingestion, regular exercise, smoking cessation, decreased dietary sodium, and increased
dietary potassium. Adequate dietary calcium and magnesium may also be beneficial.
Biofeedback, stress management techniques, and relaxation therapies may also be
of some benefit, particularly for the aviator with borderline, labile, or white coat
hypertension (discussed below). However, much of the literature does not support a
role for these modalities in treating fixed hypertension. Because of the increased risk
for cardiovascular disease, other risk factors such as lipid abnormalities should also
be aggressively pursued. A trial of lifestyle modification should be attempted for 6
months. Continuation of unrestricted flying during this nonpharmacologic trial is
recommended. If control is not achieved within that time, then therapy with a medication approved by the appropriate licensing authority should be instituted. This
should include a nonflying observation period to assess for adverse reactions and
side effects to the medication.

Initial treatment with both lifestyle modification and approved medical therapy
is recommended for the aviator with verified hypertension with systolic pressure
≥160 or diastolic pressure ≥100 mm Hg. Flying should be discontinued until blood
pressure control is achieved or at least until blood pressure is consistently below
160/100 mm Hg. Again, an appropriate nonflying observation period is warranted
after beginning medical therapy.

The reader is also referred to the discussion below of left ventricular hypertrophy
for aeromedical recommendations regarding this target organ complication.

White Coat Hypertension

White coat, office, or clinic hypertension is an entity of aeromedical interest, as it is
often seen in aviators presenting for routine flight or other examinations. It is estimated to occur in 20%-40% of patients with presumed mild hypertension based on
elevated blood pressure measurements recorded in the office. White coat hypertension may be defined as elevated blood pressure in a medical environment with normal follow-up 3-5 day blood pressure checks, home blood pressure checks, or
ambulatory blood pressure monitoring. Numerous studies have documented elevated blood pressures in the medical office compared to normal home or ambulatory recordings, and this effect is more exaggerated in the presence of a physician
compared to a nurse or technician.

The questions for the AME/FS are: What is the best method to document white
coat hypertension in an aviator, and should it be considered a normal variant or
potentially a prehypertensive condition? Twice daily (morning and afternoon) blood
pressure checks every 3-5 days in the flight medicine clinic are standard procedure
and often yield blood pressure readings within the normal range. But this is still a

medical environment and may not be adequate follow-up for all susceptible patients. Manual home blood pressure recordings are reportedly accurate and correlate well with ambulatory monitoring. If such a course is pursued, clinic personnel should validate the individual aviator's home device and technique. One also should consider the possibility of reporting bias on the part of the aviator. Although too expensive for routine use, 24-hour ambulatory blood pressure monitoring is an option for individual cases, and most studies in the literature use readings from this method compared to office readings to define white coat hypertension.

The second question is of greater impact: Is white coat hypertension normal or abnormal? The AME/FS may tend to consider white coat hypertension as a normal variant in aviators, an almost automatic response to occupational anxiety. The decision not to treat white coat hypertension pharmacologically is probably appropriate and most authorities agree with this recommendation. But it is not advisable to consider it normal and subsequently neglect to follow the individual closely for development of hypertension or fail to institute lifestyle modification therapy.

Ten-year follow-up was reported for 126 white coat hypertensives and 353 sustained hypertensives.[172] There were significantly fewer cardiovascular events in the white coat hypertensives, as well as less left ventricular hypertrophy and carotid wall thickening by echocardiography and carotid ultrasound (target organ effects). However, most patients in both groups were treated with antihypertensive therapy and there was no normotensive control group. In another study, 1187 hypertensive subjects (19.2% were white coat hypertensives) and 205 normotensive controls were followed for a mean of 3.2 years.[173] Cardiovascular morbidity did not differ between the controls and white coats, but was significantly higher in sustained hypertensives. Other investigators found no difference in carotid wall thickness by ultrasound in a group of sustained hypertensives compared to a group of untreated white coat hypertensives, but both groups had significantly thicker carotid walls than a normotensive control group.[174] Also, in two different studies left ventricular mass measurements by echocardiography were significantly greater in white coat hypertensives than in normotensive controls.[175,176]

White coat hypertension does seem to have a more benign clinical prognosis than sustained hypertension, at least for relatively short follow-up, but it also has evidence of target organ effects. Whether this should be pharmacologically treated is unclear; many of the white coat subjects in these and other studies were in fact treated medically as mild hypertension. As stated earlier, most authorities would probably agree that medical therapy is not warranted and it is not presently recommended for aviators. But to consider white coat hypertension a normal variant or a normal physiologic response is inappropriate. Nonpharmacologic therapy via lifestyle modification and careful follow-up of blood pressure is indicated.

Blood Pressure Control—Target Levels

This issue of white coat hypertension and target organ effects raises the question of what should be the appropriate target blood pressure for hypertension therapy. JNC VI defines control as maintaining a blood pressure <140/90 mm Hg, but JNC VI also recognizes pressures of 130-139/85-89 mm Hg as high normal or borderline and recommends lifestyle modification therapy for this range. Lower target levels are recommended for certain subsets of high-risk patients. JNC VI also defines blood pressure <120/80 mm Hg as optimal and <130/85 mm Hg as normal. Blood pressure readings by ambulatory monitoring are lower than routine cuff measurements, and normal is usually considered an average pressure during waking hours of <130-135/85 mm Hg.

Several studies demonstrate that ambulatory pressure readings are better predictors of target organ effects than are office blood pressure readings. In 688 hypertensive patients, ambulatory pressures were also more predictive of first cardiovascular event than were clinic pressures.[177] An opposite group of patients has also been studied—white coat normotensives, who are hypertensive patients with normal office pressures but abnormal ambulatory pressures.[178] These patients had increased left ventricular mass, thicker carotid artery walls, and more carotid artery plaques compared to normotensive controls, but had values comparable to those seen in patients with sustained hypertension (abnormal office and ambulatory readings).

After obtaining baseline ambulatory blood pressure recordings, 1542 healthy subjects over age 40 were followed for a mean of 6.2 years.[179] Based on mortality, optimal blood pressure was 120-133/65-78 mm Hg. Values >134/79 and values <119/64 mm Hg were associated with increased cardiovascular and noncardiovascular mortality, respectively. The Hypertension Optimal Treatment (HOT) trial reported on 18,790 hypertensive patients randomized to diastolic blood pressure treatment goals of ≤90, ≤85, or ≤80 mm Hg and followed for a mean of 3.8 years.[180] Treatment goals were reached in the three groups. The lowest risk for cardiovascular events occurred at a pressure of 138.5/82.6 mm Hg.

Practice with aviators often seems to involve using the lowest dose of medication possible to barely achieve the desired control. This makes some sense in that it minimizes side effects and does satisfy aeromedical requirements. However, treating an aviator to a target blood pressure of 139/89 mm Hg may satisfy JNC VI and licensing authority criteria for blood pressure control, but it may represent only adequate or minimal rather than preferred or optimal control for long-term health benefits.

Left Ventricular Hypertrophy

Left ventricular hypertrophy (LVH) by electrocardiogram or echocardiography has repeatedly been shown to be a strong, independent predictor of morbidity and mortality, including suddenly incapacitating events such as sudden cardiac death, myocardial infarction, and stroke. Much of this awareness has come from the Framingham Heart Study. The mechanism is unclear and probably multifactorial. Antihypertensive medications, including diuretics, have been shown to regress LVH. Superior LVH regression of one class of medication over others for the same level of blood pressure reduction has not been clearly demonstrated, except that direct vasodilators may not cause LVH regression.

Some studies suggest that ACE inhibitors, with or without diuretic, have the most potent LVH regression effect. In one study, significant reduction of left ventricular mass was demonstrated after 1 year of therapy for mild to moderate hypertension with captopril, atenolol, or hydrochlorothiazide, but not with clonidine, diltiazem, or prazosin.[181] In a metaanalysis of 39 randomized, double-blind trials, and a meta-analysis update of 50 trials, it was reported that LVH was reduced 13% and 12% by ACE inhibitors, 9% and 11% by calcium channel antagonists, 7% and 8% by diuretics, and 6% and 5% by beta-blockers, respectively.[182,183] Even some lifestyle modifications, such as sustained weight reduction and reduced dietary sodium, have been shown to cause LVH regression.

Efficacy of blood pressure control, duration of successful therapy and greater pretreatment LVH may be more related to LVH regression than medication selection. Improved prognosis has been demonstrated with reversal of electrocardiographic or echocardiographic LVH, and failure of therapy to achieve regression of LVH has been associated with increased cardiovascular events. However, it has not been shown that regression of LVH reverses the increased risk associated with LVH *independent* of the risk reduction effected by lowering and controlling blood pressure and other beneficial cardiovascular effects of the medication (eg, the antiarrhythmic effect of some drugs).

Aeromedical Recommendation. Nevertheless, because of the increased risk independently associated with LVH and the clear benefit of therapy and possible coincident benefit of LVH regression, it may be appropriate to discontinue or restrict flight duties in a hypertensive aviator with LVH until regression has been documented by echocardiography. Careful attention must then be given to future blood pressure control to prevent recurrence of LVH.

Antihypertensive Medications

Finally, the use of acceptable or appropriate antihypertensive medications in aviators must be considered. JNC VI generally recommends diuretics and beta-blockers as first line therapy, but gives other first choice options for certain patient subsets such as diabetics. However the AME/FS may be caught in the dilemma of wanting to follow clinical guidelines for medical therapy, yet being limited to those medications that are aeromedically approved by the licensing authority. Cardiac medications, including antihypertensives, are discussed further in a later section of this chapter.

Other Aeromedical Issues

Effects on $+G_z$ tolerance should always be a concern with antihypertensive therapy. Statistically significant reductions of $+G_z$ tolerance for relaxed and straining gradual-onset centrifuge runs were demonstrated in 7 normotensive subjects taking 25 mg captopril bid versus placebo and acting as their own blinded controls.[184] But these were normotensive volunteers, not hypertensive patients, and the reductions in $+G_z$ tolerance were small in absolute terms and might not be considered operationally significant. Another lisinopril study found no significant reduction of $+G_z$ tolerance in 15 hypertensive aviators compared to 434 normal aviator controls.[185] A more ideal protocol would have included centrifuge testing of these hypertensive aviators before and after lisinopril therapy, but this was not performed. Centrifuge assessment is an option when considering return to flight status of high-performance aviators taking antihypertensive medications.

Another $+G_z$-related question is whether chronic exposure to a high $+G_z$ cockpit environment causes elevated blood pressure. Systolic blood pressure at baseline and after 12-15 years of service was reported on 112 fighter pilots and 112 transport/helicopter pilots.[186] Mean entry systolic pressure was 122 ± 12 and 124 ± 12 mm Hg, respectively, and at the end of the study was 118 ± 12 mm Hg in both groups. The stress of the fighter (and nonfighter) aviation environment did not seem to pose an increased risk for development of hypertension.

Screening for coronary heart disease may be a consideration in selected high-risk hypertensive aviators. Recognizing the increased risk in hypertensives, the lisinopril study in 62 military aviators described above included screening for coronary heart disease.[185] Ten of 62 (18%) had measurable coronary heart disease, 7 with significant and 3 with nonsignificant disease.

Finally, a plea to the AME/FS who obtains an elevated blood pressure measurement on an aviator. There may be a practice of placing the aviator in a dim, quiet room and repeating measurements until an acceptable reading is obtained, or a 5-day blood pressure check with an average of 139/89 mm Hg may be accepted as normal even though several readings are above 140/90 mm Hg. See the above discussion about white coat hypertension and the recommendation by JNC VI of the high-risk or borderline blood pressure category of 130-139/85-89 mm Hg. Hypertension has serious health consequences and should not be underdiagnosed or inadequately treated in the interest of furthering a flying career.

Cardiac Medications

Introduction

The topic of medication use in aviators is difficult and widely discussed in aviation medicine circles. How should medical therapy affect flying eligibility? In one sense, this is a philosophical or administrative issue for licensing authorities. Each licensing agency must develop policy guidelines for aeromedical acceptability of medications for its own unique aviation and aeromedical setting. The guidelines may vary widely among the various types of flight operations and environments. Unfortunately, most licensing authorities are unable to perform long-term medication studies with large numbers of aviators and use this data to formulate their own regulations for medication use.

The basic problem is striking a balance between offering the aviator the best available medical care versus the inherent risk of medication use in an aviation environment. One must consider the potential effect of each medication on flying performance. Subtle side effects that might cause significant performance decrements must be considered, as well as more common clinical side effects. Side effect profiles applicable to the general population are usually available in the literature. The unique factors affecting aeromedical disposition are the subtle effects on performance, and such data are often not clinically important, and therefore not readily available in the literature. Also, in spite of clinical trials done prior to approval of a medication, it often requires several years of use in the general population before some significant adverse effects become known.

One must also consider the use of a medication within the context of the particular cardiac disorder being treated. For example, beta-blocker therapy for hypertension might be considered acceptable for some types of flying, but beta-blocker therapy for suppression of symptomatic, exercise-induced ventricular tachycardia might not be considered acceptable for any flight duty.

Universally allowing special issuance for an entire class of medications is probably unwise. Individual medications within a class may have widely different adverse effects. Licensing agencies should develop policies that allow safe but timely consideration of a medication. On the other hand, not every new medication released necessitates prompt immediate review. Unless it offers some significant or unique advantage, older medications with long-term published data on side effects should be used. Should there be special consideration for the individual aviator who cannot take, or is not adequately treated by, the medications allowed for a given disorder? This is a decision for each licensing agency to make according to its own unique flight operation and experience with these medications.

A few practical considerations are worth mentioning. To minimize side effects, the lowest possible dose should be used, without sacrificing efficacy and good control of the condition being treated. Combination therapy is a means to obtain good control while minimizing dose-dependent side effects, but both agents and their combined use must be acceptable to the licensing authority. Patient compliance is always a concern, perhaps more so in aviators than in the general population, so once-daily dosing should be used as much as possible.

In addition to the use of research and testing data about side effect profiles as an aid in determining choice and dose of medication, the aviator may serve as his or her own control. Most licensing authorities require a period of nonflying observation after starting a medication to monitor for both efficacy and side effects. The aviator should be evaluated and questioned carefully by the AME/FS during this observation period and during subsequent follow-up. Side effects can develop gradually and the aviator patient may not realize they may be caused by the medication without careful questioning. Abbreviated reassessment should be performed after dosage increases and after changing to a new medication within the same drug class.

Specific Cardiac Medications

Appropriate categories of cardiac medications for the cardiac diagnoses discussed above include antihypertensives, antianginals, lipid-modifying agents, and antiarrhythmics. In many instances, the same medications will have several uses. For example, some calcium channel antagonists may be used to treat angina, hypertension, or supraventricular tachycardias. Medications for treatment of congestive heart failure or left ventricular dysfunction are not considered here, because disorders of such significance requiring medical therapy are unlikely to allow return to flying.

Antihypertensives

JNC VI recommends diuretics and beta-blockers as first line therapy for most patients.[171] However, this hierarchy of therapy may not be acceptable for all aviation situations and licensing authorities. Thiazide and potassium-sparing diuretic therapy has been the traditional approach in aviation medicine for years, but some licensing authorities, especially for military aviation, may not consider beta-blocker therapy acceptable for flying. ACE inhibitors offer an aeromedically acceptable alternative or addition to diuretics.

Agents considered below are thiazide and potassium-sparing diuretics, beta-blockers, ACE inhibitors, and calcium channel antagonists. Other agents are not considered due to unacceptable side effect profiles. These include more potent diuretics (eg, furosemide), peripherally and centrally acting agents (eg, reserpine, clonidine), alpha blockers (eg, prazosin), and direct vasodilators (eg, hydralazine). Angiotensin II receptor blockers are promising for future considerations. They have hemodynamic effects similar to ACE inhibitors, but without the side effect of dry cough. Long-term data are currently insufficient for aeromedical consideration.

Diuretics. Thiazide diuretics gained early aeromedical acceptance without the scrutiny currently given to newer medications. Commonly reported side effects are decreased sexual function in men, dizziness, orthostasis, nausea, and headache. Photosensitivity is uncommon and resolves after discontinuing therapy. Electrolyte abnormalities include decreased sodium, potassium, and magnesium, and increased uric acid. Other laboratory abnormalities include elevated cholesterol and glucose. Volume depletion with possible adverse effects on $+G_z$ tolerance, and dehydration on long flights or in military flight operations is possible.

Past reports of increased risk of sudden or arrhythmic death associated with diuretic use have involved higher doses than are currently used, and/or involved patients with extant or probable underlying heart disease. Dosages equivalent to 25 mg of hydrochlorothiazide daily are currently recommended, and are effective for controlling blood pressure while minimizing electrolyte and other metabolic side effects. Doses higher than 25-50 mg daily are not recommended clinically or aeromedically; any additional antihypertensive benefit is slight or nonexistent, and adverse effects are more likely. Adequate dietary potassium and magnesium are helpful lifestyle modifications for hypertensive patients, and are especially important for the patient on diuretics. Using a combination of a thiazide and a potassium-sparing agent can minimize the hypokalemic effects.

The use of diuretic therapy in aviators has stood the test of time, and it can be used safely in most aviators, including those in high-performance flight operations.

Beta-blockers. Physical and mental depressive effects are the primary concerns in the use of beta-blockers. Lethargy, fatigability, decreased exercise tolerance, orthostatic symptoms, insomnia, nightmares, mental depression, and sexual dysfunction are commonly reported. Blunted heart rate and blood pressure response to stress is a consideration, as is possible bronchospasm. Adverse effects on physical endurance and performance may be especially important concerns for the military aviator.

One report reviewed different classes of cardiac medications from the perspective of possible occupational effects, focusing on symptom categories such as lightheadedness, paresthesias, incoordination, mental status changes, and fatigability, as well as psychiatric effects and sleep disturbances.[187] There is helpful information in the literature regarding beta-blockers, probably due to concerns regarding their overall depressive effect and their possible adverse impact on various measures of performance. Reported effects of beta-blockers on psychomotor performance depend on the particular study, the specific beta-blocker evaluated, and the parameters measured. However, concerns about the overall depressive effects of beta-blockers are generally unwarranted. For example, one review of the literature concluded that beta-blockers improved cognitive function in 16%, worsened function in 17%, and had no significant change in 67%. In several studies, performance of complex tasks was actually improved during beta-blocker therapy, probably due to its anxiolytic effect. One investigator reviewed 24 studies of the effects of beta-blockers on psychomotor performance, finding no effect in 15, improved performance in 6, and impaired performance in 3.[188] Others studied 13 hypertensive patients on atenolol, and demonstrated improved vigilance and no effect on reaction time and concentration.[189]

ACE Inhibitors. The most common complaint is a persistent, dry cough that resolves after discontinuing therapy. Hypotensive or orthostatic complaints are unusual and the side effect profile is otherwise quite benign. A review that addressed antihypertensive therapy for military aviators briefly reviewed diuretics, beta-blockers, and ACE inhibitors from an aeromedical perspective, including their "cerebral effects."[190] Several studies were cited that showed no significant effects of ACE inhibitors on psychiatric and emotional well being or neurologic function. In another study, 62 hypertensive military aviators were evaluated after achieving blood pressure control with lisinopril (maximum allowed dose of 80 mg daily).[185] Audiologic, vestibular, ophthalmologic, and laboratory testing disclosed no significant or disqualifying problems, and long-term follow-up did not reveal any new side effects. ACE inhibitors and diuretics are probably the most acceptable antihypertensives from an aeromedical viewpoint.

Calcium Channel Antagonists. Common side effects include headache, ankle edema, flushing, dizziness and orthostasis, fatigue, muscle cramps, nausea, and constipation. Many of these symptoms resolve over time with continued therapy or can be lessened or avoided by a slow dose titration. These agents are potent vasodilators; therefore decreased $+G_z$ tolerance would definitely be a concern for high-performance flying. Some of these agents have overall negative effects on myocardial contractility and conduction pathways, but these are unlikely to be a problem in the otherwise healthy hypertensive aviator.

Calcium channel antagonists have often been authorized for use in civilian aviation, but appropriate long-term safety profile data are insufficient to warrant approval by many military aviation licensing authorities.

Antianginal Medications

General considerations regarding antianginals were discussed in the section on coronary heart disease. In that discussion, medical therapy for the treatment of ischemic symptoms was not recommended for any categories of flying. The use of medications to treat ischemic symptoms implies underlying active ischemia. However, as also discussed earlier, some allowance should be made for use of these medications for indications other than the treatment of angina. For example, beta-blockers and calcium channel antagonists might be appropriately used for treatment of coexisting hypertension. Also, most treatment guidelines recommend routine use of beta-blockers, and possibly ACE inhibitors, after myocardial infarction for prognostic indications. Antianginals include beta-blockers and calcium channel antagonists (discussed above with antihypertensives), as well as nitrates.

Nitrates. Long-acting nitrates are administered orally or cutaneously to treat or prevent ischemic symptoms. Short-acting nitrates are administered sublingually as tablets or spray for the acute relief of angina. It may be desirable to prescribe short-acting nitrates to aviators with asymptomatic coronary artery disease for possible future use. Commonly reported side effects include headaches, lightheadedness, orthostatic symptoms, hypotension, flushing, and weakness, and are usually dose-related. Of the three types of antianginals mentioned here, nitrates are the least desirable for use in aviators.

Lipid-Modifying Agents

Primary and secondary prevention of coronary heart disease are significant health issues in aviators as well as in the general population. Aggressive risk factor modification is indicated for high-risk aviators and aviators with known coronary heart disease. Lipid modification by drug therapy is an important aspect of risk factor modification. A report of lipid-lowering therapy in military aviators included a review of lipid-lowering drugs from an aeromedical perspective, and some recommended treatment initiation and target lipid levels adopted from published guidelines.[63] While directed at military aviators, it is a useful discussion for all aviation environments. The 3-hydroxy-3-methylglutaryl coenzyme A (HMG-CoA) reductase inhibitors (statins) are currently the primary lipid management medications, although nonsystemic resin binding agents have traditionally been the aeromedical agents of choice due to their lack of systemic effects.

Statins (HMG-CoA Reductase Inhibitors). These are the most potent agents currently available, lowering LDL cholesterol by 25%-50%.[63,64] They also lower total cholesterol and triglycerides and increase HDL cholesterol. Their primary mechanism of action is interference with cholesterol synthesis. Reported side effects include various gastrointestinal complaints, muscle cramps and myalgia, fatigue, insomnia, headache, blurred vision, and dizziness. Skeletal myopathy and rhabdomyolysis are rare, and early concerns about statins causing cataracts have not been borne out in subsequent studies. Laboratory abnormalities include elevated transaminases and skeletal muscle enzymes.

Although decreased cognitive function was suggested by at least one small study, larger studies with longer follow-up have not confirmed this. In another study, 81 U.S. Navy aviators with hypercholesterolemia were randomized to lovastatin, pravastatin, or placebo after a trial of dietary management. After 4 weeks of therapy, no significant adverse effects were observed. Baseline cognitive testing showed no difference between treatment groups or from published norms. Repeat cognitive testing after drug therapy also showed no difference between the treatment groups or from baseline.[191] The long-term safety of these agents has been well documented.

Bile Acid Sequestrants. These agents have often been used in aviators because of their nonsystemic action. They bind bile acids in the intestine, interrupting their enterohepatic circulation and thereby increasing the conversion of cholesterol into bile acids in the liver. LDL cholesterol is lowered 10%-30% and HDL cholesterol is increased somewhat, but triglycerides are variably increased.[63,64] Side effects are limited to the gastrointestinal tract, but are common, including abdominal fullness, bloating, constipation, and gas. Patients are often unable to tolerate these agents in doses sufficient to allow their use as monotherapy. They are best used in moderate doses to complement statin therapy and further reduce LDL cholesterol.

Fibric Acid Derivatives (Fibrates). These are the most effective triglyceride lowering agents, reducing hypertriglyceridemia by as much as 50%.[63] LDL cholesterol may be reduced significantly and HDL cholesterol increased modestly. The most common side effects are gastrointestinal and headache, and in men, sexual dysfunction. These agents are generally well tolerated and are most useful for significant hypertriglyceridemia or combined hyperlipidemia.

Nicotinic Acid. These agents lower both triglycerides and cholesterol and significantly increase HDL cholesterol. Flushing is the most common and bothersome side effect and can be lessened by taking aspirin. Nausea, loose bowel movements, indigestion, and nasal congestion are other adverse effects. Elevated transaminases and glucose may occur.

Antiarrhythmics

General considerations regarding medication use for control of arrhythmias were discussed in the section on tachyarrhythmia but deserve reemphasis. Approval of antiarrhythmic medication in an aviator will depend on both the type of arrhythmia and the medication used, as well as the symptoms experienced during the arrhythmia. Maintenance of sinus rhythm and controlling ventricular rate response are the goals of medication use for atrial fibrillation and atrial flutter, whereas preventing the arrhythmia is the goal of medication use for SVT. Medical suppression of ventricular arrhythmias is not recommended for return to any category of flight operation. Perfect control with medication is not realistically possible, and one must accept that the arrhythmia may "break through" and recur. Another clinical and aeromedical concern is the prorrhythmic effect of many antiarrhythmics (ie, some antiarrhythmics also cause arrhythmias, usually ventricular). Compliance of the aviator in taking the medication is also a potential problem.

An aeromedical review of this topic concluded that antiarrhythmic medication might be acceptable in aviators without underlying cardiac disease, if the arrhythmia has been well tolerated from a physical, mental, and performance standpoint.[125] Also, the medication selected must have documented efficacy without prorrhythmic effects or significant side effects, and the aviator must be compliant with the dosing regimen. It was concluded that only hydrophilic beta-blockers, calcium channel antagonists, and digitalis met these requirements. (Beta-blockers and calcium channel antagonists are discussed above with antihypertensive medications.) As recommended in this referenced review, many other antiarrhythmics are available, but they have side effect profiles that are unacceptable for flight operations, and most are known to have prorrhythmic effects.

Digitalis. Toxicity is well known and includes some serious effects such as bradycardia, varying degrees of heart block, atrial tachycardia with block, atrioventricular dissociation with junctional rhythm, and complex ventricular arrhythmias, including ventricular tachycardia. Symptoms of toxicity include gastrointestinal complaints, visual disturbances, weakness, dizziness, headache and confusion, or other mental state alterations. However, in the absence of toxic serum and tissue levels, digitalis is quite well tolerated. Although the therapeutic/toxic ratio is low, relatively young and otherwise healthy individuals with normal renal function are very unlikely to develop digitalis toxicity.

References

1. Bennett G. First European workshop in aviation cardiology. Medical-cause accidents in commercial aviation. *Eur Heart J.* 1992;13(suppl H):13-15.

2. Tunstall-Pedoe H. First European workshop in aviation cardiology. Cardiovascular risk and risk factors in the context of aircrew certification. *Eur Heart J.* 1992;13(suppl H):16-20.

3. Joy M. First European workshop in aviation cardiology. Cardiological aspects of aviation safety—the new European perspective. *Eur Heart J.* 1992;13(suppl H):21-26.

4. Chamberlain D. Second European workshop in aviation cardiology. Attributable and absolute (polymorphic) risk in aviation certification: Developing the 1% rule. *Eur Heart J.* 1999;1(suppl D):D19-D24.

5. Averill KH, Lamb LE. Electrocardiographic findings in 67,375 asymptomatic subjects: I. Incidence of abnormalities. *Am J Cardiol*. 1960;6(1):76-83.

6. Hiss RG, Lamb LE. Electrocardiographic findings in 122,043 individuals. *Circulation*. 1962;25(6):947-961.

7. Kruyer WB. Aeromedical evaluation and disposition of electrocardiographic abnormalities. In: *Short Course on Cardiopulmonary Aspects of Aerospace Medicine, Advisory Group for Aerospace Research and Development (NATO) Report #758*. Loughton, Essex, UK: Specialized Printing Services Limited; March 1987:1-1 to 1-8.

8. Celio PV. Aeromedical disposition of arrhythmias and electrocardiographic findings in aircrew. In: Lecture Series 189: Cardiopulmonary Aspects in Aerospace Medicine, AGARD-LS-189 (NATO). Loughton, Essex, UK: Specialized Printing Services Limited; October 1993: 5-1, 5-9.

9. Schlant RC. Guidelines for electrocardiography. A report of the American College of Cardiology/American Heart Association task force on assessment of diagnostic and therapeutic cardiovascular procedures (Committee on Electrocardiography). *J Am Coll Cardiol*. 1992;19(3):473-481.

10. Barrett PA, Peter CT, Swan HJ, et al. The frequency and prognostic significance of electrocardiographic abnormalities in clinically normal individuals. *Prog Cardiovasc Dis*. 1981;23(4):299-319.

11. Zehender M, Meinertz T, Keul J, Just H. ECG variants and cardiac arrhythmias in athletes: Clinical relevance and prognostic importance. *Am Heart J*. 1990;119(6):1378-1391.

12. Gray GW, Salisbury DA, Gulino AM. Echocardiographic and color flow Doppler findings in military pilot applicants. *Aviat Space Environ Med*. 1995;66(1):32-34.

13. Palka P, Lange A, Fleming AD, et al. Differences in myocardial velocity gradient measured throughout the cardiac cycle in patients with hypertrophic cardiomyopathy, athletes and patients with left ventricular hypertrophy due to hypertension. *J Am Coll Cardiol*. 1997;30(3):760-768.

14. Rotman M, Triebwasser JH. A clinical and follow-up study of right and left bundle branch block. *Circulation*. 1975;51(3):477-484.

15. Armstrong CR, Erikson NS. Right axis deviation as a criterion for echocardiographic evaluation of aircrew candidates. *Aviat Space Environ Med*. 1998;69(9):833-836.

16. Tamura T, Komatsu C, Asukata I, et al. Time course and clinical significance of marked left axis deviation in airline pilots. *Aviat Space Environ Med*. 1991;62(7):683-686.

17. Richardson LA, Celio PV. The aeromedical implications of supraventricular tachycardia. In: The clinical basis for aeromedical decision making, AGARD conference proceedings 553. Hull, Quebec, Canada: Canada Communication Group; September 1994:25-1 to 25-5.

18. Gardner RA, Kruyer WB, Pickard JS, Celio PV. Nonsustained ventricular tachycardia in 193 U.S. military aviators: Long-term follow-up. *Aviat Space Environ Med*. Accepted for publication.

19. Sox HC Jr, Garber AM, Littenberg B. The resting electrocardiogram as a screening test: A clinical analysis. *Ann Intern Med*. 1989;111(6):489-502.

20. Joy M, Trump DW. Significance of minor ST segment and T wave changes in the resting electrocardiogram of asymptomatic subjects. *Br Heart J*. 1981;45(1):48-55.

21. Gibbons RJ. Guidelines for exercise testing. A report of the American College of Cardiology/American Heart Association task force on practice guidelines (committee on exercise testing). *J Am Coll Cardiol*. 1997;30(1):260-315.

22. Schlant RC. Guidelines for exercise testing. A report of the American College of Cardiology/American Heart Association task force on assessment of cardiovascular procedures (subcommittee on exercise testing). *J Am Coll Cardiol*. 1986;8(3):725-738.

23. Macintyre NR, Kunkler JR, Mitchell RE, et al. Eight-year follow-up of exercise electrocardiograms in healthy middle-aged aviators. *Aviat Space Environ Med*. 1981;52(4):256-259.

24. Froelicher VF, Thomas MM, Pillow C, Lancaster MC. Epidemiologic study of asymptomatic men screened by maximal treadmill testing for latent coronary artery disease. *Am J Cardiol*. 1974;34(12):770-776.

25. Allen WH, Aronow WS, Goodman P, Stinson P. Five-year follow-up of maximal treadmill stress test in asymptomatic men and women. *Circulation*. 1980;62(3):522-527.

26. Hickman JR Jr. Noninvasive methods for the detection of coronary artery disease in aviators—A stratified Bayesian approach. In: *Short Course on Cardiopulmonary Aspects of Aerospace Medicine, Advisory Group for Aerospace Research and Development (NATO) Report #758*. Loughton, Essex, UK: Specialized Printing Services Limited; March 1987:2-1 to 2-11.

27. Loecker TH, Schwartz RS, Cotta CW, Hickman JR Jr. Fluoroscopic coronary artery calcification and associated coronary disease in asymptomatic young men. *J Am Coll Cardiol*. 1992;19(6):1167-1172.

28. O'Malley PG, Taylor AJ, Gibbons RV, et al. Rationale and design of the prospective Army coronary calcium (PACC) study: Utility of electron beam computed tomography as a screening test for coronary artery disease and as an intervention for risk factor modification among young, asymptomatic active-duty United States Army personnel. *Am Heart J*. 1999;137(5):932-941.

29. Schwartz RS, Jackson WG, Celio PV, et al. Accuracy of exercise Tl-201 myocardial scintigraphy in asymptomatic young men. *Circulation*. 1993;87(1):165-172.

30. Nagueh, SF, Zoghbi WA. Stress echocardiography for the assessment of myocardial ischemia and viability. *Curr Probl Cardiol*. 1996;21(7):445-520.

31. Detrano R, Froelicher VF. A logical approach to screening for coronary artery disease. *Ann Intern Med*. 1987;106(6):846-852.

32. Kruyer WB. Screening for asymptomatic coronary heart disease. In: Lecture Series 189: Cardiopulmonary aspects in aerospace medicine, AGARD-LS-189 (NATO). Loughton, Essex, UK: Specialized Printing Services Limited; October 1993:2-1 to 2-5.

33. van Leusden AJ, Prendergast PR, Gray GW. Permanent grounding and flying restrictions in Canadian Forces pilots: A 10-year review. *Aviat Space Environ Med*. 1991;62(6):513-516.

34. Booze CF Jr, Staggs CM. A comparison of postmortem coronary atherosclerosis findings in general aviation pilot fatalities. *Aviat Space Environ Med*. 1987;58(4):297-300.

35. Underwood Ground KE. Prevalence of coronary atherosclerosis in healthy United Kingdom aviators. *Aviat Space Environ Med.* 1981;52(11, pt 1):696-701.

36. Kaji M, Tango T, Asukata I, et al. Mortality experience of cockpit crewmembers from Japan Airlines. *Aviat Space Environ Med.* 1993;64(8):748-750.

37. Osswald S, Miles R, Nixon W, Celio P. Review of cardiac events in USAF aviators. *Aviat Space Environ Med.* 1996;67(11):1023-1027.

38. Lichtlen PR, Bargheer K, Wenzlaff P. Long-term prognosis of patients with anginalike chest pain and normal coronary angiographic findings. *J Am Coll Cardiol.* 1995;25(5):1013-1018.

39. Proudfit WL, Bruschke VG, Sones FM Jr. Clinical course of patients with normal or slightly or moderately abnormal coronary arteriograms: 10 year follow-up of 521 patients. *Circulation.* 1980;62(4):712-717.

40. Radice M, Giudici V, Marinelli G. Long-term follow-up in patients with positive exercise test and angiographically normal coronary arteries (syndrome X). *Am J Cardiol.* 1995;75(8):620-621.

41. Celio PV. Aeromedical disposition for coronary artery disease. In: Lecture Series 189: Cardiopulmonary aspects in aerospace medicine, AGARD-LS-189 (NATO). Loughton, Essex, UK: Specialized Printing Services Limited; October 1993:3-1 to 3-6.

42. Kemp HG, Kronmal RA, Vlietstra RE, et al. Seven year survival of patients with normal or near normal coronary arteriograms: A CASS Registry Study. *J Am Coll Cardiol.* 1986;7(3):479-483.

43. Papanicolaou MN, Califf RM, Hlatky MA, et al. Prognostic implications of angiographically normal and insignificantly narrowed coronary arteries. *Am J Cardiol.* 1986;58(12):1181-1187.

44. Bruschke AVG, Van Der Wall EE, Cats VM. First European workshop in aviation cardiology. The natural history of angiographically demonstrated coronary artery disease. *Eur Heart J.* 1992;13(suppl H):70-75.

45. CASS principal investigators. Coronary Artery Surgery Study (CASS): A randomized trial of coronary artery bypass surgery. Comparability of entry characteristics and survival in randomized patients and nonrandomized patients meeting randomization criteria. *J Am Coll Cardiol.* 1984;3(1):114-128.

46. Weiner DA, Ryan TJ, McCabe CH, et al. Comparison of coronary artery bypass surgery and medical therapy in patients with exercise-induced silent myocardial ischemia: A report from the Coronary Artery Surgery Study (CASS) registry. *J Am Coll Cardiol.* 1988;12(3):595-599.

47. Chaitman BR, Ryan TJ, Kronmal RA, et al. Coronary Artery Surgery Study (CASS): Comparability of 10 year survival in randomized and randomizable patients. *J Am Coll Cardiol.* 1990;16(5):1071-1078.

48. Hueb WA, Bellotti G, de Oliveira SA, et al. The Medicine, Angioplasty or Surgery Study (MASS): A prospective, randomized trial of medical therapy, balloon angioplasty or bypass surgery for single proximal left anterior descending artery stenoses. *J Am Coll Cardiol.* 1995;26(7):1600-1605.

49. Marchandise B, Bourassa MG, Chaitman BR, Lesperance J. Angiographic evaluation of the natural history of normal coronary arteries and mild coronary atherosclerosis. *Am J Cardiol.* 1978;41(2):216-220.

50. Moise A, Theroux P, Taeymans Y, Waters DD. Factors associated with progression of coronary artery disease in patients with normal or minimally narrowed coronary arteries. *Am J Cardiol.* 1985;56(1):30-34.

51. Kereiakes DJ, Topol EJ, George BS, et al. Myocardial infarction with minimal coronary atherosclerosis in the era of thrombolytic reperfusion. *J Am Coll Cardiol.* 1991;17(2):302-312.

52. Raymond R, Lynch J, Underwood D, et al. Myocardial infarction and normal coronary arteriography: A 10 year clinical and risk analysis of 74 patients. *J Am Coll Cardiol.* 1988;11(3):471-477.

53. Hoiberg A. Longitudinal study of cardiovascular disease in U.S. Navy pilots. *Aviat Space Environ Med.* 1986;57(5):438-442.

54. Khan M, Amroliwalla F. Flying status and coronary revascularization procedures in military aviators. *Aviat Space Environ Med.* 1996;67(11):165-170.

55. Moorman DL, Kruyer WB, Jackson WG. Percutaneous transluminal coronary angioplasty (PTCA): Long-term outcome and aeromedical implications. *Aviat Space Environ Med.* 1996;67(10):990-996.

56. Webb-Peploe MM. Second European workshop in aviation cardiology. Late outcome following PTCA or coronary stenting: Implications for certification to fly. *Eur Heart J.* 1999;1(suppl D):D67-D77.

57. Pocock SJ, Henderson RA, Rickards AF, et al. Meta-analysis of major randomised trials comparing coronary angioplasty with bypass surgery. *Lancet.* 1995;346:1184-1189.

58. Cameron AA, Davis KB, Green GE, Schaff HV. Coronary bypass surgery with internal-thoracic-artery grafts—effects on survival over a 15-year period. CASS subset. *N Engl J Med.* 1996;334(4):216-219.

59. Cameron AA, Green GE, Brogno DA, Thornton J. Internal thoracic artery grafts: 20-year clinical follow-up. CASS subset. *J Am Coll Cardiol.* 1995;25(1):188-192.

60. Dargie HJ. First European workshop in aviation cardiology. Late results following coronary artery bypass grafting. *Eur Heart J.* 1992;13(suppl H):89-95.

61. Chua TP, Sigwart U. Second European workshop in aviation cardiology. What is acceptable revascularization of the myocardium in the context of certification to fly? *Eur Heart J.* 1999;1(suppl D):D78-D83.

62. Chaitman BR, Davis KB, Dodge HT, et al. Should airline pilots be eligible to resume active flight status after coronary bypass surgery?: A CASS Registry study. *J Am Coll Cardiol.* 1986;8(6):1318-1324.

63. Khan MA, Amroliwalla FK. Lipid lowering therapy and military aviators. *Aviat Space Environ Med.* 1996;67(9):867-871.

64. Knopp RH. Drug treatment of lipid disorders. *N Engl J Med.* 1999;341(7):498-511.

65. Gotto AM Jr. Lipid-lowering therapy for the primary prevention of coronary heart disease. *J Am Coll Cardiol.* 1999;33(7):2078-2082.

66. Keech A, Sleight P. First European workshop in aviation cardiology. Lipid screening in aircrew: Pros and cons. *Eur Heart J*. 1992;13(suppl H):50-53.

67. Pedersen TR. Second European workshop in aviation cardiology. Lipid abnormalities in aircrew: Definition and impact on cardiovascular event rate. *Eur Heart J*. 1999;1(suppl D):D37-D41.

68. Lavalee PJ, Fonseca VP. Survey of USAF flight surgeons regarding clinical preventive services, using CHD as an indicator. *Aviat Space Environ Med*. 1999;70(10):1029-1037.

69. Stefanick ML, Mackey S, Sheehan M, et al. Effects of diet and exercise in men and postmenopausal women with low levels of HDL cholesterol and high levels of LDL cholesterol. *N Engl J Med*. 1998;339(1):12-20.

70. Goldman L, Coxson P, Hunink MGM, et al. The relative influence of secondary versus primary prevention using the National Cholesterol Education Program Adult Treatment Panel II guidelines. *J Am Coll Cardiol*. 1999;34(3):768-776.

71. Hardy JC. Screening echocardiography in USAF pilot candidates (abstract). *Aviat Space Environ Med*. 1998;69(3):205.

72. Hardy JC. Echocardiographic screening in USAF pilot candidates (abstract). *Aviat Space Environ Med*. 1996;67(7):716.

73. AGARD Aerospace Medical Panel Working Group 18. Echocardiographic findings in NATO pilots: Do acceleration (+G_z) stresses damage the heart? *Aviat Space Environ Med*. 1997;68(7):596-600.

74. Lester SJ, Heilbron B, Gin K, et al. The natural history and rate of progression of aortic stenosis. *Chest*. 1998;113(4):1109-1114.

75. Bonow RO. ACC/AHA guidelines for the management of patients with valvular heart disease. A report of the American College of Cardiology/American Heart Association task force on practice guidelines (committee on management of patients with valvular heart disease). *J Am Coll Cardiol*. 1998;32(5):1486-1588.

76. Cheitlin MD, Douglas PS, Parmley WW. 26th Bethesda conference: Recommendations for determining eligibility for competition in athletes with cardiovascular abnormalities. Task force 2: Acquired valvular heart disease. *J Am Coll Cardiol*. 1994;24(4):874-880.

77. Horstkotte D, Loogen F. The natural history of aortic valve stenosis. *Eur Heart J*. 1988;9(suppl E):57-64.

78. Otto CM, Burwash IG, Legget ME, et al. Prospective study of asymptomatic valvular aortic stenosis. Clinical, echocardiographic and exercise predictors of outcome. *Circulation*. 1997;95(9):2262-2270.

79. Otto CM, Pearlman AS, Gardner CL. Hemodynamic progression of aortic stenosis in adults assessed by Doppler echocardiography. *J Am Coll Cardiol*. 1989;13(3):545-550.

80. Kennedy KD, Nishimura RA, Holmes DR, Bailey KR. Natural history of moderate aortic stenosis. *J Am Coll Cardiol*. 1991;17(2):313-319.

81. Turina J, Hess O, Sepulcri F, Krayenbuehl HP. Spontaneous course of aortic valve disease. *Eur Heart J*. 1987;8(5):471-483.

82. Dujardin KS, Enriquez-Sarano M, Schaff HV, et al. Mortality and morbidity of aortic regurgitation in clinical practice: A long-term follow-up study. *Circulation*. 1999;99(14):1851-1857.

83. Padial LR, Oliver A, Vivaldi M, et al. Doppler echocardiographic assessment of progression of aortic regurgitation. *Am J Cardiol*. 1997;80(3):306-314.

84. Bonow RO, Lakatos E, Maron BJ, Epstein SE. Serial long-term assessment of the natural history of asymptomatic patients with chronic aortic regurgitation and normal left ventricular function. *Circulation*. 1991;84(4):1625-1635.

85. Borer JS, Hochreiter C, Herrold EM, et al. Prediction of indications for valve replacement among asymptomatic or minimally symptomatic patients with chronic aortic regurgitation and normal left ventricular performance. *Circulation*. 1998;97(6):525-534.

86. Vivaldi MT, Giugliano RP, Sagie A. What is the prognosis of trace aortic regurgitation (abstract)? *J Am Coll Cardiol*. 1994;23(2, suppl A):192A.

87. Chung KY, Hardy JC. Aortic insufficiency and high performance flight in USAF aircrew (abstract). *Aviat Space Environ Med*. 1996;67(7):688.

88. Scognamiglio R, Rahimtoola SH, Fasoli G, et al. Nifedipine in asymptomatic patients with severe aortic regurgitation and normal left ventricular function. *N Engl J Med*. 1994;331(11):689-694.

89. Freed LA, Levy D, Levine RA, et al. Prevalence and clinical outcome of mitral valve prolapse. *N Engl J Med*. 1999;341(1):1-7.

90. Marks AR, Choong CY, Chir MBB, et al. Identification of high-risk and low-risk subgroups of patients with mitral valve prolapse. *N Engl J Med*. 1989;320(16):1031-1036.

91. Nishimura RA, McGoon MD, Shub C, et al. Echocardiographically documented mitral valve prolapse: Long-term follow-up of 237 patients. *N Engl J Med*. 1985;313(21):1305-1309.

92. Zuppiroli A, Rinaldi M, Kramer-Fox R, et al. Natural history of mitral valve prolapse. *Am J Cardiol*. 1995;75(15):1028-1032.

93. Osswald SS, Gaffney FA, Kruyer WB, et al. Analysis of aeromedical endpoints and evaluation in USAF aviators with mitral valve prolapse. *Aviat Space Environ Med*. 1998;69(3):250.

94. Osswald SS, Gaffney FA, Hardy JC, Jackson WG. Mitral valve prolapse in 404 military members: Long-term follow-up and clinical risk analysis. *Aviat Space Environ Med*. 1997;68(7):628.

95. Gilon D, Buonanno FS, Joffe MM, et al. Lack of evidence of an association between mitral-valve prolapse and stroke in young patients. *N Engl J Med*. 1999;341(1):8-13.

96. Stoddard MF, Prince CR, Dillon S, et al. Exercise-induced mitral regurgitation is a predictor of morbid events in subjects with mitral valve prolapse. *J Am Coll Cardiol*. 1995;25(3):693-699.

97. Fenster MS, Feldman MD. Mitral regurgitation: An overview. *Curr Probl Cardiol*. 1995;20(4):193-280.

98. Ling LH, Enriquez-Sarano M, Seward JB, et al. Clinical outcome of mitral regurgitation due to flail leaflet. *N Engl J Med*. 1996;335(19):1417-1423.

99. Hardy JC, Leonard F. Aortic valve replacement in a United States Air Force pilot: Case report and literature review. *Aviat Space Environ Med.* 1997;68(3):221-224.

100. Doty JR, Salazar JD, Liddicoat JR, et al. Aortic valve replacement with cryopreserved aortic allograft: Ten-year experience. *J Thorac Cardiovasc Surg.* 1998;115(2):371-380.

101. Parker DJ. Second United Kingdom workshop in aviation cardiology. Long-term morbidity and mortality after aortic and mitral valve replacement with tissue valves and certification to fly. *Eur Heart J.* 1988;9(suppl G):153-157.

102. Murday A. Second European workshop in aviation cardiology. Mitral valve repair and replacement: Requirements for certification to fly. *Eur Heart J.* 1999;1(suppl D):D129-D131.

103. Enriquez-Sarano M, Schaff HV, Orszulak TA, et al. Valve repair improves the outcome of surgery for mitral regurgitation. A multivariate analysis. *Circulation.* 1995;91(4):1022-1028.

104. Gramaglia B, Imazio M, Checco L, et al. Mitral valve prolapse. Comparison between valvular repair and replacement in severe mitral regurgitation. *J Cardiovasc Surg.* 1999;40(1): 93-99.

105. Gillinov AM, Cosgrove DM, Blackstone EH, et al. Durability of mitral valve repair for degenerative disease. *J Thorac Cardiovasc Surg.* 1998;116(5):734-743.

106. Orejarena LA, Vidaillet H, DeStefano F, et al. Paroxysmal supraventricular tachycardia in the general population. *J Am Coll Cardiol.* 1998;31(1):150-157.

107. Epstein EA, Miles WM. Personal and public safety issues related to arrhythmias that may affect consciousness: Implications for regulation and physician recommendations. A medical/scientific statement from the American Heart Association and the North American Society of Pacing and Electrophysiology. *Circulation.* 1996;94(5):1147-1166.

108. Dhala A, Bremner S, Blanck Z, et al. Impairment of driving abilities in patients with supraventricular tachycardias. *Am J Cardiol.* 1995;75(7):516-518.

109. Wood KA, Drew BJ, Scheinman MM. Frequency of disabling symptoms in supraventricular tachycardia. *Am J Cardiol.* 1997;79(2):145-149.

110. Wang Y, Scheinman MM, Chien WW, et al. Patients with supraventricular tachycardia presenting with aborted sudden death: Incidence, mechanism and long-term follow-up. *J Am Coll Cardiol.* 1991;18(7):1711-1719.

111. Zipes DP, Garson A. The 26th Bethesda conference: Recommendations for determining eligibility for competition in athletes with cardiovascular abnormalities. Task force 6: Arrhythmias. *J Am Coll Cardiol.* 1994;24(4):892-899.

112. Zipes DP. Wolff-Parkinson-White. In: Braunwald E, ed. *Heart Disease: A Textbook of Cardiovascular Medicine.* 5th ed. Philadelphia: Saunders; 1997:667-675.

113. Smith RF. The Wolff-Parkinson-White syndrome as an aviation risk. *Circulation.* 1964;29:672-679.

114. Zipes DP, Ritchie JL. Guidelines for clinical intracardiac electrophysiological and catheter ablation procedures. A report of the American College of Cardiology/American Heart Association task force on practice guidelines (committee on clinical intracardiac electrophysiologic and catheter ablation procedures) developed in collaboration with the North American Society of Pacing and Electrophysiology. *J Am Coll Cardiol.* 1995;26(2):555-573.

115. Munger TM, Packer DL, Hammill SL, et al. A population study of the natural history of Wolff-Parkinson-White syndrome in Olmsted County, Minnesota, 1953-1989. *Circulation.* 1993;87(3):866-873.

116. Berkman NL, Lamb LE. The Wolff-Parkinson-White electrocardiogram. A follow-up of five to twenty-eight years. *N Engl J Med.* 1968;278(9):492-494.

117. Kopecky SL, Gersh BJ, McGoon MD, et al. The natural history of lone atrial fibrillation. A population-based study over three decades. *N Engl J Med.* 1987;317(11):669-674.

118. Onundarson PT, Thorgeirsson G, Jonmundsson E, et al. Chronic atrial fibrillation—epidemiologic features and 14 year follow-up: A case control study. *Eur Heart J.* 1987;8(5): 521-527.

119. Neutel JM, Smith DH, Jankelow D, et al. The aeromedical implications of atrial fibrillation. *Aviat Space Environ Med.* 1990;61(11):1036-1038.

120. Brand FV, Abbot RD, Kannel WB, Wolf PA. Characteristics and prognosis of lone atrial fibrillation: 30-year follow-up in the Framingham Study. *JAMA.* 1985;254(24):3449-3453.

121. Kulbertus HE. First European workshop in aviation cardiology. Implications of lone atrial fibrillation/flutter in the context of cardiovascular fitness to fly. *Eur Heart J.* 1992;13(suppl H):136-138.

122. Benjamin EJ, Wolf PA, D'Agostino RB, et al. Impact of atrial fibrillation on the risk of death: The Framingham Heart Study. *Circulation.* 1998;98(10):946-952.

123. Scardi S, Mazzone C, Pandullo C, et al. Lone atrial fibrillation: Prognostic differences between paroxysmal and chronic forms after 10 years of follow-up. *Am Heart J.* 1999;137(4, pt 1):686-691.

124. Frustaci A, Chimenti C, Bellocci F, et al. Histologic substrate of atrial biopsies in patients with lone atrial fibrillation. *Circulation.* 1998;96(4):1180-1184.

125. Gorgels APM, Wellens HJJ, Vos AA. First European workshop in aviation cardiology. Aviation and antiarrhythmic medication. *Eur Heart J.* 1992;13(suppl H):144-148.

126. Campbell RWF. First European workshop in aviation cardiology. Ventricular rhythm disturbances in the normal heart. *Eur Heart J.* 1992;13(suppl H):139-143.

127. Kay GN, Plumb VJ. The present role of radiofrequency catheter ablation in the management of cardiac arrhythmias. *Am J Med.* 1996;100(3):344-356.

128. Calkins H, Yong P, Miller JM, et al. Catheter ablation of accessory pathways, atrioventricular nodal reentrant tachycardia, and the atrioventricular junction: Final results of a prospective, multicenter clinical trial. The Atakr Multicenter Investigators Group. *Circulation.* 1999;99(2):262-270.

129. Plumb VJ. Catheter ablation of the accessory pathways of the Wolff-Parkinson-White syndrome and its variants. *Prog Cardiovasc Dis.* 1995;37(5):295-306.

130. Kadish A, Goldberger J. Ablative therapy for atrioventricular nodal reentry arrhythmias. *Prog Cardiovasc Dis.* 1995;37(5):273-294.

131. Obel OA, Camm AJ. Second European workshop in aviation cardiology. Atrioventricular nodal reentry: Prevalence, presentation, management, and new strategies for intervention in the context of aviation. *Eur Heart J.* 1999;1(suppl D):D98-D104.

132. Feld GK. Catheter ablation for the treatment of atrial tachycardia. *Prog Cardiovasc Dis.* 1995;37(5):205-224.

133. Olgin JE, Lesh MD. The laboratory evaluation and role of catheter ablation for patients with atrial flutter. *Cardiol Clin.* 1997;15(4):677-688.

134. Miller JM, Cossu SF, Chmielewski IL, et al. Primary ablation of atrial flutter and atrial fibrillation. *Cardiol Clin.* 1996;14(4):569-584.

135. Viskin S, Barron HV, Olgin JE, et al. The treatment of atrial fibrillation: Pharmacologic and nonpharmacologic strategies. *Curr Probl Cardiol.* 1997;22(2):37-108.

136. Teo WS, Kam R, Lim YL, Koh TH. Curative therapy of cardiac arrhythmias with catheter ablation—a review of the experience with the first 1000 patients. *Singapore Med J.* 1999;40(4):284-290.

137. Klein LS, Miles WM. Ablative therapy for ventricular arrhythmias. *Prog Cardiovasc Dis.* 1995;37(5):225-242.

138. Toff WD, Edhag OK, Camm AJ. First European workshop in aviation cardiology. Cardiac pacing and aviation. *Eur Heart J.* 1992;13(suppl H):162-175.

139. Mitrani RD, Simmons JD, Interian A Jr, et al. Cardiac pacemakers: Current and future status. *Curr Prob Cardiol.* 1999;24(6):341-420.

140. Hull DH. Recurrent loss of consciousness in an aircrew member—a controllable cause. *Aviat Space Environ Med.* 1994;65(9):866-868.

141. Groh WJ, Boschee SA, Engelstein ED. Interactions between electronic article surveillance systems and implantable cardioverter-defibrillators. *Circulation.* 1999;100(4):387-392.

142. Hoit BD. Pericardial heart disease. *Curr Probl Cardiol.* 1997;22(7):353-404.

143. Lorell BH. Pericardial diseases. In: Braunwald E, ed. *Heart Disease: A Textbook of Cardiovascular Medicine.* 5th ed. Philadelphia: Saunders; 1997:1478-1534.

144. Wynne J, Braunwald E. The cardiomyopathies and myocarditides. In: Braunwald E, ed. *Heart Disease: A Textbook of Cardiovascular Medicine.* 5th ed. Philadelphia: Saunders; 1997:1404-1463.

145. Maron BJ, Isner JM, McKenna WJ. The 26th Bethesda conference: Recommendations for determining eligibility for competition in athletes with cardiovascular abnormalities. Task Force III: Hypertrophic cardiomyopathy, myocarditis and other myopericardial diseases and mitral valve prolapse. *J Am Coll Cardiol.* 1994;24(4):880-885.

146. Codd MB, Sugrue DD, Gersh BJ, Melton LJ. Epidemiology of idiopathic dilated and hypertrophic cardiomyopathy. A population-based study in Olmsted County, Minnesota. *Circulation.* 1989;80(3):564-572.

147. Kopecky SL, Gersh BJ. Dilated cardiomyopathy and myocarditis: Natural history, etiology, clinical manifestations, and management. *Curr Probl Cardiol.* 1987;12(10):571-647.

148. Dec GW, Fuster V. Idiopathic dilated cardiomyopathy. *N Engl J Med.* 1994;331(23):1564-1575.

149. Sugrue DD, Rodeheffer RJ, Codd MB, et al. The clinical course of idiopathic dilated cardiomyopathy. A population-based study. *Ann Intern Med.* 1992;117(2):117-123.

150. Follath F, Cleland JGF, Klein W, Murphy R. Etiology and response to drug treatment in heart failure. *J Am Coll Cardiol*. 1998;32(5):1167-1172.

151. Redfield MM, Gersh BJ, Bailey KR, Rodeheffer RJ. Natural history of incidentally discovered, asymptomatic idiopathic dilated cardiomyopathy. *Am J Cardiol*. 1994;74(7):737-739.

152. Schlant RC. The cardiomyopathies and myocarditis. *ACC Curr J Review*. 1998;3:36-41.

153. Maron BJ. Hypertrophic cardiomyopathy. *Curr Probl Cardiol*. 1993;18(11):637-704.

154. Stewart JT, McKenna WJ. First European workshop in aviation cardiology. Relationship of left ventricular hypertrophy to risk of cardiovascular events and its relevance to medical certification of aircrew. *Eur Heart J*. 1992;13(suppl H):96-102.

155. Grosgogeat Y, Webb-Peploe MM. First European workshop in aviation cardiology. Cardiomyopathy and aircrew fitness. *Eur Heart J*. 1992;13(suppl H):103-110.

156. Spirito P, Rapezzi C, Bellone P, et al. Infective endocarditis in hypertrophic cardiomyopathy: Prevalence, incidence, and indications for antibiotic prophylaxis. *Circulation*. 1999;99(16):2132-2137.

157. Takagi E, Yamakado T, Nakano T. Prognosis of completely asymptomatic adult patients with hypertrophic cardiomyopathy. *J Am Coll Cardiol*. 1999;33(1):206-211.

158. Cecchi F, Olivotto I, Montereggi A, et al. Hypertrophic cardiomyopathy in Tuscany: Clinical course and outcome in an unselected regional population. *J Am Coll Cardiol*. 1995;26(6):1529-1536.

159. Hecht GM, Panza JA, Maron BJ. Clinical course of middle-aged asymptomatic patients with hypertrophic cardiomyopathy. *Am J Cardiol*. 1992;69(9):35-40.

160. Brembilla-Perrot B, Jacquemin L, Houplon P, et al. Increased atrial vulnerability in arrhythmogenic right ventricular disease. *Am Heart J*. 1998;135(5, pt 1):748-754.

161. Daliento L, Turrini P, Nava A, et al. Arrhythmogenic right ventricular cardiomyopathy in young versus adult patients: Similarities and differences. *J Am Coll Cardiol*. 1995;25(3):655-664.

162. Kaplan S. The 22nd Bethesda conference. Congenital heart disease after childhood: An expanding patient population. Natural adult survival patterns. *J Am Coll Cardiol*. 1991;18(2):319-322.

163. Murphy JG, Gersh BJ, McGoon MD, et al. Long-term outcome after surgical repair of isolated atrial septal defect. Follow-up at 27 to 32 years. *N Engl J Med*. 1990;323(24):1645-1650.

164. Agny M, Cobanoglu A. Repair of partial atrioventricular septal defect in children less than five years of age: Late results. *Ann Thorac Surg*. 1999;67(5):1412-1414.

165. Bergin ML, Warnes CA, Tajik AJ, Danielson GK. Partial atrioventricular canal defect: Long-term follow-up after initial repair in patients greater than or equal to 40 years old. *J Am Coll Cardiol*. 1995;25(5):1189-1194.

166. Deanfield JE. First European workshop in aviation cardiology. Adult congenital heart disease with special reference to the data on long-term follow-up of patients surviving to adulthood with or without surgical correction. *Eur Heart J*. 1992;13(suppl H):111-116.

167. Cohen M, Fuster V, Steele PM, et al. Coarctation of the aorta. Long-term follow-up and prediction of outcome after surgical correction. *Circulation.* 1989;80(4):840-845.

168. Presbitero P, Demarie D, Villani M, et al. Long-term results (15-30 years) of surgical repair of aortic coarctation. *Br Heart J.* 1987;57(5):462-467.

169. Vetter VL. The 22nd Bethesda conference. Congenital heart disease after childhood: An expanding patient population. Electrophysiologic residua and sequelae. *J Am Coll Cardiol.* 1991;18(2):3331-3333.

170. Levy D, Merz CNB, Cody RJ, et al. Hypertension detection, treatment and control. A call to action for cardiovascular specialists. *J Am Coll Cardiol.* 1999;34(4):1360-1362.

171. The Joint National Committee on Prevention, Detection, Evaluation and Treatment of High Blood Pressure. The sixth report of the Joint National Committee on Prevention, Detection, Evaluation and Treatment of High Blood Pressure (JNC VI). *Arch Intern Med.* 1997;157(21):2413-2446.

172. Khattar RS, Senior R, Lahiri A. Cardiovascular outcome in white-coat versus sustained hypertension: A 10-year follow-up study. *Circulation.* 1998;98(18):1892-1897.

173. Verdecchia P, Porcellati C, Schillaci G, et al. Ambulatory blood pressure. An independent predictor of prognosis in essential hypertension. *Hypertension.* 1994;24(6):793-801.

174. Zakopoulos N, Papamichael C, Papaconstantinou H, et al. Isolated clinic hypertension is not an innocent phenomenon: Effect on the carotid artery structure. *Am J Hypertens.* 1999;12(3):245-250.

175. Owens PE, Lyons SP, Rodriguez SA, O'Brien ET. Is elevation of clinic blood pressure in patients with white coat hypertension who have normal ambulatory blood pressure associated with target organ changes? *J Hum Hypertens.* 1998;12(11):743-748.

176. Palatini P, Mormino P, Santonastaso M, et al. Target-organ damage in stage I hypertensive patients with white coat and sustained hypertension: Results from the HARVEST study. *Hypertension.* 1998;31(1):57-63.

177. Khattar RS, Swales JD, Banfield A, et al. Prediction of coronary and cerebrovascular morbidity and mortality by direct continuous ambulatory blood pressure monitoring in essential hypertension. *Circulation.* 1999;100(10):1071-1076.

178. Liu JE, Roman MJ, Pini R, et al. Cardiac and arterial organ damage in adults with elevated ambulatory and normal office blood pressure. *Ann Intern Med.* 1999;131(8):564-572.

179. Okhubo T, Imai Y, Tsuji I, et al. Reference values for 24-hour ambulatory blood pressure monitoring based on a prognostic criterion: The Ohasama Study. *Hypertension.* 1998;32(2):255-259.

180. Hansson L, Zanchetti A, Carruthers SG, et al. Effects of intensive blood-pressure lowering and low-dose aspirin in patients with hypertension: Principal results of the Hypertension Optimal Treatment (HOT) randomised trial. HOT Study Group. *Lancet.* 1998;351(9118):1755-1762.

181. Gottdiener JS, Reda DJ, Massie BM, et al. Effect of single-drug therapy on reduction of left ventricular mass in mild to moderate hypertension: Comparison of six antihypertensive

agents. The Department of Veterans Affairs Cooperative Study Group on Antihypertensive Agents. *Circulation.* 1997;95(8):2007-2014.

182. Schmieder RE, Martus P, Klingbeil AU. Reversal of left ventricular hypertrophy in essential hypertension: A meta-analysis of randomized double-blind studies. *JAMA.* 1996;275(19):1507-1513.

183. Schmieder RE, Schlaich MP, Klingbeil AU, Martus P. Update on reversal of left ventricular hypertrophy in essential hypertension (a meta-analysis of all randomized double-blind studies until December 1996). *Nephrol Dial Transplant.* 1998;13(3):564-569.

184. Paul MA, Gray GW. The effect of captopril on +G_z tolerance of normotensives. *Aviat Space Environ Med.* 1992;63(8):706-708.

185. Rhodes DB, Howe B. Lisinopril for the treatment of hypertension in USAF aircrew (abstract). *Aviat Space Environ Med.* 1997;68(7):628.

186. Froom P, Gross M, Barzilay J, et al. Systolic blood pressure in fighter pilots after 12-15 years service. *Aviat Space Environ Med.* 1986;57(4):367-369.

187. Kruyer WB, Hickman JR Jr. Medication-induced performance decrements: Cardiovascular medications. *J Occup Med.* 1990;32(4):342-349.

188. Glaister DH. Effects of beta-blockers on psychomotor performance—a review. *Aviat Space Environ Med.* 1981;52(11, pt 2):S23-S30.

189. Schenk GK, Lang E, Anlauf M. Beta-receptor blocking therapy in hypertensive patients—effects on vigilance and behavior. *Aviat Space Environ Med.* 1981;52(11, pt 2):S35-S39.

190. Amroliwalla FK. Angiotensin converting enzyme (ACE) inhibitors in hypertensive aircrew. *Aviat Space Environ Med.* 1994;65(11):1054-1057.

191. Bower EA, Baney RN, Holmes PM, et al. Lack of measurable effect of HMG-CoA reductase inhibitors on cognitive performance (abstract). *Aviat Space Environ Med.* 1998;69(3):250.

Chapter 8
Genitourinary

Medical waivers for genitourinary (GU) diseases probably represent a relatively small proportion of all waived conditions. This is explained in part by the large number of GU disorders (eg, UTIs or passage of a small renal or ureteral stone) that are either self-limiting or may be cured with appropriate therapy in a few days or weeks. Perhaps the growing number of women in the cockpit will create an increase in incidence of GU disease among aviators, as well as broaden the scope of these disorders challenging today's AME/flight surgeon. For now, however, the AME/FS will most frequently encounter renal-ureteral stones and prostatitis, so this section will primarily discuss these entities, followed by brief comments about some less common GU conditions seen in the aviation population.

Urinary Tract Calculi

Urinary tract calculi are of particular interest to aviation medicine for several reasons. First, their peak incidence is in individuals between 20 and 30 years of age, and thus they are seen most often in young aviators. Second, urinary tract calculi have the potential to cause excruciating pain that can be partially or completely incapacitating. And finally, at least under some flight conditions, the aviation environment may be conducive to calculi formation. Although not documented, it is the impression of some military flight surgeons that urinary tract stones occur with greater frequency in tropical areas such as Southeast Asia. This is probably true, and this higher incidence may be caused by the dehydrating effects of a tropical climate encountered by aviators not only in day-to-day life, but also while sitting for long periods in the hot cockpits of their aircraft before takeoff and after landing. In any event, a few cases of some degree of in-flight incapacitation have been reported.[1,2]

The vast majority of all upper urinary tract stones are composed of calcium or magnesium in combination with oxalate, phosphate, and carbonate, although stones made up of cystine or uric acid are sometimes seen. In spite of extensive research, the pathophysiology of stone formation is not entirely clear, but factors which appear to play a role include urinary pH, solute load, urinary stasis, and metabolic derangement. While the exact causes of stone formation have not been clearly defined, there is often an association with a variety of diseases, some of which cause hypercalcemia (eg, hyperparathyroidism, sarcoid, and malignancies), and others that are associated with hyperuricemia or cystinuria; however, in most cases stone formation is idiopathic. Renal stones can cause mild to moderate low back or flank pain with constitutional symptoms, but stones in the ureter can cause the abrupt onset of severe, incapacitating pain, usually in the lower paravertebral areas or flanks. There may also be hematuria and urinary symptoms of frequency, urgency, and dysuria. Regardless of the type of stone, the diagnosis can be made by this history along with plain film and ultrasound. A full investigation is necessary to determine if there is an underlying cause of stone formation. The great majority of aviators with stones have calcium or magnesium calculi without underlying disease, and treatment modalities for these patients are discussed in the following paragraphs.

There are several treatment options available to the AME/FS. First, the patient may be given a trial period to see if the stone will pass spontaneously (assuming there is no evidence of impending serious renal damage). Analgesics, antispasmodics, and adequate hydration are the hallmarks of this approach. The urine should be kept dilute by drinking about 4 quarts of fluids per day, in combination with oral thiazides or phosphates. In most cases, stones less than 5 mm in diameter will pass spontaneously within a few days to a few weeks.[3] On the other hand, if the stone does not pass, major complications such as obstruction, infection, and eventual destruction of the kidney may occur, and removal of the retained stone should be considered for these patients.

Due to the potential for severe incapacitating pain, an aviator who develops a renal or ureteral stone that is treated medically should be disqualified from flight duty until the stone passes spontaneously. If the stone does pass, and there is restoration of normal renal function as determined by serum creatinine, urinalysis, and IVP, with no evidence of underlying disease, the patient could be recertified for flying. But if the stone does not pass in a reasonable length of time and surgical intervention becomes necessary, a medical waiver could be requested after surgery, as long as the patient has a normal postoperative course with full restoration of normal renal function.

If the calculus must be removed surgically, there are several modalities including basket, extracorporeal shock wave lithotripsy (ESWL), percutaneous nephrolithotomy (PN), and open surgery. The choice of procedure depends on the clinical circumstances such as size and location of the stone(s). Consequently, the AME/FS must have an understanding of these procedures and be particularly mindful of their complications.

ESWL is performed by directing ultrasonic shock waves at the calculus resulting in its fragmentation. If the treatment is successful, the patient can go home the following day and return to the cockpit within a few weeks. Complications are usually minor and may include bleeding (usually self-limiting and of 24 hours' duration), perinephric hematoma, and infrequent and self-limiting gastrointestinal symptoms; another complication occasionally reported is ureteral obstruction due to the lodgment of a large fragment. There has also been recent evidence, although tenuous, that ESWL is associated with hypertension.[4] The AME/FS should be mindful that lithotripsy when used alone incompletely removes stones in 35%-54% of cases.[3]

PN is performed by introducing a percutaneous needle followed by a nephroscope into the renal calyx. The stone is removed either with forceps, a basket, or ultrasonic lithotripsy, and reported success rates range as high as 95%-99%.[5] Although complications are uncommon, some patients do develop infection and hemorrhage following the procedure. The incidence of bleeding is 1% and it may occur immediately or be delayed for as long as several weeks.[6] Although most bleeding stops spontaneously, transfusions may be required, as well as selective arterial embolization with gelfoam. PN has much lower morbidity compared to open surgery, the hospital stay is normally only a few days, and the patient can usually resume most normal activities in 1-2 weeks with return to the cockpit shortly thereafter.

With PN and ESWL, aviators with upper urinary tract stones will not only have decreased morbidity, but will also leave the hospital sooner, recover faster, and return to the cockpit much sooner than aviators who undergo open surgery. Although each case must be treated individually, in the absence of postprocedure complications, most patients should be able to return to the cockpit in 2-4 weeks. The AME/FS should ensure that no stone fragments remain in the urinary tract and that the patient is free of complications, particularly bleeding.

Patients who have had a urinary tract stone should be followed closely because there is a significant recurrence rate, therefore preventive measures are advisable. These include high fluid intake and reduction of consumption of foods rich in oxalate (rhubarb, spinach, tea, cola drinks, and citrus). In addition, thiazides reduce risk of stone formation by decreasing intestinal absorption of calcium and increasing reabsorption in the kidney.

A difficult aeromedical disposition decision arises if an aviator has a retained renal or ureteral calculus or nephrocalcinosis. In the former case disqualification would be the prudent course of action, mainly because of the risk of severe pain.

Many types of flight operations would be conducive to growth and movement of a stone because of the dehydrating effects of hot weather and low humidity cockpit environments in flight. Thus it is possible that the stone may move at any time, causing significant discomfort particularly if it is in the ureter. Besides the danger of incapacitation secondary to pain, there would be the ever-present threat of urinary tract obstruction, secondary infection, and renal damage.

Renal parenchymal calcifications or nephrocalcinosis may be due to a number of underlying diseases (hyperparathyroidism, sarcoid, malignancies, pyelonephritis, and glomerulonephritis being outstanding examples) or may be idiopathic. In the former cases, flight status must be determined primarily by the underlying condition. For idiopathic cases, the major determinant of aeromedical disposition is the position of the calcific deposit. Medical waivers may be granted without threat to flight safety if there is reasonable certainty, as demonstrated by imaging, that the calcifications are totally within the renal parenchyma or within cysts (such as in medullary sponge kidney), with no possibility of migration into the collecting system. In this situation there is little risk for the stone to move and cause incapacitating pain. Occasionally the radiologist finds it difficult to determine if a calcific density is within the parenchyma or in some part of the collecting system. Because this determination is extremely important in aeromedical disposition, the AME/FS, urologist, and radiologist in joint consultation should review all the clinical data and arrive at a decision based on their best judgment and experience.

Urinary tract stones may present yet another challenge to the AME/FS: If an aviator, with no apparent underlying disease and otherwise normal renal function, passes calcium or magnesium stones periodically despite preventive measures, at what point should he or she be removed from flight status? There are good arguments on both sides of this issue, and at present there is no single easy answer to this question. As in similar dilemmas facing the AME/FS, he or she must make such determinations on a case-by-case basis based on the circumstances of each individual patient.

Prostatitis

There are 4 types of prostatitis: acute bacterial, chronic bacterial, nonbacterial, and prostatodynia.[7] The acute form is usually caused by gram-negative organisms, with the patient complaining of dysuria, urethral discharge, backache, urgency and frequency, and often fever. The complications of acute bacterial prostatitis include abscess formation, acute urinary retention, pyelonephritis, and chronic prostatitis. Prescription of an appropriate antibiotic (usually trimethoprim-sulfamethoxazole or fluoroquinolones), sitz baths, bedrest, and fluids is the recommended treatment regimen.

Chronic prostatitis is an entity with a poorly defined pathogenesis for which effective therapy remains elusive. The disease is believed to be due to a number of organisms, particularly *E coli* and other gram-negative bacteria. It is also attributed to inadequate treatment of the acute form. Some patients may have asymptomatic bacteriuria, while others have urethral discharge and vague complaints of pain referred to the low back, suprapubic area, or genitalia. It is sometimes associated with recurring urinary tract infections. The diagnostic tests most commonly ordered are urinalysis, bacteriologic studies, and the three-glass test, although these procedures are of questionable reliability in diagnosing chronic prostatitis. Furthermore, rectal examination may reveal a nontender prostate of normal size or one that is boggy and enlarged. The treatment is particularly difficult because most antibiotics are unable to adequately penetrate the prostate gland, although fluoroquinolones and trimethoprim-sulfamethoxazole are exceptions. In any event, chronic prostatitis is difficult to eradicate and often requires long-term antibiotic therapy. Prostatic massage and sitz baths can also be helpful.

Other forms of this illness include nonbacterial prostatitis and prostatodynia. In the former the symptoms may mimic chronic prostatitis but there are no identifiable organisms. Nevertheless, antibiotics such as those used to treat acute and chronic prostatitis are often prescribed along with sitz baths and NSAIDs. Prostatodynia is even more vexing in that patients have symptoms of prostatitis, but no organisms, no history of UTI, and normal prostatic secretions. Alpha-adrenergic blockers such as terazosin are sometimes effective.

Prostatitis is of aeromedical interest for two reasons in particular. First, because trauma can aggravate the condition (or even cause it according to some), and vibration in the cockpit can traumatize the perineal area, temporary restriction from flying may have a salutary effect on therapy. Second, because many patients with prostatitis do not respond well to treatment, they may have to endure symptoms for months, until remission occurs either spontaneously or after long-term therapy. Medical waivers may be granted for aviators requiring long-term antibiotic maintenance therapy, but the AME/FS should be aware that undesirable side effects, particularly gastrointestinal and allergic reactions, are commonly reported with trimethoprim-sulfamethoxazole, and alpha-adrenergic blockers can cause postural hypotension, a concern for aviators in high-performance aircraft operations.

Varicoceles, Hydroceles, and Spermatoceles

Because examination of the testes may be part of an aviator's flight physical examination, the AME/FS will occasionally detect a varicocele, hydrocele, or spermatocele. The prevalence of varicocele among adults is 15%.[8] Varicoceles are formed from the venous pampiniform plexus of the testes and are almost always seen on the left side. This is probably due to the greater prevalence of incompetent valves on the left as well as the effects of gravity on venous drainage. The lesion is usually painless and located superior-posterior to the left testis. In most cases a left varicocele, if it is causing no pain and is not unduly large, can be considered an incidental finding requiring no treatment.

However, there are occasional patients with left varicocele who would benefit from varicocelectomy. For example, an aviator with a large painful varicocele or one who has an infertility problem may require surgical intervention. (For unknown reasons, individuals with a varicocele have low sperm counts with a high percentage of immature forms. If the *left* spermatic vein is ligated, the sperm count will improve.)

In contradistinction to left varicocele, a *right* varicocele is rare and far more ominous. In most cases, a right varicocele develops because of occlusion of the right internal spermatic vein by a tumor or some other retroperitoneal process; metastatic cells from a renal tumor must be highly suspect in the differential diagnosis. For this reason, patients with a right varicocele must be thoroughly investigated.

Hydroceles are cystic lesions usually lying anterior to the testes. They are of unknown etiology but occasionally develop secondary to trauma or infection. Because they are benign and rarely cause symptoms, treatment is not necessary in most cases. Indications for hydrocelectomy are discomfort and hernia.

The spermatocele is also a cystic lesion, usually quite small, located superior to the testis. Like the hydrocele, it is benign and requires no surgical treatment unless the patient is experiencing severe discomfort.

Aviators with a spermatocele, hydrocele, or left varicocele can safely continue with flying without treatment or after recovery if surgical correction becomes necessary. Those with a *right* varicocele may require temporary restriction from flying while the underlying cause is investigated. Any underlying disease should be identified and its seriousness ascertained before determination of aeromedical disposition.

Horseshoe Kidney

The anomalous development of the kidneys in utero may result in their fusion, usually at the lower poles, giving them a horseshoe-like appearance. Although many patients remain asymptomatic throughout life, a significant number will eventually complain of abdominal pain and urinary tract symptoms. One reason is the well known association of horseshoe kidney with other developmental anomalies of the genitourinary system such as polycystic kidney, ectopic kidney, reduplication and stricture of the ureter, and absence of the adrenal gland. Due to the frequent presence of these associated anomalies and because of the peculiarities of the horseshoe kidney anatomy, such individuals have a propensity for ureteral obstruction, hydronephrosis, urinary tract infection, and stone formation, with their attendant symptoms and morbidity. Treatment of horseshoe kidney may be deferred if the patient has no symptoms; otherwise, surgical correction may be indicated.

Aviators with asymptomatic horseshoe kidney pose no threat to flight safety. However, if there is recurrent stone formation, infection, or discomfort, the risk of severe pain in flight due to a stone and the need for frequent treatment of these complications would compel the AME/FS to consider surgery. Too much missed flight duty due to treatment of such complications would be unacceptable in many military and commercial operations. If normal urologic function were restored via surgical correction and the aviator remained free of stones and infection, a medical waiver could be granted with the understanding that close patient follow-up is required.

Determination of aeromedical disposition is most difficult in aviators with horseshoe kidney who develop frequently recurring complications. Because surgical correction may not be indicated, the AME/FS can only weigh the merits of each case when deciding whether or not a waiver should be granted.

Polycystic Kidney Disease

Polycystic kidney is a congenital disease with a high familial incidence. The diseased kidneys tend to be enlarged, with many cysts of varying sizes found throughout the renal parenchyma. Because the cysts are ubiquitous and have a tendency to enlarge, pressure is exerted on the various structures of the kidney causing progressive renal impairment, uremia, and death. Polycystic kidney manifests itself either in early infancy (in which case survival is rare) or after age 40. For unknown reasons, if individuals with polycystic kidney disease survive infancy without urologic problems, they usually remain symptom free until middle adulthood. But once symptoms appear, the patient will have intermittent flank pain, pyuria, hematuria, and proteinuria. Furthermore, complications such as pyelonephritis, infection of the cysts, calculus formation, and anemia can occur as the disease progresses. End-stage renal disease occurs in 45% of patients by age 60.[9]

The disease process can affect other organs including the liver (34%-78% have cysts), heart (26% have mitral valve prolapse with chest pain and palpitations), colon (diverticuli and perforation), and pancreas and spleen (cysts).[9] In addition, about 60% will develop hypertension and 5%-10% will have cerebral aneurysms. Treatment includes dialysis and renal transplant, the latter offering normal function for as long as 10 years.[9]

Because so many patients with polycystic kidney disease will develop hypertension, the diagnosis should be considered, especially in younger aviators who are hypertensive but are otherwise healthy. Unfortunately, blood pressure control in these patients is often difficult, placing them at higher risk for myocardial infarction, congestive heart failure, and stroke. Another disturbing factor is the high prevalence of cerebral aneurysms. Because this could be the harbinger of a cerebral hemorrhage, allowing these individuals to fly single seat or high-performance aircraft becomes questionable. The AME/FS must exercise extreme caution when determining the aeromedical disposition of aviators with polycystic kidney disease. If the disease was found by chance, for example by IVP in the course of a hypertension evaluation, and the patient has been asymptomatic with a normal urinalysis, a medical waiver may be appropriate. Even though polycystic disease exists, the patient may remain asymptomatic without renal impairment for years to come. However, when symptoms occur or when renal impairment is signaled by pyuria, hematuria, or proteinuria, continued flight certification must be questioned. At what point in the course of the disease (the period from the onset of signs and symptoms to the occurrence of severe uremia) an aviator should be permanently disqualified from flying must be judged on an individual basis. The early presence of mild anemia or proteinuria should not pose a threat to flight safety, but when renal impairment increases or the patient has frequent discomfort or urinary tract infections requiring treatment, continued flight certification becomes problematic. Blood pressure must be carefully monitored and controlled.

A case in point is that of a military aviator who developed hypertension at age 22.[10] He was eventually diagnosed with polycystic kidney disease and prescribed lisinopril which controlled his hypertension. Because his blood pressure was normal and no other evidence of disease was found (valvular abnormalities, berry aneurysm, cysts in other organs), he was granted a waiver. However, because of the risk of progression of the disease, this pilot requires very close following.

Medullary Sponge Kidney

Medullary sponge kidney is a relatively common congenital defect believed by some investigators to be a form of polycystic kidney disease in which there is dilatation of the tubules with cyst formation. This results in urinary stasis which creates a predisposition to calculus formation and infection. Although most patients with medullary sponge kidney remain asymptomatic without impairment of renal function, some will be afflicted with occasional infections or will pass small stones. Approximately 10% of patients have a poor prognosis and will develop ureterolithiasis, infection, and renal failure.[11] For patients with disease of one kidney who develop complications, a nephrectomy or partial nephrectomy is sometimes recommended. A medical waiver could be requested for an aviator with medullary sponge kidney if he or she is asymptomatic or only infrequently indisposed by its attendant complications. The aeromedical disposition for renal calculi is discussed elsewhere in this chapter.

Absent Kidney

In general, the absence of a kidney is not a contraindication to flight certification as long as the remaining kidney is functioning normally and there is no evidence that its continued normal function is being threatened by underlying disease. Occasionally, renal agenesis or hypoplasia is discovered incidentally when a KUB, retrograde urogram, or IVP is ordered during an evaluation for some unrelated medical problem. Furthermore, there are some cases in which a pilot has donated one of his or her kidneys to a recipient (usually a relative) in urgent need of a kidney transplant. Once the donor has fully recovered from surgery, a request for medical waiver would be appropriate. Individuals with one kidney can have normal lives and longevity and should be at no greater risk of incapacitation than individuals with two kidneys.[12]

Gynecological Issues

Pregnancy

With the increasing number of women in aviation, the aeromedical disposition of pregnant aviators must be determined by the AME/FS. The questions in disposition of the pregnant aviator are: Is it safe for a pregnant aviator to fly and if so, at what point in the pregnancy should she be temporarily disqualified?

Addressing the first question requires a review of the major stresses of flight: hypoxia, decompression, and acceleration. Because most commercial aircraft maintain a cabin altitude up to 8000 ft (2400 m), every passenger is mildly hypoxic although certainly not symptomatic. Even with an alveolar pO_2 of 64 mm Hg at 8000 ft cabin altitude, most passengers feel no effects whatsoever. Furthermore, even at that cabin altitude there is no serious effect on fetal oxygenation due to the fetal hemoglobin dissociation curve. In one study of over 500 flight attendants there was no evidence that they were at an increased risk for adverse outcomes of pregnancy,[13] and other studies reached similar conclusions.[14]

Today's aircraft commonly fly at altitudes of 30,000-40,000 ft (9100-14,000 m), and there is always the possibility of cabin decompression, therefore a primary concern would be formation of nitrogen bubbles and their possible effects on the fetus. Although there have been animal experiments indicating that decompression causes a higher rate of fetal (hamster) abnormalities, there are almost no data on human fetuses.[15,16] Of course cabin decompression is an inherent risk of flight, not only for a fetus but for passengers and crew alike. Although rapid decompression does occasionally occur in commercial and military aircraft, it is a relatively uncommon event, and the risk to the mother and fetus is probably extremely small. In most cases, the potential danger from rapid decompression can be discounted as a reason to disqualify a pregnant crew member.

High-performance aircraft, mainly military, routinely impose accelerative forces on the aircrew. Although the physiology of acceleration and its effects on pilots is well understood, we know practically nothing about the possible effects on a fetus. Military flight surgeons would agree that such forces are often sudden, violent, and frequent enough in military operations to pose an unacceptable risk to a fetus. Even though we have no empirical data to support this, and we may never have such data, such violent accelerative forces should never intentionally be imposed on a pregnant woman.

Hypoxia, decompression, and acceleration are only some of the stresses of flight. One should also consider temperature and humidity, vibration, fatigue, and circadian rhythm, among others. Certainly the physical demands placed on crew members is also an important factor. For instance, a flight attendant's or load master's tasks would be far more physically demanding than those of a pilot. In any event, for conventional flying it would seem that a pregnant crew member can continue flying with minimal risk at least early in the pregnancy. The responsible AME/FS must take into account all aspects of the type of flight duty in question (ie, aircraft type and mission) when determining aeromedical disposition of the pregnant aviator. The one case where temporary disqualification is always advisable is the pregnant crew member who is assigned to high-performance aircraft.

As for exactly when pregnant aviators should be temporarily removed from duty, different flight organizations have differing policies based on their respective operations. In some cases aviators are removed upon confirmation of pregnancy, while others allow continued flying well into the pregnancy. There is certainly no hard and fast rule as to when disqualification becomes mandatory. It can only be said that pregnant crew members with duties on conventional aircraft can safely continue flying for at least a portion of the pregnancy. Exactly when in the pregnancy the AME/FS should temporarily disqualify the individual depends on the aircraft type, the type of the operation, and the nature of the cockpit duties.

Dysmenorrhea

Dysmenorrhea is the most common problem of menstruating women, with a prevalence rate as high as 90% and absenteeism ranging from 34%-50%.[17] Dysmenorrhea can cause a host of symptoms including lower abdominal pain, nausea and vomiting, diarrhea, backache, headache, and fatigue. In its more severe form, patients might also have nervousness, dizziness, and even syncope. The most common symptom, lower abdominal pain, usually begins just before or after the menstrual flow begins and lasts 24-48 hours, with the degree of discomfort ranging from very mild to quite severe. There are primary and secondary types of dysmenorrhea. Primary dysmenorrhea occurs in the absence of any identifiable pelvic disorders, while the secondary type is associated with underlying disease such as endometriosis, ovarian cysts, congenital malformations, and pelvic inflammatory disease. Hence, these disorders must be sought by an appropriate diagnostic evaluation and treated accordingly.

The most commonly prescribed treatment regimens, oral contraceptives and NSAIDs, are extremely effective, affording patients 90% and 64%-100% relief from symptoms respectively.[17] Although NSAIDs can cause side effects such as gastrointestinal ulcers, headache, visual disturbances, and drowsiness among others, their advantage is that they need only be taken for a few days during the menstrual cycle when symptoms are present. Thus in the vast majority of cases the medication should be well tolerated.

Primary dysmenorrhea can be of consequence in aviation if symptoms are severe and an unacceptable number of work days are lost, however this should be obviated because of the availability of effective medications. Whatever medication is prescribed, the AME/FS should ensure not only its effectiveness, but also the absence of significant side effects. Although the aeromedical disposition of women with dysmenorrhea must be determined on an individual basis, one would expect that the great majority could fly safely.

Endometriosis

Endometriosis is a disease in which there is functioning endometrial tissue somewhere in the pelvic region or in distant organs such as the colon, lungs, and kidney. Sites in the pelvis may include the region of the ovaries, the uterosacral ligaments, and the rectovaginal septum. The disease is fairly prevalent as evidenced by the finding of endometrial implants in about 10% of women undergoing laparotomy.[18] Although endometriosis is a benign disease it can cause mild to severe discomfort, depending on which organs are involved. A common complaint is lower abdominal or suprapubic pain due to bleeding, irritation, and distention at the site of the implant, usually just before or during the early phase of menstruation. In more serious cases in which implants are found at distant sites, fibrosis can develop, eventually resulting in obstruction and organ dysfunction. The diagnosis of endometriosis can be confirmed by ultrasonography, MRI, and laparoscopy.

Depending on the severity of the disease and the patient's desire to have children, there are several medical and surgical treatment options.[18,19] In some cases relief can be had with mild analgesics or NSAIDs taken as needed at the time of menses. Birth control pills and progestational drugs such as medroxyprogesterone can also be effective in relieving pain and discomfort, as can gonadotropin-releasing hormone (GnRH). Danazol, a synthetic steroid that inhibits endometrial growth, is another medication sometimes prescribed. Although it may be effective, it does cause side effects such as headaches, hot flashes, edema, weight gain, and virilization. If surgery becomes necessary, options range from excision of the lesion to hysterectomy with bilateral salpingo-oophorectomy.

The prognosis of patients with endometriosis varies considerably with some women having spontaneous remission. Many others obtain relief with analgesics or hormonal therapy, although relief may be only partial and temporary. Patients undergoing conservative surgery will enjoy relief in 66% of cases over 5 years.[18] Continued flying should not be problematic for patients with symptoms well controlled by mild analgesic or birth control pills. Likewise, those who have undergone conservative or radical surgery and have had a successful outcome could safely continue flight duties. The difficult cases will be those patients with moderate to severe pain who may be somewhat incapacitated for several days per month. In addition, if danazol is prescribed, its side effects and their impact on the patient must be taken into account. Thus in many cases the AME/FS in consultation with the gynecologist will have to weigh a number of factors in determining aeromedical disposition for aviators with endometriosis.

Premenstrual Syndrome

Premenstrual syndrome (PMS) occurs during the several days to a week prior to the onset of menses, after which the symptoms remit. Patient complaints are nonspecific, may be physical and/or emotional, and are experienced by up to 8% of women in their reproductive years.[20] The emotional component includes depression, irritability, anxiety, and mood swings; bloating, headache, poor coordination, and general body aches comprise the physical component. The etiology of this illness, although investigated for years, remains elusive. Because there are no definitive diagnostic tests available, the diagnosis must be made by history. Other illness must be ruled out, and the differential diagnosis of PMS includes many other illnesses with overlapping symptoms. There are many treatment modalities for PMS, none of proven efficacy. Among them are birth control pills, progesterones, tricyclics, anxiolytics, SSRIs, diuretics, and NSAIDs. This wide array of pharmaceutical options speaks to the ineffectiveness of therapy for PMS. Because of the broad spectrum of possible symptoms, the variability of their severity, the many medications prescribed for PMS, and their uncertain effectiveness, aeromedical disposition must be individualized according to these variables and the type of flight duty in question.

References

1. Keefer KM, Johnson R. Spontaneous resolution of retained renal calculi in USAF aviators. *Aviat Space Environ Med*. 1995;66:1001-1004.

2. McCormick TJ, Lyons TJ. Medical causes of inflight incapacitation: USAF experience 1978–1987. *Aviat Space Environ Med*. 1991;62:882-887.

3. Coe FI, Packs JH, Asplin JR. The pathogenesis and treatment of kidney stones. *N Engl J Med*. 1992;327(16):1141-1152.

4. Martin TV, Sosa RE. Shock wave lithotripsy. In: Walsh PC, Retik AB, Vaughan ED, Wein AJ, eds. *Campbell's Urology*. 7th ed. Philadelphia: Saunders; 1998:2743.

5. Segura JW. Role of percutaneous procedures in management of renal calculi. *Urol Clin North Am*. 1990;17(1):207-216.

6. Crowley AR, Smith AD. Percutaneous ultrasound lithotripsy. *Postgrad Med*. 1986;79(8):57-64.

7. Prostate Disease. American Family Physician Monograph. American Academy of Family Physicians. Kansas City, Mo: 1994.

8. Rozanski T, Bloom DA, Colodny A. Surgery of the scrotum and testis in children. In: Walsh PC, Retik AB, Vaughan ED, Wein AJ, eds. *Campbell's Urology*. 7th ed. Philadelphia: Saunders; 1998:2204.

9. Beebe DK. Autosomal dominant polycystic kidney disease. *AFP*. 1996;53(3):925-931.

10. Fox KA, Rudge FW. Autosomal dominant polycystic kidney disease and hypertension in the aviator. *Aviat Space Environ Med*. 1996;67:376-378.

11. Glassberg KI. Renal dysplasia and cystic disease of the kidney. In: Walsh PC, Retik AB, Vaughan ED, Wein AJ, eds. *Campbell's Urology*. 7th ed. Philadelphia: Saunders; 1998:1796.

12. Bauer SB. Anomalies of the kidney and ureteropelvic junction. In: Walsh PC, Retik AB, Vaughan ED, Wein AJ, eds. *Campbell's Urology*. 7th ed. Philadelphia: Saunders; 1998:1714-1715.

13. Daniell WE, Vaughan TL, Millies BA. Pregnancy outcomes among female flight attendants. *Aviat Space Environ Med*. 1990;61:840-844.

14. Scholten P. Pregnant stewardess—should she fly? *Aviat Space Environ Med*. 1976;47(1): 77-81.

15. Jennings RT. Women and the hazardous environment: When the pregnant patient requires hyperbaric oxygen therapy. *Aviat Space Environ Med*. 1987;58:370-374.

16. Gilman SC, Bradley ME, Greene KM, et al. Fetal development: Effects of decompression sickness and treatment. *Aviat Space Environ Med*. 1983;54(11):1040-1042.

17. Coco AS. Primary dysmenorrhea. *AFP*. 1999;60(2):489-496.

18. Olive DL, Schwartz LB. Medical progress: Endometriosis. *N Engl J Med*. 1993;328(24):1759-1769.

19. Witt BR, Barad DH. Management of endometriosis in women older than 40 years of age. *Obstet Gynecol Clin North Am*. 1993;20(2):349-360.

20. Barnhart KT, Freeman EW, Sondheimer SJ. A clinician's guide to the premenstrual syndrome. *Med Clin North Am*. 1995;79(6):1457-1469.

Chapter 9
Dermatology

I n general, diseases of the skin are not particularly significant aeromedically because most dermatologic conditions encountered by the AME/flight surgeon are transient, cause no incapacitation whatsoever, and can usually be managed with a short course of topical medication. Thus even brief removal from flight duty is not necessary in most cases.

But not all dermatologic conditions are entirely benign. In some cases, flight safety is threatened and the AME/FS must recommend that the aviator be restricted from flying. Examples include conditions which tend to recur frequently and require periodic courses of systemic medications such as steroids. Also, skin lesions severe enough to interfere with the wearing of cockpit equipment would be disqualifying in some military operations. For instance, cystic acne might prevent complete sealing of an oxygen mask against a pilot's face, which could result in hypoxia. Following is a discussion of dermatologic diseases frequently encountered in office practice for which aeromedical disposition can be problematic.

Psoriasis

Psoriasis is a recurrent dermatosis of unknown etiology, usually involving the elbows, knees, scalp, and lumbosacral area. The lesions have been described as silvery-gray scaling papules or plaques which are usually not pruritic. They occur singly or may number as many as 100, involving extensive areas of the skin. Besides involving the skin, psoriasis can affect the nails as well as the joints of the hands or feet, simulating rheumatoid arthritis. Medications most commonly prescribed are not curative, providing at best partial and temporary relief. These include various topicals containing corticosteroids and calcipotriene (a vitamin D analog) and systemic medications including methotrexate, retinoids, and cyclosporine.[1] In addition, some patients respond to PUVA (oral psoralen, a photosensitizing agent, and ultraviolet light exposure). The course of psoriasis is extremely variable in that remissions and exacerbations are unpredictable as is the extent of the skin lesions.

The aeromedical disposition of aviators with psoriasis must be determined on an individual basis. Because of the wide range of its clinical manifestations and severity, there can be no universally applicable policy. For aviators with mild symptoms requiring topicals, flight certification is in order. However, patients being treated with other therapeutic modalities must be given special consideration. For example, patients on a PUVA regimen may require 20-30 treatments, with some complaining of pruritus, nausea, headaches, and dizziness. Methotrexate, a folic acid antagonist, can cause gastrointestinal symptoms, headaches, and malaise; it is also myelotoxic and hepatotoxic. Other strong medications prescribed for difficult cases of psoriasis and their side effects include retinoids (myalgias, corneal opacities, and abnormal liver function) and cyclosporine (gastrointestinal symptoms, headaches, paresthesias, and tremors).

Acne

Although acne is primarily a skin disease of adolescence, it is sometimes seen in younger aviators. For a full description of acne and its effects the reader is referred to any standard textbook of dermatology. Here let it suffice to say that in the vast majority of cases the disease itself as well as the various treatments used present no contraindications to flying. Frequently prescribed treatments include long-term, low-dosage tetracycline or erythromycin, topical antibiotics (clindamycin, erythromycin), and comedolytic agents such as benzoyl peroxide and tretinoin. Overall these medications do not cause significant side effects that would preclude flight certification. Isotretinoin, used to treat severe acne, may be an exception because it can cause epistaxis, photosensitivity, and impaired night vision.[2] Severe cystic acne that interferes with proper fit of cockpit equipment would be another consideration for military operations.

Lichen Planus

Lichen planus is a skin disease of unknown etiology which causes characteristic lesions—scaly, violaceous, polygonal, umbilicated papules—on the flexor surfaces of the forearms and wrists, shins, thighs, and lower back, as well as the mucous membranes of the oral cavity. The lesions are extremely pruritic and the disease runs a course of remissions and exacerbations. The course is unpredictable with some episodes lasting 1-2 years, and relapses occur in 15%-20% of cases.[3] There is no specific treatment available; transient relief can be obtained with local and systemic corticosteroids, tretinoin, PUVA, and cyclosporine.

Because of the severe pruritus seen with lichen planus, its course of remissions and exacerbations, the lack of specific therapy, and significant side effects of some medications, disqualification of some aviators may be necessary. In selected cases a medical waiver can be considered if the lesions cause only mild symptoms, exacerbations are infrequent and mild, and therapy is well tolerated.

Urticaria

Acute urticaria may be caused by foods, medication, infection, insects, heat, and cold, among other factors. The rash can be very pruritic but usually subsides within a few days if treated with antihistamines and topicals. Occasionally, systemic steroids must be prescribed. Because it is self-limiting, of short duration, and requires only a short course of treatment, restriction from flight duty may only be necessary for a few days if at all. Longer restriction would be advisable if the skin lesions were extensive, extremely pruritic, and drowsiness-inducing antihistamines were necessary for control.

There is an occasional patient who has recurring or chronic urticaria that can last for months at a time. Like the acute form, foodstuffs, medications, infection, and inhalants might trigger the illness, but the vast majority of cases are idiopathic.[4,5] If the cause can be found, its removal is curative. Treatment of the chronic form is similar to that for acute urticaria but for a longer course. Antidepressants such as tricyclics may also be necessary for long-term treatment.

The aeromedical disposition of aviators with the recurring or chronic form can be difficult. Factors to consider include the frequency of the episodes, the extent and severity of the lesions, and the type and amount of medication necessary to control the illness.

Atopic Dermatitis

Atopic dermatitis is a chronic, recurrent eczema of unknown etiology usually found in families with a strong history of allergy such as asthma, hay fever, or urticaria. It can also be triggered by irritants, allergens, foods, infection, climate, and stress. The skin lesions are pruritic and most often involve the face, neck, and antecubital and popliteal fossae. The disease occurs in early infancy with remission until adolescence or early adulthood, at which time it may recur. Studies indicate that over half of children with this disease will have a recurrence in adulthood.[6] The course thereafter tends to be one of remissions and exacerbations until about 30 years of age when the disease apparently disappears. Few individuals have outbreaks after age

30, although the atopy recurs in some patients. There is no known cure for atopic dermatitis. Relief is only partial and temporary with the use of topical steroids, antihistamines, cyclosporine, interferon, and ultraviolet light.[7]

Complications of atopic dermatitis include eczema vaccinatum, lichenification, disseminated herpes, and secondary bacterial infection. The severity of the disease will dictate the aeromedical disposition. If the lesions are widespread, severe, and frequent, temporary disqualification from flight duty may be necessary. On the other hand, if the illness is mild and requires only topicals, qualification would be in order.

References

1. Phillips TJ. Current treatment options in psoriasis. *Hosp Prac.* 1996;31(4):155-166.

2. Nguyen QH, Kim YA, Schwartz RA. Management of acne vulgaris. *AFP.* 1994;50(1):89-96.

3. Daoud MS, Pittelkow MR. Lichen planus. In: Freidberg IM, Eisen AZ, Wolff K, et al, eds. *Fitzpatrick's Dermatology in General Medicine.* New York: McGraw-Hill; 1999:575.

4. Sveum RJ. Urticaria. *Postgrad Med.* 1996;100(2):77-84.

5. Greaves MW. Chronic urticaria. *N Engl J Med.* 1995;332(26):1767-1772.

6. Rothe MJ, Grant-Kels JM. Atopic dermatitis: An update. *J Am Acad Derm.* 1996;35(1):1-3.

7. Correale CE, Walker C, Murphy L, Craig TI. Atopic dermatitis: A review of diagnosis and treatment. *AFP.* 1999;60(4):1191-1198.

Chapter 10
Psychiatry

A viators' peers, supervisors, spouses, and family physicians underestimate the impact of psychiatric illness on flying performance. Flyers do not leave their problems on the ground as will be illustrated by the tragic cases described below. Flyers with an identified psychiatric disorder present the aeromedical physician with a simple disposition decision—the patient must be grounded until fully recovered. Psychiatric drugs (including anxiolytics, antipsychotics, antidepressants, mood stabilizers, and hypnotics) all impact the central nervous system with both potent therapeutic and potentially dangerous side effects. A patient not sufficiently healthy to function without psychiatric medication cannot be considered without risk and should not be returned to flying. Future susceptibility to stress and breakdown must be considered. The major aeromedical goal is the safe and effective performance of the aviator. Diagnosis and disposition become difficult when the problem cannot be quickly and clearly identified as psychiatric or when there is no prescribed psychotropic medication indicating an underlying problem. Blatant delusional psychoses and suicidal depressions are not a diagnostic and aeromedical disposition problem. However, the broad gray areas of emotional conflict, psychological upset, marital discord, and adjustment and personality disorders create a disposition problem and consequently will be discussed.

Aviators as a group are not eager to reveal mental, emotional, or personal problems to others, especially medical authorities with the power to ground them. It would not be unusual for a pilot to conceal such information during a routine visit and to overlook or underreport current medication history. Ancillary support personnel, eg, air traffic controllers, are also reluctant to have their job security threatened by admission of a psychological problem or illness.

A major recent revision of the *Diagnostic and Statistical Manual of Mental Disorders* of the American Psychiatric Association (DSM-IV)[1] provides a nomenclature unfamiliar to many physicians. DSM-IV diagnostic categories are based on descriptive (ie, symptomatic) and historical criteria. Psychodynamic structure is not considered, and the category of psychoneuroses has been eliminated. Various types of depression are found under the heading of mood disorders. Phobias, posttraumatic stress disorder, and generalized anxiety disorder are found under the heading of anxiety disorders. The advantages of this new schema are DSM-IV's compatibility with the current International Classification of Disease (ICD-10) and a straightforward cookbook approach. The AME/FS should provide a consultant with a presumptive diagnosis (ie, depression, anxiety, adjustment reaction, substance abuse) along with known history and medication use. The final formal diagnosis and prescription of psychoactive medication should usually be left to the psychiatrist consultant, preferably one with experience working with aviators and ancillary flight personnel. When an aviator refuses psychiatric consultation, it may be necessary for the AME/FS to initiate the required medication and immediately disqualify the patient from flight duty.

In the following section, discussion will focus on the strategic approach to psychiatric disorders in various aeromedical environments, case examples, special circumstances, and mental status review.

Strategy

The Military Flight Surgeon

The active duty military flight surgeon has the best opportunity to gain an accurate and complete assessment of the psychiatric status of his or her flyers. When the FS flies, deploys, and socializes with the unit, there will be opportunities to gain insights not usually available from office visits, and this may facilitate early diagnosis and prevention. However, once again, it is not usually the flyer who reports problems to the flight surgeon; fellow pilots, spouses, and supervisors are more common sources of information about an aviator's psychiatric problems. Once privy to this information, most flight surgeons will be faced with issues of confidentiality, unit morale, mission safety, and professional and personal reputation. The military flight surgeon has the authority to call the aviator into the office for an interview, further history, mental status assessment, and referral for psychiatric consultation. The standard operating procedures for this scenario should be preestablished with the unit commander and well understood by supervisory personnel. If there is any doubt about the emotional integrity of an aviator, disqualification is indicated until a final disposition is made.

When a flyer has been referred to a mental health professional for diagnosis and treatment, it should be clearly understood that the operational and safety requirements of the organization supercede the privacy of the patient. Military flyers know that their medical records are open to their unit flight surgeons and commanders. Not all mental health professionals in the military understand the psychological and physiological requirements for safe and effective flying performance, and many do not realize the potentially negative effect of psychotropic medications on flight operations. Many have been trained in civilian institutions where confidentiality of a patient's medical record is absolute. The mental health consultant (psychiatrist, psychologist, or social worker) needs to understand from the beginning the impact of psychiatric disability on an aviator's flight duties, as well as its effect on support personnel (eg, air traffic controllers, flight attendants, maintenance technicians). In our experience, mental health personnel used to dealing with very disturbed or flagrantly ill patients do not understand the impact of relatively minor (from their perspective) psychological problems on performance of flight duties.

Early recognition of psychiatric problems in flyers is facilitated by peer training. Although not characteristically oriented to or comfortable dealing with personal or psychological problems, all pilots are safety oriented. The model for this approach to peer training, the USAF Flight Commanders Program, was developed in 1983 at Bitburg Air Force Base, Germany, and was subsequently disseminated throughout the U.S. Department of Defense. Flight leaders, squadron commanders, and operations officers are mature and responsible individuals who will accept training from a mental health professional familiar with the flying environment. This program assumes that the lowest-level supervisory personnel in an organization have the best opportunity to recognize and deal with a psychiatric problem. Special training is provided to flight commanders by an aviation psychologist in a series of training seminars designed to enable these supervisors to recognize the earliest signs of psychological difficulty, discuss such problems directly with the affected aviators, and make the appropriate referral. It is extremely important that a seamless program be established, from diagnosis to grounding to treatment to reinstatement, and that it have the full support of commanders and senior officers. These programs have proven so helpful and cost effective that there is frequently a waiting list for unit training by a qualified aviation psychologist.

The Aviation Medical Examiner

The aviation medical examiner (AME) has much less opportunity than the military flight surgeon to get to know patients well. Typically, the AME sees the patient every 6 months, 1 year, or even 2 years, with little contact between certifications. If the aviator is a patient in the AME's private practice or a friend in the community, this might provide an opportunity for additional contact and insight. The AME should consider use of a mental status examination (described below) when clearing the applicant for flight certification. Personality and adjustment disorders are difficult to diagnose, and any suggestion of such problems should be referred for consultation.

The Airline Medical Director

An airline medical director is usually first informed of a flyer with a psychiatric problem by a phone call from a staff physician or personnel officer. It is unusual for the medical director to know the patient personally. Psychiatric consultation should be arranged as soon as possible and a second psychiatric opinion sought if requested. The patient's records should be complete and legible from the outset, otherwise there will be confusion and delay. When a union becomes involved in a decision regarding an aviator's return to flight status, the diagnosis and treatment process can be facilitated by a second opinion from a board certified psychiatrist familiar with the demands of flight, controller, or other aviation-related duties.

There is an opportunity for early diagnosis and prevention in the civilian arena as described above for military aviation. Principles of early recognition of psychiatric disorders can be taught in initial and recurrent training programs for airline personnel. Clear criteria for referral to a psychologist or psychiatrist familiar with the aviator's duties should be established.

Case Examples

Adjustment Reaction

Of all psychiatric problems, these are probably the disorders most commonly seen by aeromedical physicians. DSM-IV requires fulfillment of the following criteria to make the diagnosis:

- the development of emotional or behavioral symptoms in response to an identifiable stressor occurring within 3 months of the onset of the stressor(s);
- the symptoms or behaviors are clinically significant as manifested by marked distress and impaired function;
- the stress-related disturbance does not meet the criteria for another diagnosis;
- the symptoms do not represent bereavement; and
- once the stressor has terminated, the symptoms do not recur for another 6 months.

The following case is illustrative: It was accidentally discovered that a married military student pilot was undergoing marital counseling by a psychiatric social worker (PSW). The student pilot, an experienced weapons systems officer (WSO) in a dual seat fighter aircraft, was class leader and senior ranking officer (SRO) who served as the liaison between the training wing administrative staff and his student class. This additional duty was very demanding and left little spare time for his personal needs. He was also at a critical phase of advanced jet training. His wife, a very vivacious and attractive woman, was unhappy with the necessary loss of attention and time previously devoted to her. Her complaints and eventual flirtation with another pilot led to marital counseling.

Discussion with the student's instructor pilot revealed a recent decline in performance, as well as a change in the pilot's usually cheerful and positive attitude. The student pilot was called in to the flight medicine office and interviewed regarding his failure to report his consultation with the mental health care provider, the nature of the problem leading to that consultation, and the impact on his flying performance. With great relief he discussed his frustration at not being able to "keep all the balls in the air at the same time" and his personal sadness at the infidelity of his wife. He described his preoccupation with his personal problems and considerable difficulty in concentrating on both academic studies and flying.

The PSW providing marital counseling had received her training outside of the military, believed in total confidentiality regardless of the organizational setting, and knew little of the flight training program or its high pressure environment. The training program had little margin for time-outs or delays during its most critical phases. Following his interview with the wing FS and subsequent discussion of the case with the director of flight training, the patient transferred his responsibilities as class leader to another individual, dropped back one class and began a brief program of psychotherapy directed at helping him deal with his failed marriage, the first failure of his previously highly successful life. Eight weeks later, following a period of intense psychotherapy and the initiation of divorce proceedings, he resumed flight training and graduated with his new class.

The diagnosis of this case is Adjustment Reaction of Adult Life. A review of the patient's history revealed no significant past episodes of depression and his current mental status review indicated no significant vegetative signs of clinical depression. His sadness and frustration were appropriate for the situation. He commented on his infatuation with his wife's physical beauty and sophistication, and his blindness to her strong need to be admired and coddled. In light of the lack of past history or a family propensity for depression, the patient's insight regarding his mental status, and the strong support provided by peers and supervisors, along with the overall clinical picture, the treating psychiatrist decided that antidepressant medication was not indicated. Two factors contributed to the decision to not use antidepressant medication: the likelihood that the patient would respond quickly to a brief course of psychotherapy, and the side effects of psychotropic medications. Furthermore, psychoactive drugs require significant time to take effect and cannot be abruptly terminated, and while the aviator is taking them he must be grounded; thus the patient's absence from the cockpit may be unnecessarily prolonged.

There is a practical issue involved, namely the time needed by the flight surgeon to arrange a nonpharmacologic approach to treatment. Sending the flyer off to the mental health clinic will not work if the flight surgeon has not laid the groundwork for aircrew referrals, including scheduling the first interview, and the selection of a therapist who understands the aviation environment and the personality characteristics of aviators. Many flyers would be unwilling to be seen entering a mental health clinic at their base facility (though this would probably be less of a problem in a civilian setting). The initial interview should be performed in the flight medicine section, and the issue of anonymity should be discussed. It is wise to locate a psychiatrist, psychologist, and social worker who enjoy flying and associating with flyers, and to maintain that contact for possible future mental health assistance. This early planning and preparation is time well spent.

The PSW mentioned above was invited, along with several other mental health personnel, to a flying training orientation and flight line visit. Crawling in and out of cockpits and talking with both students and instructor pilots provided them the opportunity of better understanding the flying environment. Though resentful at first of the intrusion into her counseling of the patient and his wife, the PSW quickly developed an appreciation of flight safety and the danger of prematurely returning an aviator to flight duty. Mental health personnel work with comparatively sick populations and commonly use high doses of medications incompatible with flight duty with little understanding of their impact on flying performance. When referring a patient for psychiatric consultation it is perfectly appropriate to ask the consultant if he or she is familiar with flight operations and the attendant intolerance for impaired reaction time, decision making, judgment, and visual acuity.

An aviator's flight surgeon may elect to prescribe anxiolytic medication to a flyer experiencing mild to moderate anxiety in association with a transient adjustment reaction. An aviator who has suffered an adjustment reaction is at risk for a future episode. Following recovery the aviator should be observed for 3-6 months, and should remain free of psychotropic medication while working in a position that does not involve cockpit duty. If recovery remains stable, the aviator can safely be returned to flight duty.

Psychosis

This is the least commonly encountered psychiatric disorder in aviators, and DSM-IV lists the following diagnostic criteria:

- two or more of the characteristic symptoms of delusions, hallucinations, disorganized speech and behavior, and "negative" symptoms (eg, flat affect, avolition);
- social/occupational dysfunction;
- duration of symptoms of at least 6 months; and
- schizoaffective and mood disorders, substance abuse, and developmental disorder are all excluded.

This next case, from an article by Ordiway and Rayman,[2] illustrates full-blown psychosis in a pilot. The patient was the aircraft commander of a dual seat military fighter flying a combat sortie in Southeast Asia. The aircraft weapons system officer (WSO) noted that the pilot's radio communications seemed inappropriate and that subsequent high-speed high-angle dives were followed by an attempt to land on a nonexistent (imaginary) runway. The WSO convinced the pilot to return to home base to land, fought for control of the stick, and eventually successfully landed the aircraft. In a subsequent interview the pilot expressed the belief that he was Jesus Christ and revealed that he had experienced a similar unreported and undetected psychotic episode several years earlier. Prior to the onset of the current episode, the patient had been preoccupied with financial and personal problems, and had not slept or eaten the night before the incident. The patient was immediately hospitalized in a psychiatric facility and placed on antipsychotic medication. He was not returned to flying status.

In the next case, a flight attendant suffered a major psychotic episode, possibly related to recent childbirth. The patient's strange behavior was capped by her removing all her clothes and wading across several cold streams with her infant on her back. The child drowned during the river crossing and the patient was found in a delusional state. Following a brief hospitalization and the administration of antipsychotic medication, the patient was seen once weekly as an outpatient and maintained on medication. The treating physician certified the patient for return to work, although she was continued on major tranquilizing and antidepressant medications. A review of the patient's medical record by an independent consultant found that the treating psychiatrist had little appreciation of the responsibilities of flight attendants beyond the serving of meals (a common misperception), and that no consideration had been given to the impact of psychotropic medication in this patient's unique workplace. The status of the patient's recovery could not be determined from her medical record and an independent psychiatric consultation was denied. The airline refused her return, as recommended by the consultant.

Flight personnel suffering from psychotic illness should not be returned to active flight status due to the risk of recurrence. Exceptions to this policy of disqualification would be recovery from a psychosis caused by an identified toxic exposure or extreme stress, related, for example, to incarceration as a prisoner of war.

Anxiety

This broad category includes panic attack, agoraphobia, specific and social phobias, obsessive compulsive disorder, posttraumatic stress disorder, acute stress disorder, generalized anxiety disorder, anxiety due to a general medical condition, substance induced anxiety disorder, and anxiety disorder not otherwise specified. All of these disorders have apprehension and impaired function in common; however, each category of anxiety has specific DSM-IV requirements. For example, Specific Phobia requires:

- a marked and persistent fear that is unreasonable, instigated by the presence or anticipation of a specific object or situation;
- exposure to the phobic stimulus almost invariably provokes an immediate anxiety response;
- the person recognizes that the fear is excessive or unreasonable;
- the phobic situation is avoided or else is endured with intense anxiety or distress; and
- the avoidance, anxious anticipation, or distress in the feared situation(s) interferes significantly with the person's normal routine, occupational (or academic) functioning, or social activities or relationships, or there is marked distress about having the phobia.

The criteria are extensive and the reader is referred to DSM-IV, which also includes discussions of differential diagnosis.

The following example illustrates a case of Specific Phobia. The patient, an airline captain, was the 42-year-old mother of 2 young children. Her husband's profession required that he be away from home for long periods of time. Her presenting complaint was the inability to carry out her duties as a pilot due to sexual harassment resulting from the placement of sexually explicit photos in her cockpit, and the ever-increasing anxiety she suffered in anticipation of finding the offensive photographs.

Her complaints to administrative authorities did not stop the alleged harassment. When this pilot entered the cockpit, she would spend increasing periods of time prior to preflight searching for cleverly hidden pornographic material. Her mounting anxiety could only be controlled upon discovery of the offensive material. Eventually, preflight was overwhelmed by the search and the flyer became phobic for the cockpit, requiring treatment by a psychologist. The initiation of a lawsuit and union intervention precluded getting a second opinion from a psychiatrist consultant. The patient did not return to the cockpit, and assumed the full-time care of her children.

The opportunity for early intervention and resolution of the patient's conflict over her role as mother versus pilot, as well as her inability to deal with the macho environment of her airline, was missed. Harassment leads to severe personal, social, and occupational problems. Aeromedical physicians working in airline settings should review the procedures in place for dealing with such issues and should establish preemptive corrective measures.

The aeromedical disposition of flight personnel diagnosed with an anxiety disorder depends on the specific category of the disorder and phase of the illness. Although this is a large group of disorders with varied symptomatology, the underlying common problem of anxiety requires that the patient be disqualified from flight-related duties when initially diagnosed. Anxiolytic medication, often prescribed during the early phase of these disorders, may interfere with safe and effective work performance. Anxiety related to specific stressors (eg, medical illness or trauma) may improve when the stressor is removed or the individual learns to effectively deal with it. The patient is then observed in a non-flying work environment and kept off of psychotropic medications for 3-6 months, and if symptom free considered suitable for return to flight duties. More deeply rooted disorders (eg, obsessive-compulsive and phobic types) may require extended disqualification, with observation while performing duties outside of the cockpit for 6-12 months before being considered recovered by the treating psychiatrist.

Personality and Behavior Disorders

As with adjustment disorders, these are commonly seen in aviators. DSM-IV defines a personality disorder as an enduring pattern of inner experience and behavior that deviates markedly from the expectations of the individual's culture, is pervasive and inflexible, has onset in adolescence or early adulthood, is stable over time, and leads to distress or impairment. Each of the 11 personality disorders described has its unique diagnostic criteria. For example, Narcissistic Personality Disorder requires that the patient demonstrate at least 5 of the following:

- a grandiose sense of self-importance;
- preoccupation with fantasies of unlimited success, power, brilliance, beauty, or ideal love;
- belief that he or she is "special" and unique and can only be understood by or may only associate with other special high status people or institutions;
- requires excessive admiration;
- has a sense of entitlement;
- is interpersonally exploitative (ie, takes advantage of others to achieve his or her own ends);
- lacks empathy and is unwilling to recognize or identify with the feelings and needs of others;
- is often envious of others or believes that others are envious of him or her; and
- shows arrogant, haughty behaviors or attitudes.

In this next case, a USAF B-52 bomber command pilot, considered his unit's best pilot, was known to fly perilously close to the edge of safety. During a rehearsal of low-level maneuvers to be flown in an air show, the pilot attempted a 90 degree banked turn and lost wing lift. The copilot initiated ejection, but there was time for jettison of only one hatch. All aboard were killed. The tape in the cockpit voice recorder (CVR) revealed the copilot (the pilot's squadron commander) warning the pilot about his dangerously aggressive maneuvering. In response the pilot called his copilot a demeaning name and then initiated the fatal maneuver. The pilot was known as a showoff and risk taker. His excellent piloting skills were overshadowed by his poor judgment, defective decision making, and disregard for the safety of his crew and observers on the ground. He only cared about his personal sense of power and control and often flouted authority.

The postmortem diagnosis is Narcissistic Personality Disorder. The pattern of dangerous risk-taking by this pilot should have resulted in his grounding long before the fatal mishap. A problem in diagnosing this particular personality disorder is that military pilots are selected for their self confidence and aggressive nature; flying at the edge of safety is often rewarded. However, it was clear in this case that the pattern went dangerously beyond the edge. The diagnosis is made if the patient exhibits a pattern of unnecessary risk-taking behavior with the goal of self-aggrandizement rather than mission success, together with a disregard for authority or the safety of others. In fact, the unit FS had recommended to the unit commander that the pilot be grounded; that recommendation was ignored. The only remaining option was to report the case to a higher authority, an action that would put the flight surgeon's reputation, and hence future effectiveness, in jeopardy with his commander and fellow pilots. (This is a dilemma that many flight surgeons face and there is no simple remedy.) Whether in a military or civilian setting, sooner or later the aviation medicine physician will be faced with the need to recommend that a pilot or aircrew member be grounded.

Flight personnel diagnosed with personality and behavior disorders should be permanently disqualified from all flight-related duties. These disorders are considered to be an inherent and permanent part of the individual's personality; thus their associated behaviors are an unpredictable threat to flying safety.

Diagnostic Puzzles

The next two cases describe suspected but unproven psychiatric disorders.

A unit flight surgeon referred an F-111 fighter-bomber pilot to the Consult Service of the USAF School of Aerospace Medicine. The pilot, a 28-year-old captain, had been discovered walking on the outside second story ledges of the base Officers Club, apparently inebriated, with his pockets full of Club silverware. He had a history of leading a wild life, past episodes of intoxication associated with antisocial behavior, and a recent history of mood swings. His squadron commander considered the patient "a hell of a pilot," but was uncomfortable with his immaturity and worried about his reliability. During psychiatric interviews the patient was pleasant, freely discussed his drunken behavior, denied feelings of elation or depression, attributed his recent episode to stupidity and immaturity, and was fully accepting of being grounded for 6 months. He denied any knowledge of depression or mood swings in close family members, and stated unequivocally that there had been no alcoholism in his family. Psychological testing was not sufficiently illuminating to allow a diagnosis, although the testing psychologist was of the opinion that the patient was not entirely truthful.

The patient returned to his unit in Duties Not Including Flying (DNIF) status. His commander told the patient unequivocally that a repeat of his past behavior would not be tolerated if there was any chance for his return to flight status, and that a period of at least 6 months of mental health counseling was required. However, because of exemplary behavior, the patient's commander returned the pilot to flight status after just 3 months. He performed without problems during 1 year of follow-up. The patient abruptly terminated his counseling upon return to flight status, and was lost to follow-up after 1 year, making a long-term diagnosis of a possible mood (bipolar) disorder impossible. He carefully avoided contact with his unit's flight surgeon, who rotated to a new assignment before the patient's annual flight physical examination.

The patient's "hell raising" was always associated with alcohol consumption, and until the incident described above, had never seriously crossed the line into dangerously unacceptable behavior. No history could be obtained from the patient, friends, or supervisors that could identify an event precipitating his behavior. Individuals with bipolar disorder that primarily manifest a hypomanic phase usually exhibit their aberrant behavior more often than an occasional incident of "hell raising." Addiction to alcohol would present as a more persistent and frequent problem. Although the patient was able to talk his way out of trouble, the diagnosis of Antisocial Personality Disorder could not be made. The patient appeared pleasant and cooperative, and this very intelligent and successful pilot carefully controlled his behavior and the content of his psychiatric interviews. Clearly, his goal was return to flight status. He saw his referral for psychiatric consultation as a warning, and he had the personal resources to respond in a manner that would allow him to escape further psychiatric scrutiny and get back into the cockpit. Although there was some substance abuse, some immaturity, some antisocial behavior, and some occupational dysfunction, the picture wasn't sufficiently integrated to allow a firm diagnosis. Pilots are selected for their aggressive personalities and histories of success (they are frequently captains of athletic teams, class presidents, and have high academic standing) as well as their problem solving ability. They can be charismatic, disarming, and manipulative. In this case, the patient's commander made the final disposition.

In this next example, the patient was a 39-year-old first officer for a major airline and a USAF Reserve A-10 ground attack fighter pilot. While serving as flight lead during a low-level training exercise, he appeared disoriented and crashed into a mountain with fatal results. His flight mates were shocked and surprised, later commenting how little they knew the deceased pilot. The subsequent accident investigation disclosed that the pilot had attempted to postpone his reserve commitment due to a court order to appear before a judge for alleged nonsupport. His squadron commanding officer had become exasperated by several recent similar requests, and had told the pilot to "get in here and fly or you're done with this outfit." The pilot complied with his commander's order and stood in contempt of court for nonappearance, adding to the significant stress of a contested divorce.

Associates (no friends could be found) described him as unfriendly, superior, secretive, and a hustler. The unit flight surgeon knew nothing about the pilot's personal problems. Further investigation revealed that his earlier academic and military career had been highly successful, and that it was only recently that his life seemed to fall apart. There is little question that this pilot had a great deal on his mind. It was not possible to determine if he had been preoccupied with his personal problems and consequently unable to attend to the requirements of low-level flight, or if he experienced covert suicidal ideation and intentionally crashed into the mountain. No prior history of depression was discovered. Although considered arrogant and aloof by his fellow reservists, he had enjoyed a problem-free career as an airline pilot, and there was insufficient history to support a diagnosis of Narcissistic Personality Disorder. A firm psychiatric diagnosis could not be made.

The AME/FS must always be vigilant for aviators who display behaviors indicating the presence of a psychiatric disorder, yet have insufficient history or symptomatology to determine a clear psychiatric diagnosis. Without a diagnosis, flight status may have to be determined via administrative rather than medical channels.

Mood Disorders

A disturbance of mood is the common symptom for this large array of disorders. Included are major depressive disorder, dysthymic disorder, depressive disorder not otherwise specified, bipolar I disorder, bipolar II disorder, cyclothymic disorder, bipolar disorder not otherwise specified, mood disorder due to a general medical condition, and substance induced mood disorder not otherwise specified.

For example, DSM-IV lists the following criteria for a major depressive episode, the foundation required for the diagnosis of Major Depressive Disorder. Five or more of the following symptoms must be present during the same 2-week period and represent a change from previous functioning; at least one of the symptoms has to be either depressed mood or loss of interest and pleasure:

- depressed mood most of the day, nearly every day, as indicated by either subjective report or observation made by others;
- markedly diminished interest or pleasure in all, or almost all, activities most of the day, nearly every day;
- significant weight loss when not dieting or following weight gain, or decrease or increase of appetite nearly every day;
- insomnia or hypersomnia nearly every day;
- psychomotor agitation or retardation nearly every day;
- fatigue or loss of energy nearly every day;
- feelings of worthlessness or excessive or inappropriate guilt nearly every day;
- diminished ability to think or concentrate, or indecisiveness, nearly every day;
- recurrent thoughts of death, recurrent suicidal ideation without a specific plan, or a suicide attempt or a specific plan for committing suicide.

Also required:

- The symptoms do not meet the criteria for a Mixed Episode.
- The symptoms cause clinically significant distress or impairment in social, occupational, or other important areas of functioning.
- The symptoms are not due to the direct physiological effects of a substance or general medical condition.

The diagnosis of Major Depressive Disorder, Single Episode, must meet the following criteria: 1) presence of a single major depressive episode (noted above); 2) the major depressive episode is not better accounted for by schizoaffective disorder and is not superimposed on schizophrenia, schizophreniform disorder, delusional disorder, or psychotic disorder not otherwise specified (NOS); and 3) there has never been a manic episode, or a hypomanic episode.

The following case demonstrates a problem in differentiating Major Depressive Disorder from Adjustment Disorder with Depression. The patient, a 28-year-old married copilot of an H-60 Blackhawk helicopter, attended sick call and complained to his flight surgeon of headache, insomnia, and poor appetite. Physical examination revealed no evidence of any significant pathology. While the patient was at the laboratory having basic blood work and urinalysis, the flight surgeon received a phone call from the patient's wife. She had noted a personality change in her husband about 6 months prior to this office visit, when he learned that his selection for fixed-wing (fighter) training had been canceled and that he would be transferred to a special operations training unit. The patient's wife had never interfered in her husband's career, but was quite worried about his emotional state. Previously an outgoing and sociable individual, the patient had become increasingly introverted and would no longer attend squadron social events. An attentive father to their 2-year-old daughter, he had recently appeared disinterested in her and would become irritable when she demanded his attention. During the 2 weeks prior to this office visit she had found him pacing about the house in the middle of the night, complaining of being unable to sleep. On one occasion he commented on his great frustration in failing to "get into fighters," and tearfully said how disappointed his father (a retired Air Force senior noncommissioned officer) would be. Always proud of his excellent health and physical conditioning, he recently complained of various aches and pains and had stopped his daily exercise sessions at the base gym.

When the patient returned from the laboratory (results of all tests were normal) he was informed of his wife's phone call and concern for him. At first angry at her intervention, he eventually confessed his great disappointment in losing the chance to "get into fighters" and his loss of motivation to advance in his Air Force career. An Air Force "brat" (the child of a career military father), he had lived on military airbases throughout his childhood, admiring fighters and the pilots that flew them. As a line chief responsible for the maintenance of fighter aircraft, the patient's father had expressed great admiration for "his pilots," often expressing the hope that his only son, the patient, would one day become a fighter pilot.

In view of the patient's vegetative signs of an underlying depression (ie, insomnia and anorexia), and his associated depressed thought content (ie, guilt, disappointment, self-recrimination, and loss of motivation), as well as his personality change, he was deemed unsafe to fly, and was grounded and referred for psychiatric consultation. Note that the patient denied suicidal ideation and that his wife never heard him express any such thoughts. This pilot was considered an excellent teacher and was reassigned to the academic teaching staff while receiving a short course of psychotherapy. It came out in therapy that the patient had been uncomfortable in the flying environment from the beginning of flight training and had often thought of abandoning his flying career. However, he did not want to "let his dad down or disappoint all the people" that had supported him in his effort to become a fighter pilot. In truth, the pilot was most comfortable in the world of computer science and teaching. He was encouraged to discuss his problems with his father, and found much to his relief that he had an exaggerated perception of his father's need to have his son become a fighter pilot. The patient did not return to flying and fulfilled his military obligation in the field of computer science. He planned to obtain a graduate degree and teach at the college level.

The diagnosis of this case was Adjustment Disorder with Depression. It was the consulting psychiatrist's opinion that the symptoms of depression were of insufficient duration and not severe enough to merit the diagnosis of a mood disorder (eg, Major Depressive Disorder). He was also impressed with the patient's ability to understand and deal with the personal conflicts involved, and work successfully in a new environment.

An aviator experiencing a depressive disorder must be disqualified from flight duties. The psychopathology of this group of disorders extends beyond the normal personal disappointments and mood changes of everyday life. Also, aviators presenting with an initial episode of a depressive disorder are at risk for subsequent episodes of depression, and psychiatrists cannot accurately predict which patients will experience a recurrence. The pharmacotherapy of depression is complex and requires the expertise of an experienced clinical psychiatrist. Once the diagnosis has been made, the patient should be referred to a psychiatrist for continued care.

Psychoactive Medication

The appropriate use of psychoactive medications requires extensive clinical experience in the psychiatric arena during both the acute and maintenance phase of illness. As a general rule, any aviator sufficiently ill to require psychoactive medication should be evaluated and treated by a psychiatrist. Psychiatrists should provide legible follow-up notes and understand at the time of referral that patient information is shared with the referring aviation medicine physician. Responsibility for the decision of whether to return an aviator to flight duty is properly left to the aviator's AME/FS. Aviators requiring psychotropic medication must be disqualified from flight duty. Support personnel requiring psychiatric medication (traffic controllers, flight attendants, maintenance specialists) should also be disqualified from their duties. The final aeromedical disposition should be based on the underlying disorder, the patient's recovery, and an adequate period of observation (see specific DSM-IV disease categories discussed above). Although patients may initially demonstrate improvement when treated with psychoactive medications, it is not safe to return them to duty until they have fully recovered and medication has been discontinued.

The *Manual of Clinical Psychopharmacology* of the American Psychiatric Association[3] lists 21 antipsychotic agents, and describes their side effects, including sedation, autonomic effects, endocrine effects, skin and eye complications, and various other rare complications (eg, agranulocytosis). Some examples of antipsychotic drugs are the phenothiazines (eg, chlorpromazine, triflupromazine, thioridazine, fluphenazine, perphenazine), the butyrophenone-like group (eg, haloperidol, pimozide), the thioxanthenes (eg, chlorprothixene, thiothixene), the indoles (eg, molindone), the dibenzazepines (eg, clozapine, loxapine), and the benzisoxazoles (eg, risperidone).

Common side effects of antidepressants include nausea, diarrhea, cramping, emesis, insomnia, jitteriness, agitation, restlessness, headache, syncope, tremor, perspiration, and altered sexual function. Severe drug interactions can occur, particularly with monoamine oxidase inhibitors. Examples of antidepressant drugs are the tricyclics (eg, imipramine, amitriptyline, doxepin, protriptyline), the monoamine oxidase inhibitors (eg, phenelzine, trancyclopromine, isocarboxazid), the selective serotonin reuptake inhibitors (eg, fluoxetine, sertraline, paroxetine), and the 5-HT2 antagonists (eg, trazodone).

Side effects of anxiolytic agents include bradycardia, hypotension, sedation, weakness, fatigue, clouded sensorium, and impotence. Examples of anxiolytic agents are the benzodiazepines (eg, diazepam, oxazepam, triazolam, alprazolam), the barbiturates (eg, amobarbital, meprobamate, phenobarbital), the noradrenergic drugs (eg, clonidine, propanolol), and the antihistamines (eg, hydroxyzine HCl, hydroxyzine pamoate).

Side effects of mood stabilizers are tremor, dysarthria, cogwheeling, weight gain, polyuria, renal insufficiency, nausea, rashes, and various benign electrocardiographic aberrations. The most commonly prescribed mood stabilizers are lithium carbonate, carbamazepine, valproic acid, lamotrigine, and gabapentin. Mood stabilizers are now commonly used in treating bipolar (formerly known as manic-depressive) illness. Although not often used in an aviator population, it is important to realize that these potent drugs may be inappropriately prescribed in misdiagnosed patients.

Somatoform Disorders and Psychological Factors Affecting Medical Condition

Psychophysiological or psychosomatic conditions are now found in the DSM-IV categories of Somatoform Disorders and Psychological Factors Affecting Medical Condition. Headache, chronic pain with no physical cause, and irritable bowel, when not symptomatic of a well defined and diagnosed medical condition, are examples of somatoform disorders; ulcerative colitis and essential hypertension are medical conditions that can be affected by psychological factors.

Stress is considered a major contributor to these conditions. Due to the careful selection and screening of aviator candidates, few will manifest them. However, "white coat" hypertension, caused by a flyer's anxiety during the examination needed for medical certification for flight status, is not uncommon. Most pilots with initially elevated BP readings during a periodic physical will eventually achieve acceptable levels with repeated trials. For aviators continuing to demonstrate unacceptably high readings with no evidence of physical disease, a brief course of relaxation training can be highly effective. The AME/FS who is familiar with TM (transcendental meditation) and yoga breathing techniques can train pilots to lower their blood pressure to acceptable levels, or he or she can refer the flyer to a psychologist specializing in relaxation techniques. Biofeedback relaxation training involves the instrumentation of the patient with sophisticated electronic sensors and digital readouts. The science and technology orientation of this approach may be more acceptable to some aviators.

Airsickness is a special psychophysiological condition providing an excellent opportunity for active intervention by the AME/FS. Approximately 30% of all student pilots experience motion sickness in their early training; however, 70% will adapt and have no more problems with it. Susceptibility appears to run in families, with childhood histories including intolerance for riding in the back of the family car or a bus, and inevitable motion sickness on carnival rides. In hopes of preventing airsickness, student pilots will often eat crackers before flying, sprinkle aftershave lotion in their oxygen masks, try various preflight diets, and apply split shot wristbands to their wrists (which put pressure on the Chinese acupressure point for motion sickness). Experienced aviators who were previously not prone to motion sickness may become susceptible when changing flight profiles or transitioning into aircraft that impose extreme physiological stress. Some locations in certain aircraft, such as the B-52 bomber mid-deck compartment, are notorious motion sickness generators.

Exposing wrists or face to a blast of cold air at the first signs of impending airsickness may abort the episode. Some sailors and flyers have accidentally discovered that yoga breathing techniques will prevent or abort motion sickness. Desensitization programs using a Barany chair were employed by the USAF for several years. Time-limited medication regimens using combinations of dextroamphetamine sulfate and scopolamine or promethazine and ephedrine, have been employed by the military. The use of medication in the military is usually associated with other supportive techniques, including counseling by instructors and a gradual stepwise increase in motion stress. Biofeedback in combination with relaxation training has been successfully employed in the treatment of chronic airsickness in military aircrews at the USAF School of Aerospace Medicine at Brooks AFB, Texas.[4]

Civilian pilots and airline passengers have often taken anti–motion sickness drugs with varying results. Prior to flying, a pilot should ground test the anti–motion sickness drug to be sure there will be no adverse effects (eg, sedation, fatigue, slowed reaction and information processing times, memory loss). Airsickness is potentially disabling to a pilot. Aviators unable to gain control over their motion sickness are restricted to aircraft and missions that do not generate this response. Student pilots who are refractory to therapeutic measures may have to be disqualified.

Special Circumstances

Combat

Alternative Approaches to Combat Fatigue

Flyers in combat operations present a special challenge to the military flight surgeon due to the constant stress of separation from families and friends, the threat of death, erratic rest and sleep, chronic fatigue, strange climates and cultures, and the loss of comrades. Given these conditions, it is not surprising that some flyers develop disabling psychiatric problems. Psychiatric consultation is not always readily available to the troubled flyer's flight surgeon, who is faced with the responsibility for recognizing the early signs of a developing problem, of responding to the concerns of operations officers and commanders regarding the mental health of an aircrew member, of knowing when temporary grounding and a brief rest will resolve the difficulty versus removal of the afflicted flyer to a remote rest area. The most common condition encountered in all wars has been battle fatigue or "shell shock," most recently termed ***acute posttraumatic stress disorder***. The classic signs of this condition are insomnia, apprehension, repetitive dreams, nightmares, startle, difficulty with concentration and focus, fear of return to combat, feelings of guilt and shame, tachycardia, sweating, nausea and vomiting, vertigo, and other somatic symptoms. The afflicted aircrew member may have unpleasant visual images, dreams of planes on fire or exploding, or the repetition of a witnessed specific catastrophic event. The following case is described in *Personality Disturbances in Combat Fliers*,[5] a publication of the Josiah Macy Foundation that includes 5 volumes dealing with psychiatric disturbances in the U.S. Army Air Forces during World War II:

A 24-year-old P-40 fighter pilot completed 14 combat missions before being shot up by an enemy fighter, forced out of formation, and sustaining shrapnel wounds of face and eyes. He was able to make it back to his base, made a belly landing, and spent several weeks in the hospital recuperating. He returned to flight duties and training in the newly acquired P-47. During the nonoperational training period he became increasingly anxious and preoccupied with the mechanical condition of his aircraft. On one training sortie his engine failed and he accomplished his second belly landing. He soon resumed operational sorties, but experienced mounting anxiety and preoccupation with the thought that an enemy fighter would attack from his six o'clock and shoot him down. To avoid that possibility he constantly flew "all over the sky," severely compromising his ability to fly formation. His tension increased at every sighting of an enemy aircraft and he would experience excessive anxiety, palpitations, dry mouth, and an inability to think clearly.

On his twentieth mission, his flight leader called "enemy aircraft," and he lost his head, entered a spin, recovered, and returned to base alone. He then experienced intermittent nausea and vomiting, and was grounded and referred for psychiatric evaluation. His flight surgeon noted that the pilot had exhibited a marked personality change in the last month. Formerly sociable and jovial, he became reclusive, quiet, and depressed. He described his preoccupation with the hazards of combat flying and associated anxiety and tension. In his final weeks of flying he had to force himself to climb the ladder into his aircraft. He hoped he could overcome his fears and "not let the boys down," and so at first did not report his increasing disability.

The pilot was disqualified from flying and referred for treatment. Following 2 months of treatment at a rest and rehabilitation center the pilot was returned to active flight status; however, a severe shortage of instructors with combat experience resulted in his reassignment to a training squadron in the United States.

During World War II, and the conflicts in Korea, Vietnam, and Israel, there were times when military leaders did not have the option to send flyers with combat stress or fatigue to a rear echelon for treatment and recovery. These flyers were needed back in the line as soon as possible and therefore were treated at the front. This treatment, conducted immediately behind the front line, consisted of sodium amytal–induced hypnotherapy and catharsis of the battle scene, but sometimes a decidedly simpler approach was used—a warm blanket, cup of hot cocoa, 48 hours of rest, and constant reassurance from leaders and peers. Physicians in the Israeli Defense Forces found that patients with battle fatigue treated in a rear rehabilitation unit had a longer period of disability compared to patients treated at or close to the front.

Psychiatric Problems Affecting Groups

The military flight surgeon will occasionally have to deal with psychiatric problems that affect a group of flyers or an entire organization. Some illustrative cases follow.

The "Jinx"

A unit had been flying the then-new F-106 delta wing fighter for a year and had been experiencing a high accident rate. A fatal crash of two aircraft taking off in tandem was the event that led to a request from the unit flight surgeon for psychiatric consultation. The referring FS indicated that his investigation of the accidents had not revealed any significant medical factors, but the squadron's operations officer had expressed the belief that the unit had a morale problem. After a unit suffers several fatal crashes in a short time one would expect a morale problem, but what the operations officer was referring to was the widespread belief that the unit was "jinxed." Several pilots were interviewed, and they confirmed that a widely held belief among unit members was that their fate was sealed, a belief that had not been openly expressed. The unit headquarters directed the wing commander to disband the unit and regroup in an effort to dispel this perception. Shortly thereafter the accident rate declined.

Unit Reaction to a Fatal Crash

A C-141 cargo-transport aircraft with a highly rated crew aboard crashed on approach to a night landing. All aboard were killed. There was nothing unusual about the mission and no mechanical problems caused the fatal mishap. The pilot was a highly respected senior aviator, the squadron's adverse weather instructor pilot, who was soon to leave the military to fly with a major airline. The unit's squadron commander requested aeromedical assistance when several members of his crew turned in their wings in preparation for leaving the Air Force. In addition, wives of deceased crew members were distraught and needed help. The squadron stood down (suspended operations) and a series of group discussions involving supervisors were held, led by a senior psychiatrist/flight surgeon. Wives were counseled separately, as were the aircrews. Several days of uninhibited discussion allowed the crew members and their families to express their grief at the loss of spouses and friends, and to vent their anger at supervisors and leaders. Surviving crew members expressed their guilt in not being aboard the doomed aircraft and the frustration and helplessness they felt at being unable to foresee and prevent the accident. After several hours of such therapy, the flyers retrieved their wings, and the families of the deceased crew members continued their grieving process and relocated with the help of surviving crew members and their families. The squadron returned to normal operations.

Psychological Reaction of Accident Site Recovery Crew

Safety personnel at the scene of a military aircraft accident may use volunteers to help in the retrieval of human remains. These volunteers are given plastic bags and marker sticks, and told to pick up anything that looks like a body part, marking the location with a small stake and placing a location tag on the bag. Most have never seen a dismembered or mutilated body. Several will become ill at the site; many will become upset, cry, and have nightmares, insomnia, or difficulty in carrying out their normal duties. Recovery crews should be prepared for the unpleasant experience by a FS and decompressed by a mental health professional, who should meet with the group as soon as possible after they complete the recovery, and hold a follow-up meeting the next day. Similar opportunities should be provided to recovery teams working commercial and general aviation accident sites.

Fear of Flying

The generic term *fear of flying* represents a diverse group of conditions. Some airline passengers experience great anxiety in anticipation of flying and cannot board a commercial flight without the aid of tranquilizers or alcohol. Desensitization programs have been available for fearful passengers for several years. Although idealized by many, flying may be psychophysiologically threatening to some. Even among aviators, not all are initially comfortable in flight, and many experience frank anxiety when subjected to excessive pitch, roll, or yaw. This type of fear is usually seen in the naive aviator, and it may be overcome by reassurance and repeated flight. A dangerous variation of this form of fear is the response of overcompensation, in which affected individuals deal with their anxiety by immersing themselves in flying in an effort to conquer their perceived weakness by pursuing danger. Another form of fear is the realistic appreciation of the danger of military combat as demonstrated by the case of the P-40 combat pilot described above, and by the following case.

An F-4 Fighter Weapons Systems Officer with two combat tours in Southeast Asia refused to return to flying after a scheduled break from combat. During an interview at the USAF School of Aerospace Medicine the patient said he had experienced a barely controllable urge to defecate during a long flight. He had been terrified that he would be unable to control his sphincter and would soil his water immersion suit. Thereafter he refused to fly in any aircraft other than a transport with a commode. It was eventually learned that the patient's refusal to fly was in reaction to the belief that he would be killed on his next combat sortie.

The Breakoff Phenomenon

Rayman[6] and Gillingham and Previc[7] describe a rare event experienced by pilots at very high altitudes who feel they have indeed "slipped the surly bonds of the earth." The term **breakoff** covers a variety of high altitude flight experiences, from simply feeling good through euphoria to psychological detachment. As noted by Rayman, it is important to advise pilots flying at high altitudes of the phenomenon and the need to report any such unusual experience. Psychiatric consultation should be requested if the event degrades flying performance or if the pilot is negatively influenced by the experience after return to earth.

A Brief Mental Status Review

For the purpose of this clinically-oriented volume, a brief and practical mental status review for the aerospace medicine physician is described below.

The most important single facet of the practical mental status examination is your "gut feeling" and intuition. Are you uneasy or uncertain about the patient continuing to fly? Do you find yourself calling the patient's flight commander or the chief of safety after continuing or returning the patient's flight status? Do you experience anxiety or discomfort regarding a particular patient when away from the office? Do you hear yourself saying to a colleague or your spouse, "I'm not sure it was a good idea to put John back on the schedule"? If you do not have immediate access to interview the patient, does your review of the file or a discussion with a supervisor leave you with a bad feeling or a nagging worry that the patient has a serious problem that should be attended to quickly?

Attitude and General Behavior

Does the patient approach you and the interview in an accepting manner? Is the patient inappropriately or excessively angry? Are there any significant changes in sociability, working relationships, or energy level? Does the aviator have problems with authority? Is he or she having family problems? Is the patient preoccupied with thoughts of potential illness or disability? Is their motivation to fly consistent? Is the patient manifestly arrogant and condescending? Does the aviator accept and appreciate the need for the interview?

Mood and Affect

Does the aviator exhibit evidence of depression? Is the patient tearful, does he or she speak too slowly, show evidence of insomnia, or discuss suicidal ideation? Are there signs of anorexia or feelings of hopelessness, guilt, and worthlessness? Are there signs of mania, such as pressured, rapid speech? Does the aviator have difficulty sitting still? Do his or her thoughts come flooding out in a cascade of ideas?

Content of Thought

Does the patient's thinking follow a logical and reasonable path and make sense, or is it discombobulated and confused? Does the content of the patient's discourse match his or her affect? Does the aviator express diffuse anxiety or fear? Is the patient preoccupied with hypochondriacal thoughts, paranoid ideas, frank delusions, or hallucinations?

Organic Mental Phenomena

Early brain malignancies, organic neurological conditions, occupational and toxic exposures, and drug use and abuse are problems that can present with mental status abnormalities and are sometimes seen in the aviator population. Loss of orientation to time, place, or person is another symptom of organic disease; does the patient know who they are, where they are, and why they are in your office? Is their affect flat or expressive? Are there defects of memory and calculation? Is the individual's judgment compromised?

A formal and complete mental status examination is a lengthy procedure best administered by an experienced mental health professional. It is best for the AME/FS to have a general discussion with the patient rather than go through an artificial, stepwise, outline-in-hand interview. After completing the first interview, sit down and record the pertinent mental status data gleaned from your discussion, observation, and history taken from the patient. If you conclude that there are anomalies that need to be explored or gray areas that need further development, discuss the case with a psychiatrist colleague. A second interview with the patient by you or your colleague will help assure that any underlying psychiatric problem will be uncovered and treated, and prevent any future flight safety problems.

Aeromedical physicians must recognize the difficulty in quickly establishing a complete and accurate psychiatric diagnosis, as well as the need to ensure flight safety and peak performance. The appropriate initial disposition for an aviator with a potential psychiatric problem is grounding the aviator during the diagnostic workup. The aviation medicine physician is expected to make a presumptive diagnosis, with an emphasis on significant functional impairment. The performance of both aviators and support staff (ie, air traffic controllers, crew chiefs, mechanics and maintainers, and life support personnel) can be significantly impaired by minor mental health problems. Information processing, reaction time, perception, task orientation, memory, and a host of other critical functions can be adversely affected by tranquilizers, antidepressants, and any psychoactive drug. "Better safe than sorry" should be the watchwords in the initial disposition of an aviator with a suspected psychiatric problem. The specific diagnosis and final disposition should be determined by a consulting psychiatrist or clinical psychologist (when use of medications and underlying medical problems are not issues) familiar with the occupational requirements of aviation.

References

1. American Psychiatric Association. *Diagnostic and Statistical Manual of Mental Disorders*. 4th ed. Washington: American Psychiatric Press; 1994.

2. Ordiway V, Rayman R. Case report of an in-flight incident involving an aircraft commander with a psychiatric illness. *Aerospace Med*. 1974;45(3):316-317.

3. Schatzberg AF, et al. *Manual of Clinical Psychopharmacology*. Washington: American Psychiatric Press; 1997.

4. Levy RA, et al. Biofeedback rehabilitation of airsick aircrew. *Aviat Space Environ Med*. 1981;52(2):118-121.

5. Levy N. *Personality Disturbances in Combat Flyers*. Vol. 4. New York: Josiah Macy Foundation; 1945:19-20.

6. Rayman R. *Clinical Aviation Medicine*. 2nd ed. Philadelphia: Lea & Febiger; 1990.

7. Gillingham K, Previc F. Spatial orientation in flight. In: DeHart R, ed. *Fundamentals of Aerospace Medicine*. 2nd ed. Baltimore: Williams & Wilkins; 1996.

Chapter 11
Oncology

Although cancer is an emotion-laden word, long associated with despair, slow-wasting illness, and ultimately death, modern medicine offers many patients long life expectancy and in some cases cure. Thus malignancy does not necessarily signal the end of an aviator's flying career. Depending on the type of cancer, its extent, and the efficacy of therapy, some patients can continue flying indefinitely. Indeed, flying organizations throughout the world have safely returned to flight status pilots and other crew members who have been treated for cancers involving nearly every organ system of the body.

In determining aeromedical disposition of cancer patients, some basic questions must be answered regardless of the site and type of tumor, among them: Is treatment complete, be it surgical excision, radiotherapy, hormonal treatment, or chemotherapy? Is the patient free of all side effects of therapy? Flying while on medication is to be avoided not only because of potential tumor activity, but also because chemotherapeutic agents are often toxic and may adversely affect an aviator's performance. The pharmacopeia for these drugs is extensive and warns the prescribing physician of a wide array of common side effects including nausea and vomiting (often requiring antiemetics), bone marrow depression with possible pancytopenia, CNS dysfunction, and damage to major organs among others. Further complicating the picture is the need for combination therapy when treating some types of cancer, which only increases the risks of toxicity. For these reasons it is advisable for the patient to fully complete the treatment regimen before certification is considered.

Following treatment and with assurance that significant side effects are absent, the AME/FS must next be reasonably confident that a cure has been effected (or the cancer is in remission), there is no evidence of metastases, and the patient is asymptomatic. As part of the evaluation it is also advisable, particularly in aviators, to ascertain the patient's ability to cope emotionally with the illness. Careful consideration must be given to mental as well as physical health.

Finally, critical factors in the determination of aeromedical disposition are recurrence and survival rates and the risk of an incapacitating event as a harbinger of recurrence. Because recurrence and survival rates for a multitude of cancers are readily found in the literature, it comes down to a question of the flying organization's willingness to take risks. For a pilot who has been successfully treated for a cancer that has a recurrence rate of 10% within 5 years, aeromedical disposition will differ depending on how conservative or liberal the flight organization's policies are. For many cancers seemingly benign signs or symptoms may be the usual presenting features of recurrence, thus making detection more difficult; fever, weight loss, and lymphadenopathy of Hodgkin's disease being an example. But with close follow-up by the AME/FS recurrence should be detected well before the patient's disease is serious enough to threaten flight safety. On the other hand, of far greater consequence is the risk of sudden partial or complete incapacitation, for example a seizure or acute gastrointestinal bleeding. This danger should always be closely scrutinized by the waiver authority when an aviator who has been treated for cancer is being considered for return to the cockpit.

The most common cancers in the general population (all ages) are listed in Table 11-1.[1] Because the flying population in general is relatively young, some cancers would tend to be less frequent than others. For example, prostate carcinoma reaches its peak incidence in the sixth and seventh decades, whereas Hodgkin's disease is diagnosed more frequently during the third decade. Therefore, to discuss the many types of cancers and their aeromedical implications would not only be impractical, it would in many cases be irrelevant. Rather, let us examine a few general principles followed by a discussion of several cancers most likely to be found in aviators.

The AME/flight surgeon can expect to diagnose an occasional case of cancer in any aviation medicine practice, military or civilian. The treatment modalities most

Table 11-1. The Ten Most Common Cancers in Order of Decreasing Incidence

Male	*Female*
Prostate	Breast
Lung	Lung
Colorectal	Colorectal
Bladder	Uterus
Lymphoma	Ovary
Oropharyngeal	Lymphoma
Melanoma	Melanoma
Kidney	Pancreas
Leukemia	Bladder
Stomach	Kidney

commonly employed include surgery, chemotherapy, and radiotherapy, which in some cases may effect short- or long-term remission or cure. Upon completion of treatment, the AME/FS must determine whether a request for medical waiver is appropriate and consistent with flight safety. Consideration must be given to many factors, including the efficacy of treatment, recurrence rate, and the risk of an incapacitating event should an apparently eradicated cancer insidiously recur. Because of the many types of cancers and their diverse attendant variables, aeromedical disposition must usually be determined on a case-by-case basis. With that as general background, discussion of several cancers commonly seen in aviators follows.

Malignant Melanoma

Skin cancer deserves special attention since it is the most common form of malignant disease, and particularly because of its increasing prevalence. In 1935, 1 in 1500 Americans developed melanoma; in 2000, it will be 1 in 90.[2] One explanation for this alarming increase is the depletion of the ozone layer, which allows more ultraviolet light to reach the Earth's surface. The lesion is usually brown or black and may be found on any part of the body, though the primary site is most often on an extremity. Malignant melanoma can arise de novo or may develop from a harmless nevus that may suddenly become malignant and metastasize to any of a number of organ systems, including the brain, lungs, liver, and bone. Treatment includes surgical excision, lymph node dissection, radiation, and adjuvant chemotherapy with a crude 5-year survival rate of 81%.[2] Because a significant number of treated patients die within 5 years, and because the lesion can metastasize to the brain, the AME/flight surgeon faces a difficult aeromedical disposition decision when confronted by an aviator with this disease. To help resolve this issue, it is useful to examine the prognosis and the risk of a catastrophic incapacitating event secondary to metastasis.

Although melanoma is classified according to clinical stage, histopathology, anatomic site, and thickness, it is difficult to predict the posttreatment outcome. While some patients have a rapid downhill course, others live normally for many years. There are even reported cases of spontaneous regression of the tumor, as well as others with late recurrence and metastasis as long as 23 years after excision and apparent cure.[3] In spite of the diverse classifications and unclear prognosis for melanoma, the thickness of the lesion may be the best predictor of outcome. Five-year survival rates are correlated with lesion thickness as shown in Table 11-2.[4] As with some other diseases, aeromedical disposition of melanoma entails a certain amount of risk. Clearly, a lesion of 0.85 mm or less is comforting because of its 99% 5-year survival rate. As the thickness increases, the risk becomes significantly

**Table 11-2. Melanoma Thickness and
5-Year Survival**

Thickness (mm)	5-Year Survival (%)
<.85	99
.85-1.69	94
1.7-3.64	78
>3.65	42

greater, and this risk must be carefully assessed by the AME/FS. As seen in the table, a thicker lesion has a greater probability of metastasis and portends a more serious prognosis. Melanoma can metastasize to virtually any organ of the body, including the skin, soft tissues, and lymph nodes (42%-57% of cases), lungs (18%-36%), liver (14%-20%), brain (12%-20%), bone (11%-17%), and intestines (1%-7%).[4]

While the thickness of the lesion and lymph node involvement are the primary factors affecting prognosis, the anatomic site of the melanoma also has some prognostic significance. Although a melanoma can develop virtually anywhere on the body, the survival rate is lower if the lesion is on the head, neck, or trunk.[5]

In addition to these clinical considerations, the potential for sudden incapacitation must also be assessed since this is especially important in aviation medicine. It is well known that melanoma has a predilection for metastasis to the brain with an incidence of 12%-74% in autopsy series.[6] Brain metastasis from melanoma can cause a host of CNS signs and symptoms like any other brain tumor. In the largest series to date (6953 patients with malignant melanoma, of which 703 had brain metastasis), the presenting complaints for brain metastasis were focal and nonfocal neurologic symptoms (39% and 36% respectively), seizure (13%), neurological catastrophes (3%), and behavioral changes (2%); 7% were asymptomatic.[6] Conditions that favored brain metastasis included lesions on the mucous membranes, head, neck, and trunk; thick, ulcerated lesions; lymph node or visceral metastasis; and histologic findings of acral lentiginous or nodular melanoma. In this large series, 99%, 87%, and 78% were alive and free of brain metastasis at 1, 5, and 10 years respectively. In patients who developed brain metastasis, the time interval from diagnosis of the primary skin lesion to diagnosis of metastasis averaged 3.7 years.

Of particular concern is seizure activity or intracerebral hemorrhage resulting from metastasis. Although there is always the potential for such an incapacitating event, one study indicated it is rarely the initial or presenting clinical event. For example, of 712 patients with disseminated melanoma, only 4 sustained a stroke or seizure with no antecedent symptoms. Although 32 patients presented with brain metastasis, they had experienced other more innocuous symptoms such as nausea, vomiting, headache, and paresthesias which had caused no significant disability at the time.[7] The symptoms in decreasing order of frequency in patients not having a catastrophic event were anorexia, nausea, vomiting, weakness, equilibrium disturbance, headache, paresthesias, memory disturbances, visual dysfunction, and pain.

So we can see why aeromedical disposition is problematic for aviators with treated melanoma. For the aviator with a lesion less than 0.85 mm thick and negative nodes, a return to the cockpit may present only minimal risk. On the other hand, if nodes are positive or the lesion is thicker than 0.85 mm, the increased risk of recurrence and dissemination must be taken into account. Whatever the final decision, the possibility of CNS metastasis and nervous system dysfunction demands that the patient be followed at regular intervals by the AME/FS. If this is done, recurrence or metastasis may be detectable by physical signs or more benign symptoms well before an incapacitating event occurs.

Basal Cell and Squamous Cell Carcinoma

Basal cell and squamous cell carcinoma are fairly common skin cancers that the AME/flight surgeon will occasionally encounter. There are between 900,000 and 1.2 million cases of nonmelanoma skin cancers reported per year in the U.S.[8] Almost all basal cell tumors occur on the head and neck and are particularly common in fair-skinned, fair-haired people. Cumulative sun exposure is the most important risk factor. Although this tumor rarely metastasizes it can slowly enlarge, causing encroachment and destruction of nearby anatomic structures such as the eye, bone, and possibly the brain. Those that do take several years to cause symptoms, taking an average of 14 years to reach the size of over 2 centimeters.[9] However, with early recognition and treatment (surgical excision, Moh's surgery, cryosurgery, and electrocoagulation and curettage), cure is possible in virtually 100% of cases. Because the tumor rarely metastasizes and is curable, aviators can be safely returned to flight duty following therapy. There is a 10% recurrence rate.[9]

Although squamous cell carcinoma is not as common as basal cell carcinoma, it is by no means a rare tumor. Like the basal cell type, the great majority occur on exposed areas and are frequently found on the head, neck, and dorsum of the hand. They can also develop as mucocutaneous lesions of the lip. The danger from squamous cell carcinoma is its propensity to invade local tissue and to metastasize. The risk of metastasis is 2%-15% if the lesion is on the lip or ear[10] and 45.7% if the lesion is greater than 4 centimeters in thickness.[8] Tumors arising in scars are particularly aggressive. Metastases can spread to any organ of the body, although lymph nodes, lungs, and liver are primary targets. Therefore, early recognition and treatment is even more critical for this tumor than for the basal cell variety. The treatment of choice is surgical excision, although Moh's surgery and curettage and electrodesiccation are acceptable alternatives, depending on the nature and location of the lesion. The overall cure rate is 75%-90% at 5 years; with metastasis it is 25%.[8] Once the tumor has been removed and there is no evidence of metastasis, the patient can be considered cured and recertified for cockpit duty.

Testicular Cancer

Testicular tumors will occasionally be detected in aviators because these tumors are most common in men an average of 32 years of age.[11] The most common histologic types of malignancies are seminoma, embryonal cell carcinoma, teratocarcinoma, and choriocarcinoma. The most frequent presenting symptom is enlargement of the testis, often without pain. For this reason, the disease is sometimes first detected during a periodic flight physical examination rather than patient discomfort. Treatment of testicular tumors includes orchiectomy, lymph node dissection, radiotherapy, and chemotherapy, depending on the type of tumor and extent of involvement.

Although most testicular tumors are malignant, the prognosis for survival is quite favorable, particularly if the disease is found prior to widespread metastasis and an appropriate treatment regimen is immediately instituted. When metastasis occurs, it usually involves lymph nodes and lungs primarily, but can spread to other organs as the disease progresses. Nevertheless, overall cure rates of over 95% are frequently reported, mainly because of advances in chemotherapy.[12]

Seminoma is the most frequent testicular tumor. Because it is extremely radiosensitive, orchiectomy and radiotherapy afford a cure rate approaching 100%.[13] If there is spread requiring lymphadenectomy and chemotherapy the prognosis is not as good. Other testicular tumors are not radiosensitive, and are treated with orchiectomy, lymphadenectomy, and chemotherapeutic drugs such as platinum, bleomycin, and vinblastine. Cure rates of 90% can be achieved as long as the disease is not advanced. For patient follow-up, it is useful to monitor alpha-fetoprotein and human chorionic gonadotropin levels because increases in these components can herald recurrence.

With today's treatment regimens most aviators with testicular tumors should be able to return to the cockpit. If there is no evidence of widespread metastasis, such as to the lungs or liver, the chances for a normal life span are excellent. This is particularly true for seminoma which is confined to the testis. If medical waiver is granted, as with any type of treated cancer, the patient must be followed closely since there is always the possibility of recurrence or occult metastasis. It is advisable to follow patients at 3-month intervals for the first year because recurrence is highest in this period.[12]

Thyroid Cancer

Although cancer of the thyroid gland is not particularly common in the general population, it is sometimes detected during routine aviation physical examinations. Most cases present with a lump in the neck, although patients with more advanced disease may have symptoms of dyspnea, dysphonia, dysphagia, or pain. For metastatic lesions, there is a predilection for the lung and bone. Besides spontaneous development of this disease, there is also an apparent association with therapeutic x-ray of the head and neck, that in previous decades was prescribed for enlarged tonsils, adenoids, and thymus gland. For all these reasons careful palpation of the neck should be a part of any physical examination.

If a mass or nodule is palpated in the thyroid gland, it must be determined if the lesion is benign or malignant. This usually cannot be done by examination or laboratory tests alone—most patients with thyroid cancer are clinically and chemically euthyroid. Thus other tests such as echography, scanning, and needle biopsy must be done, the latter being the most reliable with more than 90% sensitivity.[14]

There are four major histologic types of thyroid cancer: papillary, follicular, medullary, and undifferentiated. The papillary and follicular types are the most common, accounting for 91% of all thyroid malignancies.[15] Both are slow-growing with excellent 5-year survival rates following therapy depending on the stage of disease. Prognosis worsens with age, particularly beyond age 45. On the other hand, the medullary and undifferentiated types, while less common are far more malignant, with a propensity to rapidly invade adjacent structures and to metastasize to distant organs: 10-year survival for the medullary type is 5%-74% depending on stage and treatment, and for the undifferentiated type death is expected within 36 months. Thus the prognosis depends largely on the histologic type, the extent of spread at the time of diagnosis, and the patient's age.

The basic treatment of thyroid cancer is surgery, ranging from simple nodule removal to thyroidectomy and radical neck dissection, depending on the extent of disease. Some patients suffer complications including hypoparathyroidism and injury to the recurrent laryngeal nerve. Other treatment modalities for the more aggressive cancers are radioactive iodine, external radiation, and chemotherapy (bleomycin, adriamycin, vinblastine). For patients receiving radiotherapy, the AME/flight surgeon should keep in mind that side effects may include bone marrow suppression with leukopenia, thrombocytopenia, and anemia, as well as pulmonary fibrosis for those with pulmonary lesions.

Aviators found to have a thyroid mass or nodule must be fully investigated to rule out a malignant lesion and treated accordingly. The criteria for determining aeromedical disposition should be the histologic type of lesion, the extent of spread, the patient's age, and the posttherapeutic course. If the lesion is successfully removed, there is no evidence of metastasis, and the patient has no significant post-treatment complications, a return to flight duty would be reasonable. Even if there is recurrence with metastasis, the risk of sudden incapacitation is very low. As with any type of malignancy, frequent follow-up is advisable with serum thyroglobulin, chest x-ray, and thyroid ultrasound or MRI for at least a few years following treatment.

Hodgkin's Disease

Hodgkin's disease is a malignant tumor involving lymphoid tissue. Although the etiology is unknown, there is some speculation that it is caused by a virus (Epstein-Barr) or by hereditary factors. Because the average age of incidence is 32, it can be expected to occur occasionally in the aviation population. Patients may be completely asymptomatic or present with complaints of fever, night sweats, pruritus, and weight loss. On occasion, more serious symptoms will occur due to obstruction of the vena cava or spinal cord compression. Asymptomatic cases are sometimes diagnosed on routine physical examination because of enlarged, rubbery, painless nodes, usually cervical or supraclavicular. The examiner might also note hepatosplenomegaly or enlarged mediastinal nodes on chest x-ray. If the patient is not treated, signs and symptoms of the disease will eventually appear. The diagnosis is usually made by clinical impression and biopsy of lymphoid tissue. Characteristic of but not pathognomonic for Hodgkin's disease is the presence of the Reed-Sternberg cell.

Histologically, Hodgkin's disease is usually classified into four types: lymphocytic predominance, nodular sclerosis, mixed cellularity, and lymphocyte depletion.

The lymphocytic predominance type has the most favorable prognosis, while lymphocyte depletion has the worst, with the other two types in between. This histologic classification is further subdivided into four clinical stages[16]:

- Stage I: disease limited to a single lymph node region or lymphoid structure;
- Stage II: disease in two or more lymph node regions on the same side of the diaphragm;

- Stage III: disease on both sides of the diaphragm; and
- Stage IV: involvement of bone marrow, lung parenchyma, pleura, liver, bone, skin, kidneys, gastrointestinal tract, or any extranodal sites.

The four stages are further classified A or B, A indicating the presence of symptoms and B the absence of symptoms. Determining the patient's anatomical involvement, or staging, allows for selection of the proper therapeutic regimen and for prediction of the course of the disease. Staging can be done by laparotomy, biopsy, x-ray, and lymphangiography.

Modern treatment regimens include radiotherapy and/or combination chemotherapy. Although new chemotherapeutic agents and combinations are always under investigation, the combinations most commonly prescribed today are MOPP (nitrogen mustard, vincristine, procarbazine, and prednisone) and its variants.

MOPP is usually given for 14 days, followed by 14 days off treatment to recover from side effects. This 28-day cycle is then repeated 6 times. Other antineoplastic agents used include thiotepa, bleomycin, and vinblastine. The literature on Hodgkin's disease is replete with controversy over which therapeutic regimen is most effective for each stage. Therefore, the treatment of Hodgkin's disease will differ to some extent depending on the patient's stage as well as the preference of the managing physician.

When determining flight status for aviators with Hodgkin's disease, the AME/FS is particularly concerned with the untoward effects of treatment, the extent of recovery, and the prognosis. The chemotherapeutic agents have myriad side effects, most of which resolve after treatment is completed. For example, MOPP therapy can cause bone marrow suppression with a susceptibility for bleeding and infection, immunosuppression, anemia, and increase the risk of developing a second malignancy such as leukemia. Following is a summary of the major effects of the most commonly used agents:

- Nitrogen mustard: nausea, vomiting, bone marrow depression
- Vincristine: hair loss, neuritic pain, numbness, weakness
- Procarbazine: neuropathies, marrow depression, nausea, vomiting
- Prednisone: Cushingoid effects, hypertension, osteoporosis, ulcer, diabetes
- Vinblastine: marrow suppression, nausea, vomiting
- Bleomycin: pulmonary fibrosis

In addition to these immediate effects of chemotherapy, there are also long-term complications, particularly second malignancies from the disease itself or from therapy. Second malignancies include acute leukemia, especially after MOPP (2%-3%); the risk is also increased for non-Hodgkin's lymphoma. Solid tumors of the breast and lung and sarcomas constitute 50% of all second malignancies found in patients with a history of Hodgkin's disease, some occurring as long as 10 years posttreatment.[17]

Radiotherapy is also not without its risks. In one review, complications reported included pulmonary effusion and fibrosis, hypothyroidism, Graves' disease, premature myocardial infarction, and lung and thyroid cancer.[16]

In spite of the seriousness of Hodgkin's disease and the frequency of complications from radiation therapy and combination chemotherapy, the prognosis has improved remarkably over the years with most patients achieving cure. Currently 90% of patients with early stage Hodgkin's disease and 75% of those with advanced disease achieve complete remission with therapy.[18] If there are recurrences, most occur within the first 3 years. Therefore, occurrence of this disease in an aviator does not necessarily terminate their career.

In light of the need for close supervision of patients undergoing treatment for Hodgkin's disease and because of the many side effects of chemotherapy and radiotherapy, aviators should not continue flight duty while being treated. Return to duty should only be considered once all medication has been discontinued, all adverse side effects have remitted, and hematologic deficits (WBCs, platelets, and hemoglobin) have reverted to normal levels. Furthermore, the disease process must be arrested and the patient free of symptoms. The AME/flight surgeon should be particularly wary if bleomycin was used for treatment because of the many patients who develop pulmonary fibrosis resulting in significant ventilation-perfusion aberrations.

In any event, once the AME/FS recommends returning the patient to the cockpit, the patient should be followed closely. This will help ensure that the patient remains symptom free, there are no delayed side effects of treatment or late complications of the disease process, and there has been no recurrence. It should also be remembered that there is a higher incidence of second malignancies in treated Hodgkin's disease patients. Once these conditions have been met, the aviator may immediately return to flying.

References

1. Rugo HS. Cancer. In: Tierney Jr LM, McPhee SJ, Papadakis MA, eds. *Current Medical Diagnosis and Treatment*. 37th ed. Stamford, Conn: Appleton-Lange; 1998.

2. Runkle GP, Zaloznik AJ. Malignant melanoma. *AFP*. 1994;49(1):91-98.

3. Sweeney WB, James LP, Ghosh BC, et al. Late recurrence of malignant melanoma. *AFP*. 1988;37(4):243-247.

4. Langley RGB, Barnhill RL, Mihm MC, et al. Neoplasms: Cutaneous melanoma. In: Freedberg IM, Eisen AZ, Wolff K, et al, eds. *Fitzpatrick's Dermatology in General Medicine*. 5th ed. New York: McGraw-Hill; 1999.

5. Stadlmann WK, Rapaport DP, Soong SJ, et al. Prognostic clinical and pathologic features. In: Balch CM, Houghton AN, Sober AJ, Soong SJ, eds. *Cutaneous Melanoma*. 3rd ed. St. Louis: Quality Medical Publishing; 1998.

6. Sampson JH, Carter Jr JH, Friedman AH, Seigler HF. Demographics, prognosis, and therapy in 702 patients with brain metastasis from malignant melanomas. *J Neurosurg*. 1998;88:11-20.

7. Mosely HS, Nizze A, Morton DL. Disseminated melanoma presenting as a catastrophic event. *Aviat Space Environ Med*. 1978;49(11):1342-1346.

8. Bernstein SC, Lim KK, Brodland DG, Heidelberg KA. The many faces of squamous cell carcinoma. *Dermatol Surg*. 1996;22:243-254.

9. Randle HW. Basal cell carcinoma. *Dermatol Surg*. 1996;22:255-261.

10. Marks R. Squamous cell carcinoma. *Lancet*. 1996;347:735-738.

11. Junnila J, Lassen P. Testicular mass. *AFP*. 1998;57(4):685-692.

12. Kinkade S. Testicular cancer. *AFP*. 1999;59(9):2539-2544.

13. Presti Jr JC, Herr HW. Genital tumors. In: Tanagho EA, McAninch JW, ed. *Smith's General Urology*. 14th ed. Norwalk, Conn: Appleton & Lange; 1995.

14. Larson PR, Davies TF, Hay ID. The thyroid gland. In: Wilson JD, Foster DW, Kronenberg HM, Larson PR, eds. *Williams Textbook of Endocrinology*. 9th ed. Philadelphia: Saunders; 1998.

15. Greenspan FS. The thyroid gland. In: Greenspan FS, Strewler GJ, eds. *Basic and Clinical Endocrinology*. 5th ed. Stamford, Conn: Appleton & Lange; 1997.

16. Weinshel EL, Peterson BA. Hodgkin's disease. *CA Cancer J Clin*. 1993;43:327-346.

17. Maireh PM, Kalish LA, Marcus KC, et al. Second malignancies after treatment for laparotomy-staged IA-IIIB Hodgkin's disease: Long-term analysis of risk factors and outcome. *Blood*. 1996;87(9):3625-3632.

18. Carbonero RG, Arez LP, Arcediano A, et al. Favorable prognosis after late relapse of Hodgkin's disease. *Cancer*. 1998;83(3):560-565.

Index

Abscesses, in pilonidal sinus, 20–21
Absence (petit mal) seizure, 98
Absent kidney, 279
Acceleration, +G$_z$
  and herniated disks, 54
  and hypertension, 251
  and pregnancy, 280
  and venous pooling, 5
Accidents
  and presbyopic pilots, 112
  and reactions of site recovery crew, 309
ACE inhibitors, 43, 169, 171, 193, 227, 250
  side effects of, 255
Acephalgic migraine, 87. *See also* Headache:
    migraine
Acetazolamide, 117
Acne, 286
Acoustic neuroma, 132
  and flight status, 134
Acquired immunodeficiency syndrome (AIDS),
    39, 63, 64. *See also* Human immunodeficiency
    virus infection
Acute otitis media, 137
Acute posttraumatic stress disorder, 307–308
Adenomas, 70
ADHD. *See* Attention deficit-hyperactivity disorder
Adjustment reaction, 292–294
  and flight status, 294
  case examples of, 293–294, 302–303
  diagnostic criteria for, 292
Anxiety, 296–297
  and flight status, 297
  case example of, 296–297
  diagnostic criteria for, 296
  fear of flying and, 309–310
AFib. *See* Atrial fibrillation
AI. *See* Aortic insufficiency
AIDS. *See* Acquired immunodeficiency syndrome
Airline medical director, role of, in psychiatric
    assessment, 291–292
Airsickness, 305–306
Alcohol
  absorption of, 41–42
  and familial/essential tremor, 74
  and micturition syncope, 96
  and role in pancreatitis, 18
  and seizures, 97, 99
  as possible cause of phorias, 114
  avoidance of
    to prevent recurrent ulcers, 12

    to treat GERD, 15
  effects of, 41
  rate of alcohol-associated fatal general
    aviation accidents, 41
  studies of performance decline in aviators
    with, 41
  subclinical drinkers of, and safety, 41
  urine screening for consumption of, 42
Alcoholism, 41–42
  success of rehabilitation programs for aviators,
    42
Allergic rhinitis, 139–140
  and flight status, 140
  symptoms of, 139
  treatment of, 139–140
Allopurinol, 10
Alpha-agonists, 95
Alpha-glucosidase inhibitors, 45
  side effects of, 46
Alpha thalassemia, 35
Alternobaric vertigo, 132–133, 134
Amantadine, 72
Amaurosis fugax, 77
Amblyopia, 114
AME. *See* Aviation medical examiner
Amitryptiline, 88
Amnesia, 89–90
  posttraumatic, 65, 66
  retrograde, 89
  transient epileptic, 90
  transient global, 89–90
    and flight status, 90
    case history of, 89–90
    differentiation of, from other forms, 90
  transient ischemic, 90
Amoxicillin, in treatment of duodenal ulcers, 12
Anemia, 31–37
  and flight status, 31–32
  glucose-6-phosphate dehydrogenase
    deficiency, 36–37
  hemoglobinopathies, 33–35
  hereditary spherocytosis, 32–33
  pernicious anemia, 32
Aneurysm, 81, 82
  aortic, 242, 243
  surgical isolation of, 83
Angiography, coronary
  noninvasive, 161–162
  normal, 165
Angioplasty, 173–174